Tra
Self-Assessment and Review, 2nd Edition

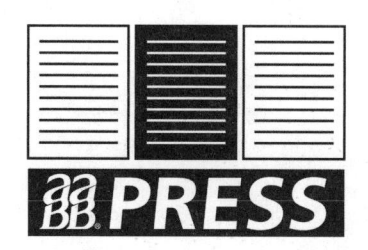

PRESS

Other related publications available from the AABB:

Technical Manual, 16th edition
Edited by John D. Roback, MD, PhD;
Martha Rae Combs, MT(ASCP)SBB; Brenda J. Grossman, MD; and
Christopher Hillyer, MD

Practical Guide to Transfusion Medicine, 2nd edition
By Marian Petrides, MD; Laura Cooling, MD; Gary Stack, MD, PhD; and
Lanne Maes, MD

**Transfusion Medicine Interactive:
A Case Study Approach CD-ROM**
By Marian Petrides, MD; Roby Rogers, MD; and
Nora Ratcliffe, MD

Look It Up! (A Quick Reference in Transfusion Medicine)
Edited by Mark E. Brecher, MD

Look This Up, Too! (A Quick Reference in Apheresis)
Edited by Mark E. Brecher, MD; Shauna Hay, MT(ASCP); and
Beth Shaz, MD

To purchase books or to inquire about other book services, including chapter reprints and large-quantity sales, please contact our sales department:
- 866.222.2498 (within the United States)
- +1 301.215.6499 (outside the United States)
- +1 301.951.7150 (fax)
- www.aabb.org>Bookstore

AABB customer service representatives are available by telephone from 8:30 am to 5:00 pm ET, Monday through Friday, excluding holidays.

Transfusion Medicine Self-Assessment and Review, 2nd Edition

Douglas P. Blackall, MD
Arkansas Children's Hospital
Little Rock, Arkansas

Priscilla I. Figueroa, MD
Cleveland Clinic
Cleveland, Ohio

Jeffrey L. Winters, MD
Department of Laboratory Medicine and Pathology
Mayo Clinic
Rochester, Minnesota

AABB Press
Bethesda, Maryland
2009

Mention of specific products or equipment by contributors to this AABB Press publication does not represent an endorsement of such products by the AABB Press nor does it necessarily indicate a preference for those products over other similar competitive products.

AABB Press authors are requested to comply with a conflict of interest policy that includes disclosure of relationships with commercial firms. A copy of the policy is located at http://www.aabb.org.

The authors have disclosed no conflicts of interest.

Efforts are made to have publications of the AABB Press consistent in regard to acceptable practices. However, for several reasons, they may not be. First, as new developments in the practice of blood banking occur, changes may be recommended to the AABB *Standards for Blood Banks and Transfusion Services*. It is not possible, however, to revise each publication at the time such a change is adopted. Thus, it is essential that the most recent edition of the *Standards* be consulted as a reference in regard to current acceptable practices. Second, the views expressed in this publication represent the opinions of authors. The publication of this book does not constitute an endorsement by the AABB Press of any view expressed herein, and the AABB Press expressly disclaims any liability arising from any inaccuracy or misstatement.

Copyright © 2009 by AABB. All rights reserved. Reproduction or transmission of text in any form or by any means, electronic or mechanical, including photocopying, recording, or by any information storage and retrieval system is prohibited without permission in writing from the Publisher.

The Publisher has made every effort to trace the copyright holders for borrowed material. If they have inadvertently overlooked any, they will be pleased to make the necessary arrangements at the first opportunity.

AABB
8101 Glenbrook Road
Bethesda, Maryland 20814-2749

ISBN NO. 978-1-56395-280-7
Printed in the United States

Library of Congress Cataloging-in-Publication Data

Blackall, Douglas P.
  Transfusion medicine : self-assessment and review / Douglas P. Blackall, Priscilla I. Figueroa, Jeffrey L. Winters—2nd ed.
     p. ; cm.
  Rev. ed. of: Transfusion medicine : self-assessment and review / Douglas P. Blackall ... [et al.]. 2002.
  Includes bibliographical references.
  ISBN 978-1-56395-280-7
  1. Blood—Transfusion—Examinations, questions, etc. I. Figueroa, Priscilla I. II. Winters, Jeffrey L. III. AABB. IV. Title.
  [DNLM: 1. Blood Transfusion—Examination Questions. 2. Blood Group Antigens—Examination Questions. WB 18.2 T772 2009]
  RM171.B57 2009
  615'.39076--dc22

2009035956

AABB Press
Editorial Board

Miguel Lozano, MD, PhD
Richard J. Davey, MD
Susan T. Johnson, MSTM, MT(ASCP)SBB
Marisa B. Marques, MD
Bruce C. McLeod, MD
Sally V. Rudmann, PhD, MT(ASCP)SBB
Clarence Sarkodee-Adoo, MD, FACP
John W. Semple, PhD

Table of Contents

Preface.. ix
About the Authors................................... xi

1. **Quality and Compliance** 1
   Questions..1
   Answers...12
   References......................................29

2. **Medical Assessment of Blood Donors, Blood Collection (Autologous and Allogeneic), and Donor Complications** ..31
   Questions.......................................31
   Answers...42
   References......................................65

3. **Blood Components: Preparation, Storage, and Characteristics** 67
   Questions.......................................67
   Answers...79
   References......................................98

4. **Carbohydrate Blood Group Antigens** 101
   Questions......................................101
   Answers..119
   References.....................................145

5. **Protein-Based Blood Group Antigens**...........147
   Questions......................................147
   Answers..159
   References.....................................181

6. **Pretransfusion Testing and Antibody Identification** 183
   Questions......................................183
   Answers..202
   References.....................................224

7. **Clinical Transfusion Practice and Effective Use of Blood Components**............................227
   Questions......................................227

Answers................................... 240
References................................ 268

8. **Hematopoietic Progenitor Cells, Cord Blood, and Growth Factors** 269
   Questions 269
   Answers.................................. 278
   References............................... 296

9. **Hemolytic Disease of the Fetus and Newborn, and Rh Immune Globulin** 299
   Questions 299
   Answers.................................. 315
   References............................... 346

10. **Noninfectious Complications of Transfusion** 349
    Questions 349
    Answers................................. 361
    References.............................. 387

11. **Infectious Complications of Transfusion and Positive Disease Markers in Blood Donors** 389
    Questions 389
    Answers................................. 401
    References.............................. 431

12. **Coagulation** 435
    Questions 435
    Answers................................. 445
    References.............................. 468

13. **Hemapheresis**.............................. 469
    Questions 469
    Answers................................. 480
    References.............................. 504

14. **The HLA System** 505
    Questions 505
    Answers................................. 515
    References.............................. 534

15. **Tissue Banking and Organ Transplantation**. 535
    Questions 535
    Answers................................. 544
    References.............................. 563

Preface

We are pleased to have participated in the preparation of this book. The first edition of *Transfusion Medicine Self-Assessment and Review* was successful, most importantly because it filled an educational niche in the field. In particular, residents and fellows training in the field of transfusion medicine have come to regard this book as an important educational resource, for both learning the field and for board examination preparation. We are confident that the second edition of this text will be even more useful to the educator and the student.

There are a number of significant changes worthy of note in the second edition of this text. Foremost, there has been a change in authors. Sadly, Dr. Pam Helekar died several years ago. A second edition was her vision, however, and we believe that she would be pleased with our efforts. She was the driving force behind the first edition, and she is missed. Although Dr. Darrell Triulzi was also unable to participate in the authorship of this edition because of other commitments, Drs. Blackall and Winters are thrilled that Dr. Figueroa has joined as an author for this edition. Her contributions have been invaluable.

On a more practical note, a number of changes have gone into the preparation of the second edition that should provide significant benefits to the learner. First, there are now 15 chapters in this edition, with the deletion of "Parentage Testing" and the additions of "Quality and Compliance" and "Tissue Banking and Organ Transplantation." These changes alone are a good reflection of the current state of transfusion medicine. Second, significant changes to the questions from both a quantitative and qualitative perspective bring the total this edition to 440 questions covering all areas of transfusion medicine, up from 379 in the first edition. The questions have been updated and revised to reflect the current state of the field. An important example of a change is that "except" questions have largely been rewritten for the sake of clarity. Finally, selected references have been included at the conclusion of each chapter.

As with the first edition, the authors' anticipate that the second edition of *Transfusion Medicine Self-Assessment and Review* will be a resource that benefits all who desire an improved understanding of transfusion medicine. We hope that our text is an effective and enjoyable tool that will enhance the reader's understanding of the field for years to come.

Douglas P. Blackall, MD
Priscilla I. Figueroa, MD
Jeffrey L. Winters, MD

About the Authors

Douglas P. Blackall, MD, is the Chief of Pediatric Pathology and Director of the Clinical Laboratories at Arkansas Children's Hospital in Little Rock. He is also a Professor of Pathology at the University of Arkansas for Medical Sciences. Previously, he was the Co-Director of Transfusion Medicine at the UCLA Medical Center and directed resident education in Clinical Pathology at UCLA.

Dr. Blackall attended medical school at the University of Arkansas and completed residency training in Clinical Pathology at the University of Pennsylvania. While in Philadelphia, he was also a postgraduate research fellow in the laboratory of Dr. Steven Spitalnik and completed fellowship training in transfusion medicine. His clinical and research interests are focused on immunohematology and transfusion practice; however, his first love is education, which is a major reason for coauthoring this book.

Jeffrey L. Winters, MD, is Medical Director of the Mayo Clinic Therapeutic Apheresis Unit and an attending physician on the Transfusion Service, Division of Transfusion Medicine, Department of Laboratory Medicine and Pathology at the Mayo Clinic. He is also an associate professor in the Mayo College of Medicine. He was formerly the Medical Director of Donor Services, being responsible for autologous and allogeneic blood collections at the Mayo Clinic.

Dr. Winters graduated magna cum laude from Centre College in Danville, KY, and with high distinction from the University of Kentucky College of Medicine in Lexington. His postgraduate training consisted of an anatomic/clinical pathology residency in the Department of Pathology and Laboratory Medicine at the University of Kentucky and a transfusion medicine/blood banking fellowship in the Division of Transfusion Medicine at the Mayo Clinic, Rochester, MN. He is certified by the American Board of Pathology in Anatomic Pathology, Clinical Pathology, and Blood Banking/Transfusion Medicine.

A member of the editorial board for the Journal of Clinical Apheresis, Dr. Winters is the president-elect of the American Society for Apheresis (ASFA). He is also currently Chair of the Mayo Clinic Human Cellular and Tissue-Based Products Committee and has responsibility for oversight of tissue collected and purchased for transplantation.

Since 2004, he has served as the Director of Mayo Clinic's ACGME-accredited Transfusion Medicine Fellowship. In 2005 and 2009, Dr Winters was awarded the Mayo Fellow's Association Clinical Pathology Teacher of the Year.

Priscilla I. Figueroa, MD, is Head of the Section of Transfusion Medicine and Director of the Hematopoietic Progenitor Cell Laboratory at Cleveland Clinic. Prior to July 2005 she was Director of the Division of Transfusion Medicine at the University of California Los Angeles Medical Center, where she was also a Clinical Associate Professor of Pathology and Laboratory Medicine at the UCLA School of Medicine. Her association with UCLA began when she was Director of Transfusion Medicine and Serology at the Los Angeles County Harbor-UCLA Medical Center.

Dr. Figueroa received her Bachelor of Arts degree from Harvard University and her medical degree from Cornell University Medical College. After an internship in Internal Medicine at Columbia-Presbyterian Medical Center in New York City, Dr. Figueroa pursued training in Anatomic and Clinical Pathology at the New York Hospital Cornell University Medical Center, followed by a fellowship in Transfusion Medicine and Blood Banking at the Mayo Clinic. Dr. Figueroa is a member of the AABB, College of American Pathologists, American Society for Apheresis, and International Society for Cellular Therapy. She is a former President of the California Blood Bank Society.

Dr. Figueroa's areas of interest include stem cell therapies, transfusion safety, blood management, quality management, and physician education.

In: Blackall D, Figueroa P, Winters J
Transfusion Medicine Self-Assessment and Review, 2nd Edition
Bethesda, MD: AABB Press, 2009

1

Quality and Compliance

QUESTIONS

Question 1: Which of the following is considered a quality assurance (QA) activity?

A. Performing a bedside, two-person verification of unit and recipient identity before transfusion.
B. Weekly review of all red cell antigen typing records.
C. Visual inspection of all blood components before release from the blood bank.
D. Monitoring the temperature of all refrigerators and freezers on a daily basis.
E. Creating a dedicated training position at a community blood center in anticipation of a large expansion necessitating the hiring of many new technologists.

Question 2: Which of these organizations is a regulatory agency?

A. The Joint Commission.
B. AABB.
C. Clinical and Laboratory Standards Institute (CLSI).
D. Food and Drug Administration (FDA).
E. College of American Pathologists (CAP).

Question 3: Product specifications are developed for the purpose of:

A. Meeting customer requirements.
B. Meeting regulatory expectations.
C. Meeting requirements of accrediting organizations.
D. Defining operational requirements.
E. All of the above.

Question 4: A laboratory wishes to implement a new automated analyzer. The instrument is expected to run 100 specimens per hour with a turnaround time of less than 30 minutes per specimen and a failure rate of ≤1%. The process that demonstrates this instrument meets customer specifications is called:

A. Calibration.
B. Quality control.
C. Performance qualification.
D. Validation.
E. Change control.

Question 5: The individual designated to oversee a blood center's quality functions should report directly to:

A. The supervisor or manager in charge of operations.
B. The board of directors.
C. The medical director.
D. The FDA.
E. Executive management.

Question 6: The individual designated to oversee a facility's quality functions must have authority to:

A. Take disciplinary action against individuals who are repeatedly noncompliant with institutional policies and procedures.
B. Initiate corrective action for processes that are noncompliant with requirements.
C. Approve and implement new or changed policies and procedures.
D. Approve deviations from established policies and procedures.
E. None of the above.

Question 7: With regard to quality oversight functions, operational staff:

A. Should not audit work they have performed.
B. May audit their own work providing they receive adequate supervision during the audit process.
C. May perform quality oversight functions providing they have additional training as certified quality specialists.
D. May not perform quality oversight functions because of a conflict of interest. Only members of the quality oversight unit may perform quality oversight.
E. None of the above.

Question 8: With regard to competency assessment (CA), which is *true*?

A. CA must be performed for each procedure or test an employee performs.
B. CA must be performed at 3 months and 6 months during the first year of employment.
C. Written evaluation and direct performance observation must be included in each CA.

D. Beyond the initial year of employment, CAs must be performed at least annually.
E. According to Clinical Laboratory Improvement Amendments (CLIA) regulation, CA must be performed by the laboratory supervisor.

Question 9: A new employee reports to the blood bank on the first day of employment. A bench technologist is assigned to train the new employee. After 7 weeks of training, consisting of watching and then performing each task under her trainer's supervision, the employee passes her CA and is allowed to work independently. Does this employee's training comply with current good manufacturing practice (cGMP) requirements for employee training?

A. Yes, because she performed each task under supervision and passed her CA before being allowed to work independently.
B. No, because cGMP requirements specify a minimum of 8 weeks of training for a new blood bank employee.
C. No, because she was not given cGMP training.
D. No, because employees may not work independently until two CAs are performed.
E. No, because cGMP requirements specify that employee training must be performed by a training specialist.

Question 10: With regard to critical supplies or services, which of the following is *true*?

A. Critical supplies are supplies that are most needed for daily operations.
B. The quality system should include processes to ensure that incoming supplies are acceptable.
C. A standing purchase order qualifies as a written agreement.
D. Vendors of FDA-approved supplies and reagents may be assumed to qualify as vendors of critical supplies.
E. The supplier must define acceptance criteria for the product or service.

QUALITY AND COMPLIANCE

Question 11: Regarding agreements with providers of supplies or services, which is *true*?

A. Agreements are not necessary as long as the provider is within the same institution.
B. Agreements must be renewed annually.
C. The contracting facility assumes responsibility for ensuring that the contractor complies with all applicable product standards and regulations.
D. The legal responsibility for the work preformed by the contractor belongs to the contractor.
E. All of the above.

Question 12: Which of the following is required for any equipment used in the collection, processing, testing, or storage of blood components and human cells, tissues, and cellular and tissue-based products?

A. Biannual preventive maintenance.
B. FDA inspection and approval before implementation.
C. Biannual recalibration.
D. Documentation of operational qualification.
E. A list of employees currently approved to use the equipment.

Question 13: A facility uses an FDA-approved antisera for red cell antigen testing. Staff have established that they can use the antisera at a 1:1 dilution without affecting the sensitivity of the test. Which of the following is *true*?

A. FDA-licensed establishments may dilute the antisera providing they have validated that dilution does not change the performance.
B. It is never acceptable to deviate from the manufacturer's instructions for product use.

C. A registered establishment may deviate from the manufacturer's instructions if the manufacturer provides data that support the decision.
D. All establishments must validate the diluted antisera, then apply for an FDA variance from the manufacturer's instructions.
E. Establishments that are not registered or licensed may use the antisera by whichever method they demonstrate to be effective.

Question 14: With regard to documents and records, which of the following is *true*?

A. The terms *documents* and *records* are used interchangeably.
B. Documents and records must be retained indefinitely.
C. Documents provide information on what should happen.
D. Accrediting agencies may review documents, but records are legally protected from outside review.
E. Records provide information on what should happen.

Question 15: Which of the following events is a biological product deviation (BPA) that must be reported to the FDA?

A. An Rh-positive Red Cell Blood (RBC) unit is incorrectly labeled as Rh negative and issued to an Rh-positive patient. The unit is returned to the blood bank.
B. An Rh-positive unit is labeled as Rh negative and is crossmatched for an Rh-negative individual with anti-D. The unit is crossmatch incompatible. There is a delay in providing blood for the patient while the explanation for the positive crossmatch is pursued.
C. While reviewing the blood donor questionnaires from the day's collections, a supervisor notices that follow-up questions were missing for 15 donors who had responded that they had traveled to a malarial risk area. Eventually all 15 collections must be discarded because of incomplete donor histories.

D. Blood bank policy requires that all neonates receive cytomegalovirus (CMV)-seronegative cellular blood products. AB CMV seronegative platelets are not available for a type AB 3-month-old infant. Leukocyte-reduced AB platelets are issued with approval of the blood bank medical director.
E. None of the above.

Question 16: Which of the following would require a product recall?

A. An internal audit reveals that the documentation of the storage, before the shipment to the final manufacturer, of source plasma used to produce a lot of 5% albumin is incomplete. There have been no adverse events or product complaints associated with use of this lot.
B. A lot of Rh Immune Globulin (RhIG) is labeled with a potency of 250 IU/dose but is actually 204 IU/dose.
C. A manufacturer of intravenous immune globulin (IVIG) receives reports of an unusual amount of urticarial reactions with a specific lot of IVIG.
D. A software manufacturer receives reports that its blood bank information system software is failing to issue QA warnings/failures when there is a mismatch between reaction results and interpretations. The problem occurs only in highly atypical situations.
E. On repeat donation, a donor provides information that he traveled to a malarial risk area within the past 12 months. A review of records reveals that he donated blood on two different occasions after that travel but had not remembered to provide the travel information.

Question 17: A 48-year-old woman receives one unit of RBCs after liposuction resulted in severe unexpected bleeding. Shortly after onset of the transfusion, she develops a fever, her blood pressure drops, and she begins to ooze from her incision sites. A transfusion reaction workup reveals that she received an ABO-incompatible unit. Despite supportive measures, she develops disseminated intravascular coagulation (DIC) and acute circulatory collapse, leading to death. Which of the following is correct?

A. The FDA must receive initial notification of the death within 7 days of occurrence.
B. The FDA must receive written notification of the death within 14 days of occurrence.
C. The transfusion center is always responsible for reporting a transfusion-associated death.
D. If different from the transfusion facility, the facility that performed the compatibility testing is required to make an FDA report only when the fatality was the result of an error on its part.
E. FDA reporting is required only when the death is the result of a blood bank error.

Question 18: With regard to FDA licensure and registration, which is correct?

A. Hospital transfusion services are required to register if they transfuse more than 100 products per year.
B. Hospital blood banks must be licensed if they collect or manufacture blood components.
C. Community blood banks must be licensed.
D. Neither registration or licensure is required for hospital blood banks.
E. Hospital blood banks must be registered if they collect or manufacture blood components.

Question 19: With regard to complying with cGMP requirements to perform quality assessments, which of the following is *true*?

A. Peer review is not an acceptable form of assessment.
B. Proficiency testing may not be counted as an assessment.
C. An assessment should focus on one process.
D. Self-assessment tools are not adequate for performing assessments.
E. Assessments may be internal or external.

QUALITY AND COMPLIANCE   9

Question 20: A hospital hematopoietic progenitor cell (HPC) laboratory uses CD34 cell counts to assess the quality of HPC products. The CD34 counts are performed by the hospital flow cytometry laboratory. The stem cell laboratory participates in proficiency testing (PT), which includes CD34 cell counting. When the PT specimens arrive, they are carried to the flow cytometry laboratory supervisor who personally performs the CD34 analyses and repeats them to make sure they are correct before giving the results to the HPC laboratory. Which is *true*?

A. Proficiency testing may not be performed in duplicate.
B. The flow cytometry laboratory may not perform proficiency testing that is reported by the HPC laboratory.
C. Proficiency testing is required only for CLIA-regulated tests.
D. The laboratory may compare its results with other laboratories' results before reporting the results.
E. If a laboratory fails a PT survey, it must discontinue performing that test until corrective action is implemented.

Question 21: Deviation management reports at a given facility reveal several examples of technologists' having dispensed blood components without first issuing them in the information system, as required by operating policies and procedures. These errors were discovered when the units could not be accounted for during inventory reconciliation. On reviewing these errors, management decides that at the end of each shift a technologist must review the retained compatibility slip copies for all components issued, and, if necessary, correct their computer status. This is an example of:

A. Preventive action.
B. Remedial action.
C. Corrective action.
D. Process improvement.
E. None of the above.

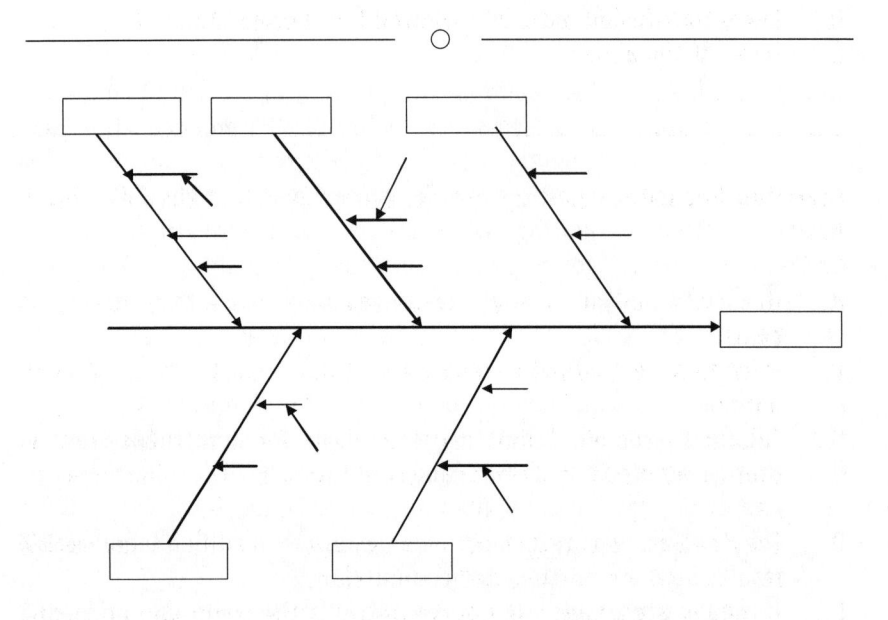

Figure 1.1.

Question 22: The diagram shown in Fig 1-1:

A. Is an outline of a cause-and-effect diagram.
B. Is an outline of a Pareto diagram.
C. Is intended to document personnel involved in a nonconformance.
D. Is a diagrammatic representation of a procedure.
E. Is an outline of a process map.

Question 23: The Joint Commission hospital accreditation requirements specify that:

A. Ten percent of all transfusions must be reviewed for appropriateness.
B. All ABO-incompatible transfusions must be reported to The Joint Commission.
C. Blood and blood component use is a high-risk process.

D. Every transfusion must be reviewed for appropriateness.
E. None of the above.

Question 24: With regard to sentinel events, which of the following is *true*?

A. A sentinel event is any unexpected occurrence that results in death.
B. Hospitals are required to report a sentinel event to The Joint Commission.
C. Failure to submit a root cause analysis for a reported sentinel event may result in denial of accreditation by The Joint Commission.
D. Only deaths resulting from medical errors qualify as reviewable sentinel events by the Joint Commission.
E. A root cause analysis is not necessary if the event can be clearly attributed to an error on the part of an individual or group of individuals.

Question 25: Which of the following is an essential element of the management of nonconforming events?

A. Event classification.
B. Data analysis.
C. Implementation of corrective action.
D. Reporting to regulatory agencies.
E. All of the above.

ANSWERS

Question 1: B

Explanation:

- Quality control (QC) is performed for the purpose of evaluating a process in progress. QC assesses the suitability of inputs to determine whether the output meets specifications. Outputs may be products or services. The following are examples of QC functions: reagent QC, storage condition monitoring, measuring product properties (eg, measuring supernatant hemoglobin after RBC deglycerolization, or cell counts after leukocyte reduction), and visual inspections. Answers A, C, and D are examples of QC.
- QA activities are not directly tied to the performance of a process. The purpose of QA is to control processes, detect unwanted shifts or trends that may require correction, and identify opportunities for process improvement.
  - QA activities include reviewing procedures and policies for compliance with regulatory and accrediting agency expectations, reviewing operational performance data, reviewing records for completeness and accuracy, performing audits, and monitoring quality indicators.
- Quality management encompasses an organization's entire system for ensuring quality throughout the organization. Answer E is an example of an important element of quality management—planning.

Question 2: D

Explanation:

- Regulatory agencies act under authority of law to enforce compliance with law. Regulations are the rules under which the requirements of law are enforced. Federal agencies such as the FDA and the Center for Medicare and Medicaid Services (CMS) are regulatory agencies.
  - The FDA regulates blood establishments under the authority of the Food, Drug, and Cosmetics Act of 1938 (under which blood compo-

nents are considered drugs) and the Public Health Service Act of 1944.
  - Applicable regulations are listed in the Code of Federal Regulations (CFR), Title 21, Parts 200-299 (labeling, current good manufacturing practice), 600-680 (biological products), and 800-898 (medical devices, adverse events).
 ○ Human cells, tissues, and cellular and tissue-based products (HCT/Ps) are regulated under The Public Health Service Act of 1944, Section 361.
  - Applicable regulations are found in 21 CFR 1270-1271.
 ○ FDA guidances address the agency's thinking and expectations with regard to items that have not yet been codified, or they provide further clarity on existing regulations. Although expectations that are not yet codified can be issued only as recommendations, few establishments fail to heed them.
 ○ CMS regulates US medical laboratories under the authority of the Public Health Service Act of 1944, Section 353, and the Clinical Laboratory Improvement Amendments of 1988 (CLIA '88).
  - CLIA regulations are found in 42 CFR 493.
- In addition to federal regulatory agencies, there may be state and local-level regulatory agencies that have jurisdiction over blood and tissue establishments.
- Accreditation is certification that an establishment has met the quality standards set forth by an agency recognized as an authority in the industry or service being accredited. Participation in accreditation programs is voluntary. Accreditation assessments are usually performed by peers.

Question 3: E

Explanation:

- Product and service specifications are necessary for meeting customer, operational, regulatory, and accrediting organization requirements.
- Developing product and service specifications is a critical step in the planning of a new product or service. Other critical steps include the following:
 ○ Establishing quality goals.

- Identifying customers and determining the customer's needs and expectations.
- Developing policies and procedures.
- Securing necessary resources.
- Developing process controls.
- Validating processes.

Question 4: C

Explanation:

- Equipment qualification (previously referred to as equipment validation) demonstrates that the equipment is capable of fulfilling specified requirements within the operational setting and conditions in which it will be used. Equipment qualification consists of the following:
  - Installation qualification.
  - Operational qualification.
  - Performance qualification.

  (See explanation for Question 12 for definitions of these terms.)
- Calibration is a comparison of measurements by one instrument to those of a more accurate instrument or standard for the purpose of identifying and eliminating errors in measurement.
- Change control refers to adhering to established policies and processes for preventing unplanned, unapproved, and unmonitored changes to infrastructure, processes, products, or services.
- See Question 1 for explanation of quality control.

Question 5: E

Explanation:

- The person charged with oversight of the quality system must report directly to executive management.
- Executive management is the individual or group with responsibility and authority over operations; this group has the ability to establish or make changes to the quality system and has responsibility for

compliance with applicable accreditation and regulatory requirements.
  - Each establishment may define the composition and structure of its executive management.
- Under a quality system, manufacturing units and quality units should remain independent. In limited circumstances, such as a very small facility, a single individual may perform both production and quality functions.

Question 6: B

Explanation:

- The person with responsibility for oversight of the quality system should have the authority to recommend and initiate corrective action when appropriate.
- Other quality oversight functions include the following:
  - Review and approval of:
    - Standard operating procedures.
    - Training plans.
    - Validation and qualification plans.
    - Document control and recordkeeping systems.
    - Suppliers.
    - Product specification.
  - Review of nonconformances.
  - Analysis of operational data.
- The medical director must approve all medical and technical policies and procedures. The quality oversight officer may not implement new or changed policies or procedures without the medical director's approval.
- Exceptions to policies, processes, and procedures must be warranted by clinical situations, require justification, and must be preapproved by the medical director on a case-by-case basis.

Question 7: A

Explanation:

- Operational staff may perform quality oversight functions, but they should not provide oversight for operational work they have performed. Special certification is not required to provide quality oversight functions, but staff involved in such activities should be adequately trained and sufficiently knowledgeable to perform these functions.
- The purpose of this restriction is to avoid conflicts of interest that may interfere with the reporting of nonconformances and corrective action development.

Question 8: D

Explanation:

- CA is required for any staff members whose functions may affect the quality of testing, the provision of services, or the manufacture of products.
- CA methods may include the following:
  - Written tests.
  - Direct observation.
  - Review of completed work.
  - Testing of unknown samples.
- It is up to the employer to determine which methods will be used for performing CA.
- Assessments may be targeted at techniques or methods that are applicable to several procedures. CA for each procedure or test that an employee performs is not required.
- CMS requires that CA be performed a minimum of twice in the first year of employment and at least yearly thereafter. The assessment completed at the end of training may serve as one of the first year's assessments.
- CLIA regulations specify that the laboratory supervisor is responsible for ensuring that staff maintain competency, but they do not specify

that only the supervisor may perform CA. Each establishment may determine who is eligible to perform CAs. Criteria for eligibility should be described in the establishment's quality system.

Question 9: C

Explanation:

- 21 CFR Part 211 requires that personnel engaged in the manufacture, processing, packing, or holding of a drug product (blood products included) be trained in cGMP. These requirements also apply to personnel engaged in the manufacture, processing, packaging, or holding of HCT/Ps.
- cGMP refers to the methods used in, and the facilities or controls used for, the manufacture, processing, packing, or holding of a drug (including blood products) to ensure that the product meets regulatory (FDA) requirements for potency, purity, and safety.
- cGMP training should be provided with the employee's initial training, whenever a change in responsibilities warrant additional training, and as part of continuing education.

Question 10: B

Explanation:

- Critical supplies are those materials, supplies, or services that affect the quality of products produced or services provided.
- A list must be maintained of critical materials, supplies, and services and approved suppliers.
- The quality system should include policies and processes that address the following:
  - Supplier qualification.
  - Agreements.
  - How incoming supplies are received and qualified for use.
- Vendors of FDA-approved products must be qualified to serve as suppliers of critical supplies. The criteria used to qualify the vendor are determined by the establishment.

Question 11: C

Explanation:

- Blood banks and transfusion services must have agreements with vendors of critical materials, supplies, or services. These agreements are for purposes of defining the expectations and responsibilities of both the contractor and contracting facility.
- Agreements should address the following:
  - The specifications of the product or services provided.
  - The availability of products or services.
  - How products will be shipped.
  - Requirements for notifying the facility about product nonconformances, or changes that affect the safety or quality of the product.
  - The contracting facility's responsibilities with regard to the vendor.
  - Other issues as identified by the facility or contractor.
- Agreements should be reviewed annually to verify that they still meet the establishment's needs. However, agreements do not have to be renewed on a yearly basis.
- Agreements are necessary whenever the supply or service is from a source that is managed independently from the facility using the supply or service. In a hospital, services provided by an independently managed laboratory require an agreement between the two laboratories. Agreements are also necessary between hospitals within the same health-care system. Agreements may be as simple as a memorandum of understanding.
- The contracting facility bears responsibility for the finished product and for ensuring that the contractor has complied with all product standards and regulatory requirements.
- The contracting facility shares legal responsibility for work performed by the contractor.
- Examples of services that may be performed by contractors include compatibility testing, blood product irradiation, and blood donor infectious disease testing.

QUALITY AND COMPLIANCE 19

Question 12: D

Explanation:

- All equipment used in the collection, processing, testing, or storage of blood components or HCT/Ps must be qualified for use before implementation and after modifications or repairs that may affect its function.
- Qualification is demonstrating that the equipment is capable of fulfilling specified requirements.
- There should be written procedures for installation, operational, and performance qualification.
  - Installation qualification (IQ) verifies that the equipment and all components have been installed and activated in accordance with the manufacturer's specification and any cGMP requirements that may be applicable.
    - IQ includes ensuring that the equipment is assigned a unique identification number and entered into a preventive maintenance program.
  - Operational qualification (OQ) verifies that the functionality of the equipment conforms with the manufacturer's specifications.
  - Performance qualification (PQ) verifies that the equipment meets the user's specifications. PQ tests should be designed to verify the satisfactory performance of the equipment or system in the organization's processes. PQ is performed under the user's operating conditions, by user personnel, with real process materials. PQ is performed after IQ and OQ.
- Employees must be trained on equipment use before being allowed to operate a piece of equipment. Employee training records should provide evidence of this training and should document satisfactory results on CA. A specific list of employees authorized to use the equipment is not required but may be desirable for complex pieces of equipment.

Question 13: D

Explanation:

- FDA regulations specify that reagents used in the testing of blood components must be used in accordance with the manufacturer's instructions. Those instructions reflect the test conditions for which the reagents received FDA approval.
- Establishments desiring to vary from the manufacturer's instructions are required to apply for an FDA variance. Requests for variances must be supported by data that validate the requested change. The modified protocols may not be implemented without specific FDA approval. Variances are seldom granted.
- FDA requirements are also applicable to nonregistered establishments.

Question 14: C

Explanation:

- Documents are written policies, procedures, process descriptions, labels, work instructions, and forms. They describe the activities of the establishment and the expectations for how things should happen. Documents may be in paper or electronic format.
- Records provide evidence that what should have happened has happened. Forms become records when data are added to them. Records may be in paper or electronic format.
- The quality system should include a document management system that ensures that documents are current and comprehensive and that both current and obsolete documents are available. The system should also ensure records are accurate and complete.
- There should be defined processes for developing, approving, distributing, and maintaining documents.
- Distribution of documents should be controlled so copies of obsolete documents may be reliably retrieved and replaced with current documents.
- Documents must be reviewed, modified, and reapproved periodically. Review should be performed on an annual basis.

- Documents must be protected from unintended alterations or destruction.
- The required retention period for documents and records is determined by the purpose of the documents and records and is established by regulatory and accrediting organizations.

Question 15: A

Explanation:

- Manufacturing events that affect the safety, purity, or potency of blood components that have been distributed must be reported to the FDA. These events constitute BPDs.
  - Manufacturing encompasses testing, processes, packing, labeling, storage, and distribution steps.
  - Distribution of a product that does not meet known patient specifications also constitutes a BPD when this is a result of an error and not a therapeutic decision.
- Reporting is required only when the manufacturer has lost control of the product; ie, it has distributed the product. BPDs discovered before the establishment loses control of the product need not be reported, but they should be thoroughly investigated and addressed by the quality unit.
  - Reporting is required regardless of whether the product was administered or whether it resulted in an adverse event.
- A BPD report (BPDR):
  - Must be submitted within 45 days of discovering information that would reasonably suggest that a BPD has occurred.
  - May be submitted on paper or electronically using a standardized form available from the Center for Biologics Evaluation and Research (CBER) Web site.
  - Deviation codes are used to classify events according to the type of error that occurred.
  - The requirement to report BPDs also applies to HCT/Ps. HCT/P deviations are defined as events that are in violation of regulatory and established specifications for the prevention of communicable disease transmission or contamination, or unexpected or unforeseeable events that may result in disease transmission or contamination.

Question 16: B

Explanation:

- The RhIG lot in question deviates from the manufacturer's potency specifications, is incorrectly labeled, and is unsafe for patients requiring the higher dose specified on the label. These deviations require product recall.
- Manufacturers of blood and tissue products and pharmaceutical manufacturers are required to monitor and investigate product problems, including those detected after distribution. When appropriate, defective products should be corrected or removed from use.
- Recalls are a firm's removal or correction of a marketed product that the FDA considers to be in violation of the laws it administers and against which the agency would initiate legal action.
  - Recalls may be conducted on an establishment's own initiative, by FDA request, or by FDA order.
- Market withdrawals are an establishment's removal or correction of a distributed product involving a minor violation that would not be subject to legal action by the FDA or involving no violation.
- Answers A, C, and E are examples of market withdrawals, not recalls.
- Answer D is an example of a medical device product notification. In this example, the device defect did not warrant recall or ceasing distribution. However, notification and corrective action in the form of providing corrective software is required.

Question 17: C

Explanation:

- When a complication of blood collection or transfusion is confirmed to be fatal, the Office of Compliance and Biologics Quality, CBER, must be notified as soon as possible.
  - Initial notification may be by means of telephone, facsimile, express mail, or electronically transmitted mail as soon as possible.

QUALITY AND COMPLIANCE 23

- ○ A written report of the investigation must be submitted within 7 days after the fatality by the collecting facility, in the event of a donor reaction, or by the facility that performed the compatibility tests, in the event of a transfusion reaction.
- When compatibility testing is contracted to an outside establishment, both the compatibility testing laboratory and the transfusion facility share responsibility for reporting the fatality, regardless of whether either institution committed an error. A single combined report may be submitted, or each institution may submit a separate report.

Question 18: E

Explanation:

- All establishments that manufacture blood components must be registered with the FDA. Those that engage in interstate commerce must also be licensed.
  - ○ Manufacturing includes collection and processing, freezing, deglycerolizing, washing, and leukocyte reduction performed in the blood bank or transfusion service.
- Transfusion services that do not routinely collect or process blood or blood components and are part of a facility approved for Medicare reimbursement (CLIA certified) are exempt from registration. Transfusion services of this type are inspected under authority of CMS.
  - ○ FDA retains jurisdiction over these facilities and may conduct inspections if warranted.
  - ○ The collection and processing of blood and blood components in an emergency situation, therapeutic phlebotomies, preparation of recovered plasma, and the preparation of RBCs for transfusion are not acts requiring registration.

Question 19: E

Explanation:

- Assessments are systematic evaluations of whether laboratory activities and outputs comply with stated internal, accreditation, and regulatory expectations.
- Assessments may be internal or external. External assessments are performed by regulatory agencies or accrediting organizations. They may be used as part of the institution's quality assurance activities.
- Assessments may focus on a single process and its output, or they may address multiple related processes and outputs.
- In addition to formal audits, assessments may include peer review, self-assessments, and proficiency testing.
- Assessments should not be driven just by the detection of problems; assessments should be planned and scheduled so as to ensure periodic assessment of all critical processes.
- Assessments should be reviewed by management.
- There should be a process for corrective action implementation and monitoring of effectiveness.
- Identified problems should be tracked, trended, and analyzed.

Question 20: C

Explanation:

- As a condition of certification, laboratories must participate in an approved proficiency testing program for any CLIA-regulated testing that they perform.
- In the absence of an approved program, laboratories must have a system for determining the accuracy and reliability of test results. For example, they may test reference samples or samples from a regional pool.
- Proficiency testing samples must be handled and tested in the same manner as regular patient samples. Repeat testing is permitted providing that is also the manner in which patient specimens are tested.

- Laboratories operating under the same CLIA certificate may perform testing for each other. However, a laboratory may not send PT samples to a laboratory that operates under a different CLIA number, even if that laboratory is within the same facility and that is the manner in which patient samples are usually handled.
- Laboratories may not discuss a proficiency survey with other laboratories during the active period of a survey.
- For CAP surveys, unsatisfactory performance on a single testing event requires investigation and corrective action by the laboratory but does not require suspension of testing or reporting to the laboratory accrediting program.
- Failure to attain a satisfactory score on 2 of 3 events requires immediate corrective action or suspension of testing. The corrective action must be approved by the accrediting program.
- Failure to attain a satisfactory score on 3 of 4 events is considered critical PT performance and requires immediate suspension of testing.

Question 21: B

Explanation:

- Remedial action is an action taken to alleviate the symptoms of an existing nonconformance or problem. This supervisor did not determine why technologists did not issue the blood components properly, and therefore the solution only addresses the signs of the problem, not the cause of the problem.
- Corrective action addresses the root cause of an existing nonconformance or problem to prevent recurrences.
- Preventive action identifies ways to reduce or eliminate the potential for nonconformances or problems to occur. In this example, management's solution does nothing to prevent blood components from being incorrectly issued.
- Preventive action is proactive; corrective action is reactive.

Question 22: A

Explanation:

- The diagram is an outline of a cause-and-effect diagram, also known as a fish or Ishekawa diagram, after its originator.
- Cause-and-effect diagrams are used in root cause analysis and in process improvement to focus ideas around the component parts of a process, not individuals. Tools for generating the cause-and-effect diagrams include brainstorming, reviewing checklists, and the "repetitive why" approach.
- Cause-and-effect diagrams look at personnel, methods, policies and processes, environment, materials (reagents and supplies), and equipment as potential contributors to nonconformances.
- A Pareto diagram is a modified bar graph that identifies causes of a problem in order of decreasing frequency. The purpose is to identify those causes that account for the majority of errors so that process improvement efforts may be focused on the most common sources of error.
- Procedures are diagrammed with flow charts.
- A process map is a modified flow chart that depicts the steps of a process, the responsibility for those steps, and critical process measures.

Question 23: C

Explanation:

- The Joint Commission hospital accreditation standards specify that blood and blood component transfusion is a high-risk process, and require that hospitals collect data on the use of blood and blood components for purposes of performance improvement.
- The Joint Commission does not specify what types of data are to be collected or the number of examples to be reviewed.
- In 2007, The Joint Commission initiated the Blood Management Performance Measures Project to explore the development of blood management performance measures. The stakeholders advised identifying

priority areas for blood management that focused on activities related to blood conservation and appropriateness of transfusion and activities with a patient-centered focus. In 2008, the project technical advisory panel developed a proposed set of standardized measures to be used for assessing blood management in the hospital setting. It is expected that The Joint Commission will include at least some of those proposed measures in future accreditation requirements.
- There is no requirement to report ABO-incompatible transfusions; however, these events qualify as sentinel events and should be handled accordingly.

Question 24: C

Explanation:

- A sentinel event is an unexpected occurrence involving death or serious physical or psychological injury, or risk thereof.
  - Serious injury includes loss of limb or function.
  - "Risk thereof" includes any situation for which recurrence would carry a significant chance of a serious adverse outcome.
  - These events signal the need for immediate investigation and response.
- Hemolytic transfusion reactions caused by the administration of ABO-incompatible blood or components are sentinel events.
- The Joint Commission does not require sentinel event reporting but it does encourage reporting for purposes of:
  - Sharing "lessons learned" with other institutions.
  - Consultation with The Joint Commission staff during root cause analysis and development of corrective action.
  - Demonstrating due diligence in addressing patient safety issues.
- Once The Joint Commission is aware of a sentinel event, either through voluntary reporting or other methods, the organization must submit a thorough and credible root cause analysis and action plan within 45 days of discovering the event.
  - If more than 45 days have elapsed at the time of discovery, the organization has 15 days to submit a root cause analysis and action plan.

- Beyond the due date, opportunities are still provided for an organization to comply with the requirement to submit a root cause analysis and action plan. If the root cause analysis is not submitted within 90 days of the due date, a recommendation for denial of accreditation status is submitted to the Accreditation Committee. Even then, the organization is given the opportunity to respond.
- Root cause analysis should identify the risk factors that contribute to the probability of an event occurring. An error on the part of an individual or group of individuals may be indicative of an ineffective process. Additionally, not all sentinel events are the result of errors.

Question 25: E

Explanation:

- Nonconforming events are those that result in deviation from established policies, processes, and procedures, and in failure to comply with accreditation and regulatory requirements.
- A management system for nonconforming events is an essential component of a quality system. Event management should include the following:
    - Documentation of events.
    - Classification of events.
        - Classification is necessary for reporting purposes and for tracking and trending.
    - Assessment of how the event has affected quality.
    - Evaluation of the impact on interrelated processes.
    - Root cause analysis.
    - Corrective action.
    - Preventive action.
    - Where appropriate, market withdrawal or recall.
    - Follow-up evaluation of the effectiveness of corrective and preventive action.
    - Tracking, trending, and data analysis.

REFERENCES

1. Motschman TL, Jett BW, Wilkinson SL. Quality systems: Theory and practice. In: Roback JD, Combs MR, Grossman BJ, Hillyer CD, eds. Technical manual. 16th ed. Bethesda, MD: AABB, 2008:1-39.
2. Ramsey G. Regulatory issues in blood banking. In: Roback JD, Combs MR, Grossman BJM, Hillyer CD, eds. Technical manual. 16th ed. Bethesda, MD: AABB, 2008:91-102.
3. Price TH, ed. Standards for blood banks and transfusion services. 26th ed. Bethesda, MD: AABB, 2009.
4. Food and Drug Administration. Notification process for transfusion related fatalities and donation related deaths. Rockville, MD: Center for Biologics Evaluation and Research, 2008. [Available at http://www.fda.gov/BiologicsBloodVaccines/ResourcesforYou/Industry/default.htm (accessed June 30, 2009).]
5. Food and Drug Administration. Recalls, withdrawals, field corrections, and notifications. Rockville, MD: Center for Biologics Evaluation and Research, 2009. [Available at http://www.fda.gov/BiologicsBloodVaccines/ResourcesforYou/Industry/default. htm (accessed June 30, 2009).]
6. The Joint Commission. Comprehensive accreditation manual for hospitals. Oakbrook Terrace, IL: The Joint Commission, 2008.

In: Blackall D, Figueroa P, Winters J
Transfusion Medicine Self-Assessment and Review, 2nd Edition
Bethesda, MD: AABB Press, 2009

2

Medical Assessment of Blood Donors, Blood Collection (Autologous and Allogeneic), and Donor Complications

QUESTIONS

Question 1: A donor with which value is acceptable for whole blood donation?

A. Hemoglobin of 12 g/dL by venipuncture in a woman.
B. Hematocrit of 36% by earlobe puncture in a man.
C. Hemoglobin of 12 g/dL by venipuncture in a man.
D. Hemoglobin of 12.5 g/dL by venipuncture in a man or a woman.
E. Hematocrit of 37% by venipuncture in a woman.

Question 2: Which of the following donors is eligible to donate?

A. 18-year-old female, blood pressure 150/80 mm Hg, pulse 80 bpm, hematocrit 36%, temperature 37 C.
B. 16-year-old male, blood pressure 130/70 mm Hg, pulse 90 bpm, hematocrit 42%, temperature 37.7 C.
C. 80-year-old female, blood pressure 120/40 mm Hg, pulse 72 bpm, hemoglobin 12.5 g/dL, temperature 37.5 C.

D. 35-year-old female, blood pressure 175/101 mm Hg, pulse 86 bpm, hemoglobin 13 g/dL, temperature 36 C.
E. 27-year-old male, blood pressure 190/99 mm Hg, pulse 100 bpm, hematocrit 45%, temperature 36.7 C.

Question 3: Which of the following donors is unacceptable for whole blood donation?

A. A donor desiring to donate 2-unit red cell units by apheresis who donated whole blood 8 weeks ago.
B. An athlete with a pulse of 48 bpm.
C. A 26-year-old woman, 8 weeks after delivery of a healthy infant.
D. A 35-year-old nurse who received Hepatitis B Immune Globulin 18 months ago.
E. A 17-year-old with an oral temperature of 37.8 C.

Question 4: Donors with which of the following would be eligible to donate whole blood?

A. Aspirin ingestion in the last 24 hours.
B. Receipt of a tattoo 7 months ago at a tattoo parlor in a state that does not license such establishments.
C. Delivery of a child 4 weeks ago.
D. History of treatment for gonorrhea 9 months ago.
E. Household contact with an individual with active unknown viral hepatitis 6 months ago.

Question 5: Which of the following donors is eligible to donate?

A. Donor is taking finasteride (Propecia) for male pattern baldness.
B. Donor was taking isotretinoin (Accutane) for acne. Last dose 2 weeks ago.
C. Donor took acitretin (Soriatane) for psoriasis. Last dose 2 years ago.

D. Donor took etretinate (Tegison) for psoriasis. Last dose 10 years ago.
E. Donor took finasteride (Proscar) for prostatic hypertrophy. Last dose 35 days ago.

Question 6: Which of the following donors is eligible to donate?

A. Donor immunized against German measles (rubella) 2 weeks ago.
B. Donor who received varicella zoster immunization (Varivax) 3 weeks ago.
C. Donor immunized against rubeola 4 weeks ago.
D. Donor received an experimental, unlicensed vaccine as part of a research project 12 weeks ago.
E. Donor given oral typhoid vaccine 1 week ago.

Question 7: A 35-year-old male nurse received his first hepatitis B vaccine as a part of the hospital's safety program and an Occupational Safety and Health Administration requirement. He has had no exposures. He is eligible to donate blood:

A. Today.
B. In 24 hours.
C. In 48 hours.
D. In 6 months.
E. In 12 months.

Question 8: After receiving Hepatitis B Immune Globulin, donors are deferred for:

A. 3 months.
B. 6 months.
C. 12 months.
D. 3 years.
E. Indefinitely.

Question 9: Which of the following donors is eligible to donate?

A. Wife of a hemophilia patient; last sexual contact 2 days ago.
B. Former prostitute; married with no high-risk behavior for 10 years.
C. Male who had sex with a prostitute 9 months ago; a condom was used.
D. Male who had sex with another male 20 years ago.
E. Male jailed for 7 days, 15 months ago.

Question 10: Which of the following donors is eligible to donate?

A. Donor had surgery for a ruptured berry aneurysm 15 months ago; received 2 units of allogeneic red cells and an allogeneic dura mater graft.
B. Donor had a history of hepatitis A at age 20.
C. Donor's husband was vaccinated for smallpox; she has developed a rash after changing the bandage covering her husband's vaccination site.
D. Donor studied in Ireland for 1 year in 1993.
E. Donor has spent a total of 4 weeks in France, 2 months in Scotland, 3 months in England, and 2 months in Northern Ireland between 1988 and 1995.

Question 11: Which of the following statements regarding plateletpheresis donation is *true*?

A. Donors can donate more than 24 times per year.
B. Donors donating a triple platelet product are deferred from platelet donation for 7 days.
C. Donors must have a minimum platelet count of 100,000/µL to be eligible to donate.
D. Donors must not have ingested aspirin-containing products within 36 hours prior to donation in order to be eligible.

E. Donors donating after a whole blood donation must wait 8 weeks until they can donate platelets unless the extracorporeal volume of the apheresis instrument is less than 200 mL.

Question 12: A frequent plasma donor is defined as an individual donating plasma more frequently than every 4 weeks. Which of the following concerning this type of donor is *true*?

A. The total serum protein must be at least 10.0 g/dL.
B. A serum protein electrophoresis or quantitative immunodiffusion must be performed with every donation.
C. The donor can donate within 12 months of traveling to a malaria-endemic area.
D. If the donor weighs less than 175 lb and is undergoing manual plasmapheresis, only 1 L of whole blood can be processed every 24 hours.
E. If the donor weighs less than 175 lb and is undergoing manual plasmapheresis, only 2 L of whole blood can be processed during a 3-day period.

Question 13: Which of the following statements regarding the donation of red cells by automated methods is *true*?

A. The deferral period after the donation of a combination of a single unit of red cells and a single unit of platelets by apheresis is 16 weeks.
B. The copper sulfate method of determining hematocrit cannot be used to qualify a donor for double red cell donation.
C. Donor weight and hematocrit requirements for double red cell donation are the same as those for whole blood donation.
D. Double red cell donation is associated with a higher frequency of reactions compared to whole blood.
E. In a donor donating the maximum number of donations in a year, iron losses are greater with double red cell donation than whole blood donation.

Question 14: Which of the following statements regarding autologous donation is *true*?

A. Hemoglobin of 11 g/dL is acceptable.
B. Requirements for allogeneic donation must be met.
C. Blood must be drawn 96 hours before the anticipated surgery.
D. These units can be used (crossed over) for other patients.
E. The interval between two donations must be 7 days.

Question 15: Which of the following autologous donors is eligible to donate?

A. A 75-year-old male with prostate cancer whose hemoglobin is 10 g/dL. He is otherwise healthy and is scheduled for a prostatectomy in 3 weeks.
B. A 35-year-old paraplegic with infected decubitus ulcers over the sacrum, hemoglobin 13 g/dL, debridement and skin grafting in 14 days.
C. A 40-year-old female with degenerative joint disease. Her hemoglobin is 11 g/dL. She will undergo bilateral knee replacement in 24 hours.
D. A 16-year-old with chronic tonsillitis, hemoglobin 15 g/dL, tonsillectomy in 2 weeks. There is no physician order, but the patient's mother gives approval and insists upon donation.
E. An 86-year-old female with degenerative joint disease. Her hemoglobin is 12 g/dL. She will have a right hip replacement in 4 days.

Question 16: Which of the following diseases is treated with therapeutic phlebotomy?

A. Porphyria cutanea tarda (PCT).
B. Alagille syndrome.
C. Refsum's disease.
D. Susac syndrome
E. Cerebral autosomal dominant arteriopathy with subcortical infarcts and leukoencephalopathy (CADASIL).

Question 17: Which of the following is a *true* statement concerning the use of blood collected from therapeutic phlebotomies from hereditary hemochromatosis for transfusion?

A. Blood from therapeutic phlebotomies of hereditary hemochromatosis patients cannot be used for transfusion.
B. Eligibility criteria for hereditary hemochromatosis patients are stricter than those for whole blood donors.
C. Blood collected more frequently than every 56 days cannot be used for transfusion.
D. A prescription from the physician treating the hereditary hemochromatosis patient is required.
E. If a prescription is not available, a physician at the donor center must examine the patient and certify he or she is in good health once a year.

Question 18: Which of the following is the most common adverse event to whole blood donation?

A. Bruise or hematoma.
B. Vasovagal reaction.
C. Nerve injury.
D. Arterial puncture.
E. Thrombophlebitis.

Question 19: Which of the following statements concerning vasovagal reactions is *true*?

A. It is characterized by hypotension and tachycardia.
B. It is associated with young age.
C. It is most common in repeat donors.
D. The pathophysiology is caused by increased sympathetic activity.
E. It is more common in overweight donors.

Question 20: Which of the following is an appropriate treatment for a vasovagal reaction?

A. Apply cold compresses to the donor's neck or forehead.
B. Distract the donor.
C. Place the donor in the Trendelenburg position.
D. Change the donor's breathing patterns.
E. All of the above.

Question 21: Which of the following is *true* about arterial punctures during whole blood donation?

A. It is usually painless.
B. Bright red blood is always seen in the bag.
C. A risk factor is inexperience in the phlebotomist.
D. If no pain is present, the collection should be completed.
E. All of the above are true.

Question 22: Which of the following statements concerning nerve injuries associated with whole blood donation is *true*?

A. Onset of symptoms is usually delayed 2 to 3 days after donation.
B. It is associated with hematoma formation.
C. It is most commonly seen in male donors.
D. In the majority of cases, recovery takes greater than 4 weeks.
E. It is associated with older-than-average donors.

Question 23: Which of the following statements is *true* about acute normovolemic hemodilution (ANH)?

A. The units of blood are reinfused in the same order in which they were collected.
B. Blood is collected into a dry bag with no anticoagulant.

C. Blood is stored at room temperature.
D. ANH increases the risk of ABO-incompatible transfusion.
E. If crystalloid solutions are used to replace the removed blood, they are infused at a ratio of 1 mL for every 1 mL of whole blood removed.

Question 24: Which of the following statements is *true* about ANH?

A. According to AABB standards, the blood bank or transfusion service is required participate in the development of policies and procedures for ANH.
B. It is acceptable to use the blood collected for transfusion to other patients.
C. It is not necessary for a program that *only* performs ANH to have a quality control and quality assurance program.
D. It is not necessary to use the same arm preparation techniques employed in whole blood donation.
E. Patients with hemoglobin <12 g/dL and for whom the probability of transfusion is less than 10% are optimum candidates for ANH.

Question 25: Which of the following is *true* with regard to intraoperative blood recovery (cell salvage)?

A. Intraoperative blood recovered with processing (washing and concentration) when stored at room temperature must be transfused within 4 hours from the start of collection.
B. Intraoperative blood recovered without processing when stored at 1 to 6 C must be transfused within 24 hours of the end of collection.
C. Vacuum settings on the suction device are typically set less than 150 torr to prevent hemolysis.
D. The collection and processing of a single unit of blood is cost effective in most cases.
E. Anticoagulation of the blood is not required because it is collected from the surgical field.

Question 26: Which of the following statements is *true* of intraoperative blood recovery?

A. The storage bag need only be labeled with the patient's name.
B. The presence of bacteria in the recovered blood is associated with a high frequency of sepsis or adverse outcomes.
C. When blood is processed (washed and concentrated) it is not necessary to reinfuse the blood through a microaggregate filter.
D. Processing can occur in the operating room using cell salvage devices or at another location using a cell washer.
E. Blood is usually washed with lactated Ringer's solution or D5W.

Question 27: A 72-year-old male donor presents for whole blood donation. The donor completes the Blood Donor History Questionnaire and no unexpected answers are uncovered. Donor examination shows the donor to be afebrile with normal blood pressure and pulse. Hemoglobin is 14 g/dL. He successfully donates 450 mL of whole blood. While waiting in the donor lounge, he becomes diaphoretic and complains of crushing substernal chest pain. He collapses and becomes pulseless and apneic. Cardiopulmonary resuscitation is initiated and emergency medical service is called. Attempts to resuscitate him are unsuccessful. Subsequently, it is discovered that he had a history of severe coronary artery disease and unstable angina which he failed to mention when completing the donor questionnaire. Which of the following statements is *true* concerning actions which must be taken?

A. The Center for Biologics Evaluation and Research (CBER) must be notified of the death as soon as possible and a final complete written report must be submitted within 7 days.
B. The Center for Devices and Radiologic Health (CDRH) must be notified of the death within 24 hours and a written report must be submitted within 7 days.
C. The Center for Drug Evaluation and Research (CDER) must be notified of the death within 24 hours and a final complete written report must be submitted within 7 days.

D. CBER must be notified of the death as soon as possible and a written report must be submitted within 7 days.
E. Because the donor had an underlying health condition, the death is not related to donation and no reporting is required.

ANSWERS

Question 1: D

Explanation:

- See Question 3. Of note, CBER has stated that earlobe hemoglobin measurements are unacceptable because of substantial variation in hemoglobin values compared with concurrent values from venipuncture samples.
- There are *no* differences in hemoglobin requirements based upon donor sex.

Question 2: C

Explanation:

See Question 3.

Question 3: E

Explanation:

- Requirements for donor eligibility to donate whole blood are set forth in AABB *Standards for Blood Banks and Transfusion Services (Standards)*. See Table 2-3A.
- Acceptable criteria for whole blood donation are as follows:
  - Age:
    - Lower limit: 16 years.
    - 16- and 17-year-old donors are acceptable as permitted by state law.
    - Upper limit: None.
  - The donor should appear in good health and must be free of major organ disease (heart, liver, and lungs), cancer, or abnormal bleeding tendency.

Table 2-3A.

Criteria	Category
Age	≥16 years old as appropriate by applicable state law
Blood volume collected	Maximum of 10.5 mL/kg of donor weight, including samples; blood collection container must be approved for volume collected
Blood pressure	≤180 mm Hg systolic ≤100 mm Hg diastolic
Pulse	50-100 beats per minute <50 beats per minute acceptable if athlete
Temperature	≤37.5 C (99.5 F) if measured orally, or equivalent if measured by another method
Hemoglobin/hematocrit	≥12.5 g/dL or 38%, regardless of the donor's gender

- ○ Maximum allowable collection volume is 10.5 mL of whole blood collected per kg body weight (450 ±45 mL for a 110-lb adult, including samples).
- ○ Persons weighing less than 110 lb (50 kg) may have as little as 300 mL drawn without reducing the amount of anticoagulant in the primary bag. If it is necessary to draw <300 mL, the amount of anticoagulant must be reduced proportionately.
- Minimum donation intervals required following apheresis and whole blood donations are explained in AABB *Standards*. See Table 2-3B.
- Donors are deferred for 6 weeks after the delivery of a healthy infant.
- After Hepatitis B Immune Globulin administration, donors are deferred for 12 months.

Table 2-3B.

Donation Interval	Procedure
16 weeks	2-unit erythrocytapheresis
8 weeks	Whole blood donation
4 weeks	Infrequent plasmapheresis
2 days	Leukocytapheresis
2 days	Single apheresis platelet donation
7 days	Double or triple apheresis platelet donation

Question 4: A

Explanation:

- AABB standards for temporary deferral of whole blood donors:
  - Donors are deferred during pregnancy and for 6 weeks after the conclusion of pregnancy.
  - Completion of treatment for syphilis or gonorrhea, a history of syphilis or gonorrhea—12-month deferral.
  - Residing in a household with or sexual contact with an individual with hepatitis A, hepatitis B, symptomatic Hepatitis C, or unknown hepatitis—12-month deferral. Residing with or sexual contact with a person with asymptomatic hepatitis C is not grounds for deferral.
  - Sexual contact with an individual with human immunodeficiency virus (HIV) infection or a positive test for the HIV/AIDS virus—12-month deferral.
  - Allogeneic blood component transfusion—12-month deferral.
  - Organ, tissue, bone marrow transplant—12-month deferral.
  - Bone or skin graft—12-month deferral.
  - Sexual contact with a prostitute or anyone else who takes money, drugs, or other payment for sex—12-months.
  - Sexual contact with anyone who has ever used needles to take drugs or steroids or anything not prescribed by their doctor—12-month deferral.

MEDICAL ASSESSMENT

- Sexual contact with anyone who has hemophilia or has used clotting factor concentrates—12-month deferral.
- Female donors: Sexual contact with a male who has ever had sexual contact with another male—12-month deferral.
- Had a tattoo—12-month deferral. (In states where tattoo parlors are licensed and inspected by the state, deferral is not necessary.)
- Had an ear or body piercing—12-month deferral.
- Came in contact with someone else's blood (mucous membrane contact or needlestick)—12-month deferral.
- Incarceration in jail, juvenile detention, lockup, or prison for more than 72 hours—12-month deferral.
- Traveled to a malaria-endemic area—12-month deferral.
- Emigrated from a malaria-endemic area—3-year deferral.
- Had a history of malaria—3-year deferral.
- See Question 5 for deferrals related to medications.
- See Question 6 for deferrals related to immunizations.

• Food and Drug Administration (FDA) guidance requires that ingestion of aspirin or aspirin-containing medications within "2 full days" preceding donation or ingestion of medications that irreversibly inhibit platelet function is not a cause for deferral if the platelets from the donation are not used as the sole source of platelets for transfusion. Because plateletpheresis donors are the sole source of platelets for a patient, they are not eligible to donate if aspirin is ingested within 48 hours. This is because aspirin blocks the generation of thromboxane A_2, which inhibits the platelet release reaction and renders the platelets inactive. According to CBER guidance, donors taking clopidogrel (Plavix) or ticlopidne (Ticlid) must have 14 full medication-free days before donation. If other drugs known to inhibit platelet function have been ingested, they should be evaluated.

Question 5: E

Explanation:

- All of the following drugs are teratogens and could potentially adversely affect a child in utero if transfused to a pregnant woman:
  - Finasteride (Proscar or Propecia): 1-month deferral after last dose.
  - Isotretinoin (Accutane, Amnesteem, Claravis, and Sotret): 1-month deferral after last dose.

- Dutasteride (Avodart): 6-month deferral after last dose.
- Acitretin (Soriatane): 3-year deferral.*
- Etretinate (Tegison): permanent deferral.*

*Both are used to treat psoriasis. Acitretin reacts with alcohol to form a slowly excreted teratogen. Etretinate is never completely excreted.

Question 6: C

Explanation:

See Question 8.

Question 7: A

Explanation:

See Question 8.

Question 8: C

Explanation for Questions 6 through 8:

- Toxoid, synthetic, or killed vaccines: no deferral; accept if donor is free of symptoms [anthrax, cholera, diphtheria, hepatitis A, hepatitis B, influenza, Lyme disease, paratyphoid, pertussis, plague, pneumococcal polysaccharide, polio (Salk, injectable), rabies, Rocky Mountain spotted fever, tetanus, typhoid (injectable)].
- Recombinant vaccines: no deferral.
- Live attenuated viral and bacterial vaccines: 2-week deferral [measles (rubeola), mumps, polio (Sabin, oral), typhoid (oral), yellow fever].
- Live attenuated viral vaccines: 4-week deferral [rubella (German measles), varicella zoster (chicken pox)].
- Smallpox vaccination: 21 days from the date of vaccination or until the vaccination site scab falls off, whichever is later (if no complica-

tions have occurred), 2 months from the date of vaccination if the scab was removed (did not fall off), 14 days after resolution of complications in those with vaccine-related complications.
- Exposure to a smallpox vaccination site: no deferral if simple exposure; until the scab falls off if they have developed a skin lesion following exposure; 3 months from the time of vaccination of the person they came in contact with if they developed a skin lesion and removed the scab (did not fall off); 14 days after resolution of any complications.
- Other vaccines: 12-month deferral (Hepatitis B Immune Globulin, unlicensed vaccines).
- Hepatitis B vaccine contains hepatitis B surface antigen (HBsAg), synthesized using recombinant DNA technology or from noninfectious virions obtained from infected individuals. A series consisting of three intramuscular injections is required, with the second and the third injections given 1 month and 6 months after the first injection, respectively. In the United States, universal childhood vaccination has been implemented. All laboratory workers with possible exposure to blood and tissues should receive this vaccine.
- Hepatitis B vaccination is not required for individuals who have adequate titers of antibodies to HBsAg. Hepatitis B vaccine contains only HBsAg. Recent or remote immunization with hepatitis B vaccine does not explain the presence of antibody to hepatitis B core antigen (HBc) in a donor. Studies have shown that some sensitive HbsAg assays can detect the injected HBsAg for up to 5 days following immunization. The potential for a positive HBsAg result does exist.

Question 9: E

Explanation:

- 12-month deferral for some high-risk behavior: see Question 4.
- Permanent deferral for other high-risk behavior or situations:
  - Positive test for HIV.
  - Using needles to take drugs, steroids, or anything not prescribed by a doctor.
  - Receiving a clotting factor concentrate.
  - Males having sex with another male, even once, since 1977.
  - Receiving money, drugs, or other payment for sex.

- Being born in, having lived in, having visited and received blood products in, or having sex with someone having been born in, lived in, or who received blood products from Cameroon, Central African Republic, Chad, Congo, Equatorial Guinea, Gabon, Niger, or Nigeria. This is because of the presence of HIV-1 Group O in these countries. The HIV-1 subtype is not detected by all licensed HIV enzyme immunoassays (EIAs). If an EIA that can detect Group O is used for testing, the questions concerning sexual contact or living in Africa can be eliminated.
- With regard to males having sex with males, sexual contact with prostitutes, or sexual contact with other high-risk groups, it is irrelevant whether or not the individual involved used a barrier method or practiced "safe sex." Similarly, if the individual was a prostitute in a country or area where prostitution is legal and regulated (ie, serologic screening for sexually transmitted disease is used), the individual is still deferred.

Question 10: D

Explanation:

- Creutzfeldt-Jakob disease (CJD) and variant CJD (vCJD) deferral criteria:
  - Recipient of human-derived growth hormone or dura mater graft: permanent deferral (CJD risk).
  - One or more blood relatives with CJD: permanent deferral (CJD).
  - Recipient of bovine insulin since 1980 produced from cattle in a country where BSE is endemic: permanent deferral (vCJD).
  - Residing in Great Britain (England, Wales, Scotland, Northern Ireland, the Isle of Man, Channel Islands, Gibraltar, Falkland Islands) for a total for 3 months between 1980 and 1996: permanent deferral (vCJD).
  - Transfusion of blood or blood components in the United Kingdom or France since 1980: permanent deferral (vCJD).
  - Lived 5 or more cumulative years in Europe since 1980, including time lived in the United Kingdom: permanent deferral (vCJD).
  - Former or current US military personnel, civilian employee, or dependent who resided at US military bases in Northern Europe

(Germany, Belgium, Netherlands) for 6 months or more between 1980 and 1990: permanent deferral (vCJD).
- Former or current US military personnel, civilian employee, or dependent who resided at US military bases in Southern Europe (Greece, Turkey, Spain, Portugal, Italy) for 6 months or more between 1980 and 1996: permanent deferral (vCJD).

- Deferral criteria for individuals exposed to a smallpox vaccination site:
  - No deferral if simple exposure.
  - Until the scab falls off if they have developed a skin lesion following exposure.
  - Three months from the time of vaccination of the person they came in contact with if they developed a skin lesion and removed the scab (did not fall off).
  - Fourteen days after resolution of any complications.
  - See Question 8 for deferral criteria for those receiving the smallpox vaccine.

- Permanent deferral criteria for hepatitis, HIV, and human T-cell lymphotropic virus (HTLV):
  - History of viral hepatitis after 11th birthday (regardless of virus responsible).
  - HBsAg-positive, confirmed by neutralization.
  - Anti-HBc-reactive on more than one occasion.
  - Donor of the only unit of blood given to a patient who subsequently developed hepatitis, HIV, or HTLV.
  - Past or present laboratory or clinical evidence of hepatitis C virus (HCV), HIV, or HTLV infection.

---------------- ◯ ----------------

Question 11: B

Explanation:

- Plateletpheresis donors may donate as frequently as twice per week. They are not allowed to donate more than 24 times per year. This restriction arises from the fact that early apheresis equipment removed significant numbers of lymphocytes during plateletpheresis. This resulted in concerns that this could, with time, lead to immunodeficiency. Studies of these donors did demonstrate decreased T-lymphocyte counts and IgG levels 8 months after donation. However,

current apheresis instruments remove significantly fewer lymphocytes, and more recent studies have failed to demonstrate immunologic changes.
- Donors must have a minimum platelet count of 150,000/µL to be eligible to donate.
- CBER guidance requires that a sample for a platelet count be drawn before collection.
    - This count should be used for eligibility determination (current collection or future collections) and to set the yield parameters. The count may be completed before the procedure starts or immediately following initiation.
    - If the platelet count cannot be obtained (eg, during collections on a mobile drive), an average of previous counts from the donor or a default count can be used to program the instrument.
    - If one of these surrogate counts is used, a triple platelet collection cannot be performed.
- The instrument must be set so that there will be a platelet count of no less than 100,000/µL at the end of the procedure.
- Donors should also not have taken aspirin within "2 full days" of donation. This is interpreted to mean 48 hours. If they have taken other medications known to interfere with platelet function, these should be evaluated before accepting the donor.
- Donors should also not have taken clopidogrel (Plavix) or ticlopidine (Ticlid) for 14 days before donation and piroxicam (Feldene) for 2 days before donation.
- Donors of whole blood must wait 8 weeks to donate platelets again unless the extracorporeal volume of the instrument is less than 100 mL.
- The total plasma volume (including plasma collected on the platelet product and concurrent plasma) must not exceed 500 mL (or 600 mL if the donor is 175 lbs or greater) or the volume described in the instrument's labeling.
- Red cell and plasma losses must be monitored and are used to determine donor eligibility status. See Tables 2-11A and 2-11B.

Table 2-11A.

Initial Red Cell Loss	Second Red Cell Loss within 8 Weeks	Deferral
<200 mL	<200 mL	No deferral
<200 mL	>200 mL but <300 mL	Defer for 8 weeks from second loss
>200 mL but <300 mL	NA	Defer for 8 weeks from initial loss
<200 mL	Total loss from first and second losses >300 mL	Defer for 16 weeks from second loss
≥300 mL	NA	Defer for 16 weeks from initial loss

Table 2-11B.

Donor Weight	Plasma Loss within 12 Months
110-175 lbs	12 L
>175 lbs	14.4 L

Question 12: C

Explanation:

- Plasma can be collected by either manual methods (collecting whole blood in plastic bags, separating the plasma, and returning the cellular components) or automated methods.

- Plasma donations can also be categorized by the frequency with which the donor donates:
  - Infrequent plasma donors: the interval between donations is more than 4 weeks. These donors must fulfill whole blood donor requirements.
  - Frequent plasma donors: the interval between donations is less than 4 weeks. These donors must fulfill criteria outlined in the Code of Federal Regulations (21 CFR 640.63 and 21 CFR 640.65). These requirements are similar to those for whole blood donation but differ in the following respects:
    - Malaria risk is not a cause for deferral.
    - The total serum protein must be at least 6.0 g/dL.
    - Either a serum protein electrophoresis or quantitative immunodiffusion assay must be performed every 4 months. The plasma protein fractionation must be within normal limits.
    - The donors must undergo a physical examination once a year.
- Both frequent and infrequent plasma donors have limitations on the amount of plasma that can be donated in a 12-month period. This is given in Table 2-11B.
- See Table 2-12 for volume limits on whole blood removed for donors undergoing manual plasmapheresis. Volume limits for donors undergoing automated plasmapheresis are defined by the manufacturer of the equipment used to perform the collection.
- Frequent plasma donors must not have red cell losses greater than 200 mL within 8 weeks. If they do, they are deferred for 8 weeks from the last red cell loss.

Table 2-12.

	Weight of the Donor	
	<175 lb	≥175 lb
Whole blood withdrawn at one time	500 mL	600 mL
Whole blood withdrawn during the entire session or 2-day period	1000 mL	1200 mL
Whole blood collected in 7-day period	2000 mL	2400 mL

MEDICAL ASSESSMENT

- As with plateletpheresis, there must be at least 2 days between donations and no more than two donations within a 7-day period.

Question 13: B

Explanation:

- CBER guidance requires that a quantitative method for determining hemoglobin/hematocrit be used. The copper sulfate method is qualitative only and cannot be used.
- The deferral period for collecting a single red cell unit by automated methods would be 8 weeks. The deferral period for double red blood cell collections is 16 weeks.
- Donor weight and hematocrit requirements for double red cell donation are defined by the manufacturer of the instrument used to collect the red cells. They vary according to donor sex and are generally higher than those defined by the FDA for whole blood donation.
- Studies have found a *lower* incidence of reactions with double red cell donations compared with whole blood donations. This is thought to be because the donor is euvolemic after a double red cell donation as a result of infused anticoagulant, in contrast to a hypovolemic donor with whole blood donation.
- An individual donating whole blood regularly and one donating double red cell units regularly would have the same iron losses at the end of the deferral periods. Although double red cell donors lose twice as much iron per donation, they are deferred twice as long. Within their respective deferral periods, the two donors can only donate the same number of units.

Question 14: A

Explanation:

- A hemoglobin of 11 g/dL (hematocrit of 33%) is acceptable for autologous donation. (AABB *Standards*)
- Questions required of allogeneic donors are not required of autologous donors.

- If more than one unit is required, the phlebotomy schedule is established by the transfusion facility. The last phlebotomy must be scheduled ≥72 hours before the anticipated surgery. This is to avoid hypovolemia and attendant negative effects for the patient. (AABB *Standards*)
- Autologous units are not used (crossed over) for other patients unless exceptional circumstances warrant the transfusion. The decision must be approved and documented by the medical director of the collection facility. (AABB *Standards*)
- The donor/patient's physician and the collection facility medical director decide the interval between donations.

Question 15: E

Explanation:

- See Question 14 for additional explanation.
- Autologous donations *must* be ordered by the patient's physician.
- Blood should not be collected when the donor/patient has a bacterial infection that could be associated with bacteremia because this places him or her at risk for septic transfusion reactions at the time of transfusion of the blood component.
- Other than the criteria listed in Question 14 and those above, no other criteria exist in AABB *Standards* or CBER regulations concerning autologous blood donation. There are additional patient issues that should be considered as contraindications to autologous blood donation, including the following:
  - Presence of diseases with which the donor/patient has a fixed cardiac output (eg, aortic stenosis) or has a cardiac output that is volume dependent (eg, hypertrophic cardiomyopathy or subaortic stenosis).
  - Presence of unstable angina or severe coronary artery disease.
  - Recent myocardial infarction or stroke.
  - Cyanotic heart disease.

Question 16: A

Explanation:

- See Table 2-16 for a list of diseases treated with therapeutic phlebotomy.
- PCT is the most common porphyria.

Table 2-16.

Disease	Rationale behind Therapeutic Phlebotomy
Polycythemia vera	Reduce hyperviscosity due to increased red cell mass
Erythropoietin receptor mutations	Reduce hyperviscosity due to increased red cell mass
High oxygen affinity Hb mutations	Reduce hyperviscosity due to increased red cell mass
Polycythemia due to high-altitude residency	Reduce hyperviscosity due to increased red cell mass
Cyanotic congenital heart disease	Reduce hyperviscosity due to increased red cell mass
Respiratory disease	Reduce hyperviscosity due to increased red cell mass
Erythropoietin producing neoplasms	Reduce hyperviscosity due to increased red cell mass
Porphyria cutanea tarda	Reduce intrahepatic iron, which oxidizes porphyrinogens to porphyrins
Hereditary hemochromatosis	Reduce systemic iron overload

- It is caused by a deficiency in uroporhyrinogen decarboxylase. The result is a build up of porphyrinogens which can then be oxidized by iron to porphyrins. These result in chronic blistering of the skin in sun-exposed areas.
- Removing iron results in interruption of iron-mediated oxidation of the porphyrinogens and improvement of symptoms.
- PCT can be inherited or acquired. Acquired causes include hepatitis C infection, HIV infection, excessive alcohol consumption, estrogen use, pregnancy, and exposure to chlorinated and polycyclic aromatic hydrocarbons.
- For PCT, phlebotomy is performed weekly until ferritin levels reach the lower limit of normal. Maintenance therapy phlebotomies are performed at an interval necessary to control symptoms.
- For disorders resulting in erythrocytosis, the goal of therapy is to maintain a hematocrit less than 44%. This occurs through weekly or monthly phlebotomy until iron stores are depleted.
- For hereditary hemochromatosis, phlebotomy is performed weekly until the transferrin saturation is less than 20% to 30% of normal. Once this is reached, maintenance therapy is initiated. Some centers use a goal of a mean corpuscular volume (MCV) 5% to 10% below baseline.
- Alagille syndrome is an autosomal dominant disorder characterized by billiary hypoplasia with cholestasis, vertebral anomalies, prominent forehead, deep-set eyes, and congenital heart anomalies (pulmonic stenosis). It is not treated with therapeutic phlebotomy. Refsum's disease (phytanic acid storage disease) is a deficiency in an enzyme necessary for metabolism of dietary phytanic acid. It is treated with plasma exchange. Susac syndrome is a microangiopathic process involving the retina, cochlea, and cerebellum, which has been treated with plasma exchange. CADASIL is a rare form of inherited strokes. None of these diseases are treated with therapeutic phlebotomy.

Question 17: D

Explanation:

- In order to transfuse blood collected from patients with hereditary hemochromatosis without labeling the unit of blood with the donor's disorder, the following criteria must be met:

- The patient must meet the same eligibility requirements as other whole blood donors.
- To collect blood more frequently than every 8 weeks: 1) A physician's prescription, including instructions on the frequency of phlebotomy and hematocrit/hemoglobin limits, is required or 2) A physician must examine the patient and certify that he or she is in good health on the day of each donation.
- There must be *no* charge or fees performed on *any* hereditary hemochromatosis patients undergoing phlebotomy, including those who do not meet eligibility requirements for whole blood donation.
* If these criteria are met, a variance can be requested from CBER to allow the use of the therapeutic phlebotomy units collected without labeling them with the donor's disorder.
* The rationale behind not charging for phlebotomies for both eligible and ineligible donors is to eliminate any incentives (ie, the cost of the phlebotomy) that may encourage an individual to withhold information concerning risk factors on the donor questionnaire.
* One study estimated that if *only* the units from eligible hemochromatosis patients undergoing maintenance phlebotomy were used for transfusion, this would represent a 16% increase in the US Red Blood Cell supply.

---------------------- O ----------------------

Question 18: A

Explanation:

* Complications of whole blood donation (or any venipuncture) are given in Table 2-18.
* Risk factors associated with bruising and hematoma formation are:
  - Untrained phlebotomist.
  - Tourniquet too tight.

Table 2-18.

Reaction/Injury	Frequency
Bruising and hematoma	9 to 16%
Vasovagal reaction	2 to 5%
Local irritation/allergy to tape or antiseptic	0.5%
Vasovagal reaction with syncope	0.1 to 0.3%
Nerve injury	0.016%
Thrombophlebitis/phlebitis	0.001 to 0.002%
Arterial puncture	0.001%
Arterial psuedoaneurysm	Rare
Arteriovenous fistula	Very rare
Compartment syndrome	Very rare
Angina/myocardial infusion/cerebrovascular accident	0.0005%
Local infection	<0.0005%

Question 19: B

Explanation:

- Vasovagal reactions consist of pallor, lightheadedness, anxiety, diaphoresis, hyperventilation, irregular breathing, weakness, nausea, vomiting, hypotension, and bradycardia.
- Risk factors include:
  - Young age.
  - Low weight.
  - First-time donation.
  - Epidemic fainting.
  - Inattentive or noncommunicative phlebotomist.
- The pathophysiology of vasovagal reactions represents excessive parasympathetic outflow. During blood donation, hypovolemia leads to sympathetic activation. The parasympathetic response to counter-

act this, however, is excessive, leading to bradycardia and vasodilatation with hypotension. If someone presents with excessive sympathetic drive at the start of donation (eg, a first-time donation), the probability increases.
- Reactions can occur anytime during the donation process (even before phlebotomy) but most will occur within 15 minutes of the completion of donation.
- Vasovagal reactions with syncope occur in 0.1% to 0.3% of donations.

Question 20: E

Explanation:

- All of the answers are treatments for vasovagal reactions.
- In addition, the donation is usually discontinued and the needle removed, especially if syncope occurs. Tonic-clonic movements may occur with loss of consciousness that could lead to vascular injury. If only mild symptoms occur, the collection can be completed.
- If the donor has syncope and falls or strikes his or her head, he or she should be evaluated for secondary injuries.

Question 21: C

Explanation:

- Arterial puncture occurs when the needle passes through the vein and enters the artery underlying the vein.
- It is characterized by:
  - Severe or unusual pain.
  - Rapid filling of the bag in 92%.
  - Bright red blood in 75%.
  - Movement of the needle with each heart beat in 33%.
- Arterial punctures are associated with inexperienced phlebotomists.
- Treatment consists of immediate discontinuation of donation and firm pressure applied to the site for 10 minutes. A pressure bandage should be applied and left in place for 3 to 4 hours.

- Arterial puncture can rarely be complicated by:
  - Arterial pseudoaneurysm.
  - Arterial-venous fistula formation.
  - Compartment syndrome.

Question 22: B

Explanation:

- Nerve injuries result from irritation of small nerve branches near the phlebotomy site.
- Risk factors include:
  - Hematoma formation.
  - Female gender.
  - Younger than average age.
- Symptoms usually present on the day of donation in the majority of cases (78%).
- Treatment is usually symptomatic, with 39% recovering within 2 days and 70% within 1 month. The remaining 30% recover within 6 to 9 months. Time is the major treatment option for these patients.

Question 23: C

Explanation:

- ANH is the removal of blood from a patient and restoration of the patient's volume with the infusion of an acellular fluid. The collected whole blood can then be used to transfuse the patient during the surgical procedure.
- ANH minimizes blood loss because the blood hemorrhaged during the procedure is of lower hematocrit because of the dilution.
- The solutions used are either crystalloid (infused at a ratio of 3 mL:1 mL whole blood removed) or colloid (infused at a ratio of 1 mL:1 mL of whole blood removed).
- The blood is collected into standard blood bags containing anticoagulant. It is stored at room temperature in the operating room and reinfused according to standard fluid management.

MEDICAL ASSESSMENT 61

- In order to maximize effect, the blood is reinfused in the reverse order that it was drawn. In this way, the lower concentrations of red cells are reinfused first.
- The total amount of blood collected depends upon the patient's ability to tolerate the anemia induced by the procedure. The patient's circulating volume and perfusion status must be monitored.
- The blood is stored at room temperature in order to preserve platelet function. As a result, storage should not exceed 8 hours from the start of collection.
- The blood must be appropriately labeled with the following information: patient's full name, medical record number, date and time of collection, and "For autologous use only."
- ANH units collected by operating room staff minimize procurement and administration costs. Because the blood does not leave the operating room, the dangers of clerical errors and their results (eg, ABO-incompatible transfusion) are minimized.

Question 24: A

Explanation:

- AABB standards exist for perioperative blood collections. These require the following:
  ○ A physician to be responsible for the program.
  ○ Compliance with AABB *Standards* for *Perioperative Autologous Blood Collection and Administration*.
  ○ Establishment of written policies and procedures, to be periodically reviewed.
  ○ Participation of the blood bank or transfusion service in the development of policies and procedures related to perioperative blood recovery.
  ○ Perioperative blood shall not be transfused to other patients.
  ○ Methods of collection and reinfusion shall be safe and aseptic.
  ○ All facilities regularly collecting blood by perioperative methods should establish a program of quality control and assurance.
- Criteria for the selection of patients for ANH are as follows:
  ○ Likelihood of transfusion exceeds 10%.
  ○ Preoperative hemoglobin ≥12 g/dL.

- Absence of significant coronary artery, pulmonary, renal, or liver disease.
- Absence of severe hypertension.
- Absence of infection and risk of bacteremia.

Question 25: C

Explanation:

- Storage requirements for the various forms of perioperative blood components are given in Table 2-25.
- Vacuum settings are usually set according to the manufacturer's recommendations and are usually 150 torr. This is to prevent hemolysis

Table 2-25.

Collection	Storage Temperature	Shelf Life
Acute normovolemic hemodilution	Room temperature	8 hours from start of collection
	1-6 C	24 hours from start of collection
Intraoperative blood recovered with processing	Room temperature	4 hours from end of collection
	1-6 C	24 hours from start of collection
Intraoperative blood recovered without processing	Room temperature or 1-6 C	4 hours from end of collection
Shed blood with or without processing	NA	6 hours from start of collection

that can occur, especially if there is surface skimming because of shallow collections of blood.
- In most circumstances, in order to be cost effective, 2 or more units of blood need to be collected and processed.
- Anticoagulation, in the form of heparin or citrate, is necessary to prevent clotting of blood in the collection canister.

Question 26: D

Explanation:

- The bag should be labeled with patient name, medical record number, date and time of collection, and "For autologous use only."
- Bacteria are frequently cultured from processed blood. Reports have failed to identify adverse consequences of this. Nevertheless, intraoperative blood should not be used when the surgical field is grossly contaminated or frankly infected.
- Intraoperative blood, whether processed or not, should be transfused through a microaggregate filter.
- Processing can occur either in the operating room or at another site. If the unit of blood is processed outside of the operating room, processes and procedures must be in place to verify patient and product identity before infusion.
- Blood is usually washed using normal saline. The use of other solutions, just as during routine red cell transfusions, could result in clotting of the product or hemolysis.

Question 27: D

Explanation:

- The FDA is composed of a number of centers that regulate different areas. These include the CBER, CDER, CDRH), and the Center for Food Safety and Applied Nutrition. CBER is responsible for the regulation of blood products and biologicals.
- In the event of the death of a blood donor that *may* be related to the donation process, CBER requires notification as soon as possible after

the time that the facility becomes aware of the death. This notification can be by telephone, fax, e-mail, or express mail. CBER requires that a written report be submitted within 7 days. This report does *not* need to be the final report but should provide as much information as available.
- In the event that the report submitted at 7 days is not complete, the FDA requires that the report be amended by submitting the missing material as it becomes available.
- Materials to be included in the written report include:
  - Discharge summary and/or death certificate.
  - Autopsy report (if performed).
  - Conclusions and follow-up actions if appropriate.
- Additional information that should also be included is outlined in the CBER guidance. For blood donors, this include the following:
  - The deceased's donor record file that includes the donation just before the fatal incident and information on all donations during the past 2 years.
  - Lot numbers and expiration dates of collection sets or harnesses; if replacement fluid(s) was given during the collection, indication should be given for which fluid(s) and the unit or lot number(s) and any other relevant information, such as manufacturer's notices, contamination warnings, or replacement fluid recalls.
  - Performance log for the device and any other relevant performance logs, maintenance records, manufacturer's notices, or recalls on significant machine part(s) on the device/system during the past 2 years.
  - If the donor was hospitalized due to the reaction, any relevant documents should be provided (eg, reports of laboratory tests) that may help determine the cause of the fatality.
- Similar notification is required if a patient's death *may* be caused by transfusion, a therapeutic apheresis procedure, or a therapeutic phlebotomy. The requested information varies according to which of these the death is associated with.

REFERENCES

1. Eder AF. Allogeneic and autologous blood donor selection. In: Roback JD, Combs MR, Grossman BJ, Hillyer CD, eds. Technical manual. 16th ed. Bethesda, MD: AABB, 2008:137-88.
2. Smith JW, Burgstaler EA. Blood component collection by apheresis. In: Roback JD, Combs MR, Grossman BJ, Hillyer CD, eds. Technical manual. 16th ed. Bethesda, MD: AABB, 2008:229-40.
3. Food and Drug Administration. Guidance for Industry: Recommendations for deferral of donors and quarantine and retrieval of blood and blood products in recent recipients of smallpox vaccine (*vaccinia* virus) and certain contacts of smallpox vaccine recipients. (December 2002) Rockville, MD: CBER Office of Communication, Training, and Manufacturer's Assistance, 2002.*
4. Food and Drug Administration. Guidance for industry and FDA review staff: Collection of platelets by automated methods. (December 2007) Rockville, MD: CBER Office of Communication, Training, and Manufacturer's Assistance, 2007.*
5. Food and Drug Administration. Memorandum: Volume limits for automated collection of source plasma (November 4, 1992) Rockville, Maryland: CBER Office of Communication, Training, and Manufacturer's Assistance, 1992.*
6. Food and Drug Administration. Memorandum: Revision of FDA memorandum of August 27, 1982: Requirements for infrequent plasmapheresis donors. (March 10, 1995) Rockville, MD: CBER Office of Communication, Training, and Manufacturer's Assistance, 1995.*
7. Food and Drug Administration. Memorandum: Donor deferral due to red blood cell loss during collection of source plasma by automated plasmapheresis. (December 4, 1995) Rockville, MD: CBER Office of Communication, Training, and Manufacturer's Assistance, 1995.*
8. Code of federal regulations. Title 21, CFR Part 610.63. Washington, DC: US Government Printing Office, 2008 (revised annually).
9. Code of federal regulations. Title 21, CFR Part 610.65, Washington, DC: US Government Printing Office, 2008 (revised annually).
10. Price TH, ed. Standards for blood banks and transfusion services. 26th ed. Bethesda, MD: AABB, 2009.
11. Ilstrup S, ed. Standards for perioperative autologous blood collection and administration. 4th ed. Bethesda, MD: AABB, 2009.
12. Autologous blood donation and transfusion. In: Brecher ME, ed. Technical manual. 15th ed. Bethesda, MD: AABB, 2005:117-38.
13. Food and Drug Administration. Guidance for industry: Recommendations for collecting red blood cells by automated apheresis methods. (January

2001) Rockville, MD: CBER Office of Communication, Training, and Manufacturer's Assistance, 2001.*

14. Winters JL, Pineda AA. Hemapheresis. In: McPherson RA, Pincus MR, eds. Henry's clinical diagnosis and management by laboratory methods. 21st ed. Philadelphia: Saunders Elsevier, 2006:685-715.
15. Klein HG, Anstee DJ. Blood donors and the withdrawal of blood. In: Klein HG, Anstee DJ. Mollison's blood transfusion in clinical medicine. 11th ed. Malden, MA: Blackwell Publishing, 2005:1-18.
16. Food and Drug Administration. Guidance for industry: Variances for blood collection from individuals with hereditary hemochromatosis. (August 2001) Rockville, MD: CBER Office of Communication, Training, and Manufacturer's Assistance, 2001.*
17. Newman BH. Donor reactions and injuries from whole blood donation. Transfus Med Rev 1997;11:64-75.
18. Food and Drug Administration. Guidance for industry: Notifying the FDA of fatalities related to blood collection or transfusion. (September 2003) Rockville, MD: CBER Office of Communication, Training, and Manufacturer's Assistance, 2003.*

*Food and Drug Administration draft guidances, final guidances, and memoranda can be downloaded from the FDA Web site [Available at http://www.fda.gov/BiologicsBloodVaccines/ResourcesforYou/Industry/default. htm (accessed June 30, 2009).]

3

Blood Components: Preparation, Storage, and Characteristics

QUESTIONS

Question 1: The correct temperature for shipping Red Blood Cells (RBCs) is:

A. ≤–18 C.
B. 1 to 6 C.
C. 1 to 10 C.
D. 20 to 24 C.
E. 37 C.

Question 2: RBC storage times vary with the anticoagulant/preservative used. Which of the following is properly paired?

A. Citrate-phosphate-dextrose (CPD): 35 days.
B. Additive solution (AS): 47 days.
C. Citrate-phosphate-dextrose-adenine (CPDA)-1: 21 days.
D. Acid-citrate-dextrose (ACD): 35 days.
E. Citrate-phosphate-dextrose-dextrose (CP2D): 21 days.

Question 3: Which of the following represents a change seen in a unit of RBCs stored with CPDA-1 at the end of its shelf life?

A. Percentage of viable cells at 24 hours after transfusion decreases to 71%.
B. Supernatant K^+ (potassium ion) concentration decreases.
C. Supernatant pH increases.
D. Red cell 2,3-diphosphoglycerate (2,3-DPG) increases.
E. Supernatant hemoglobin decreases.

Question 4: A unit of RBCs is issued to the floor and returned without being transfused. How long can the blood be out of the refrigerator and still be used for transfusion?

A. 10 minutes.
B. 30 minutes.
C. 1 hour.
D. 4 hours.
E. 6 hours.

Question 5: The maximal shelf life of irradiated RBCs is:

A. 4 hours.
B. 6 hours.
C. 24 hours.
D. 21 days.
E. 28 days.

Question 6: The preferred method for generating leukocyte-reduced RBC components is:

A. Thawing and deglycerolizing a frozen unit.
B. Filtering using a leukocyte-reduction filter.

C. Irradiation.
D. Centrifugation.
E. Washing.

Question 7: The most common concentration of glycerol used in the United States for freezing RBCs is:

A. 5%.
B. 10%.
C. 20%.
D. 40%.
E. 65%.

Question 8: The rationale for deglycerolizing frozen RBCs with extensive washing is:

A. Glycerol is not approved by the Food and Drug Administration (FDA).
B. Glycerol is toxic to kidneys.
C. Glycerol can cause hemolysis.
D. Glycerol can cause anaphylaxis.
E. Glycerol can cause thrombocytopenia.

Question 9: Which of the following choices explains why a unit of blood may form an insoluble jelly-like mass during deglycerolization?

A. Inadequate deglycerolization.
B. Bacterial contamination.
C. Insufficient anticoagulant.
D. Inadvertent use of hypotonic saline for washing.
E. Red cells from a donor with sickle cell trait.

Question 10: A 20-year-old man was involved in a motor vehicle accident. He is Rh-negative, had a negative antibody screen, and received 68 RBC units, the majority of which were Rh-positive. The patient eventually recovered, but he developed six clinically significant blood group antibodies: anti-D, -C, -E, -K, -S, and -Jk^b. Two years after the accident, the patient donated 2 units of autologous blood, which were kept frozen for 8 years. The patient is now admitted for gastrointestinal bleeding and both of his autologous units are deglycerolized in preparation for possible transfusion. With fluid resuscitation, however, the patient is stabilized. His hemoglobin is 10.2 g/dL and his hematocrit is 31%. The medical director should:

A. Refrigerate the units until the expiration time and discard if not clinically needed.
B. Advise medical staff to transfuse the units because they are rare.
C. Document the value of the antigen-negative units and refreeze for up to another 10 years.
D. Extend the shelf life of the units by 24 hours.
E. Release the rare units so that they can be made available for another patient.

Question 11: Two S–, s–, U– units are deglycerolized in preparation for possible transfusion. The patient, however, is stabilized and transfusion is no longer required. The medical director should:

A. Refrigerate the units until the expiration time and discard if not clinically needed.
B. Advise medical staff to transfuse the units, because they are rare.
C. Document the value of the antigen-negative units and refreeze for up to another 10 years.
D. Extend the shelf life of the units by 24 hours.
E. Release the rare units so that they can be made available for another patient.

Question 12: According to AABB standards, the maximum allowable shelf-life of platelets without gentle agitation is:

A. 1 hour.
B. 4 hours.
C. 8 hours.
D. 24 hours.
E. 36 hours.

Question 13: According to AABB standards, 90% of the units of random-donor platelets prepared from whole blood should contain a minimum of ___ platelets per unit.

A. 5.5×10^9.
B. 5.5×10^{10}.
C. 5.5×10^{11}.
D. 3×10^{10}.
E. 3×10^{11}.

Question 14: The minimum acceptable pH of platelet units at the end of the storage period is:

A. 4.2.
B. 5.2.
C. 6.2.
D. 7.2.
E. 8.2.

Question 15: Which of the following is a change associated with platelet storage?

A. Decreased H^+ concentration.
B. Platelet activation.

C. Change in shape from round to discoid.
D. Increased swirling effect.
E. Increased expression of glycoprotein Ib and glycoprotein IIb/IIIa.

Question 16: Transfusion of 1 platelet concentrate unit (ie, the platelets present in one whole blood donation) into a hematologically stable adult of average size with no history of transfusion and/or pregnancy is expected to increase the platelet count by:

A. 1000 to 5000/µL.
B. 3000 to 5000/µL.
C. 3000 to 12,000/µL.
D. 5000 to 10,000/µL.
E. 30,000 to 40,000/µL.

Question 17: Which of the following is a theoretical advantage associated with transfusion of a whole-blood-derived pooled platelet unit compared with an apheresis platelet unit?

A. Decreased donor exposure for infectious disease transmission.
B. Decreased risk of transfusion-related acute lung injury (TRALI).
C. Decreased donor exposure for HLA alloimmunization.
D. Decreased risk of septic transfusion reaction.
E. All of the above are advantages of a pooled component compared with an apheresis component.

Question 18: Fresh frozen plasma (FFP) that has been thawed and is being stored at 1 to 6 C should be transfused within:

A. 4 hours.
B. 6 hours.
C. 12 hours.
D. 18 hours.
E. 24 hours.

Question 19: Which of the following statements is *true*?

A. To prepare FFP, plasma must be separated from red cells within 24 hours.
B. If an additive solution is used, the expiration date for RBCs stored at 1 to 6 C is 42 days after phlebotomy.
C. To prepare Cryoprecipitated Antihemophilic Factor (AHF), FFP is thawed at 20 to 24 C.
D. Platelets derived from a unit of whole blood must contain 3×10^{11} platelets in 75% of the units tested.
E. The expiration date of RBCs that are frozen and stored at ≤65 C is 5 years.

Question 20: A group B, Rh-positive patient requires fresh frozen plasma. Group B FFP is not available. The substitute component of choice is:

A. Group O FFP.
B. Group B, Rh-positive Cryoprecipitated AHF.
C. Group A FFP.
D. Group AB FFP.
E. Group A, Rh-negative Cryoprecipitated AHF.

Question 21: Which of the following statements is *true*?

A. Cryoprecipitated AHF can be produced from either cryoprecipitate-reduced plasma (CRP) or FFP.
B. CRP cannot be used in manufacturing albumin and immunoglobulins.
C. CRP and AHF cannot be prepared from FFP collected by apheresis.
D. CRP is rich in fibrinogen, Factor VIII, and von Willebrand factor (vWF).
E. CRP is deficient in ADAMTS13 (a disintegrin and metalloproteinase with thrombospondin motifs).

Question 22: Cryoprecipitated AHF should be stored at:

A. ≤–18 C.
B. 1 to 6 C.
C. 20 to 22 C.
D. 30 C.
E. 37 C.

Question 23: After thawing, Cryoprecipitated AHF should be stored at:

A. 42 C.
B. 37 C.
C. 20 to 24 C.
D. 1 to 6 C.
E. –18 C.

Question 24: According to AABB standards, each bag of Cryoprecipitated AHF must contain a minimum of how many International Units of Factor VIII?

A. 70.
B. 80.
C. 100.
D. 120.
E. 150.

Question 25: Cryoprecipitated AHF contains which of the following?

A. Factor XI.
B. Protein C.
C. Protein S.
D. Factor XIII.
E. Factor XII.

Question 26: Which one of the following statements regarding Cryoprecipitated AHF is *true*?

A. It is prepared from FFP thawed at 20 to 24 C.
B. Once thawed, it is stored at 1 to 6 C and administered within 6 hours of thawing or within 4 hours of pooling.
C. It is prepared by filtering thawed FFP at 1 to 6 C.
D. It is prepared by centrifuging thawed FFP at 1 to 6 C.
E. Thawed Cryoprecipitated AHF is stored at 1 to 6 C during transportation.

Question 27: A 71-kg patient in disseminated intravascular coagulation (DIC) has a hematocrit of 30% and a fibrinogen level of 90 mg/dL. How many units of Cryoprecipitated AHF should be administered to achieve a fibrinogen level of 200 mg/dL?

A. 3 units.
B. 10 units.
C. 14 units.
D. 25 units.
E. 30 units.

Question 28: Granulocytes are stored at:

A. 1 to 6 C without continuous gentle agitation.
B. 1 to 6 C with continuous gentle agitation.
C. 20 to 24 C without continuous gentle agitation.
D. 20 to 24 C with continuous gentle agitation.
E. 37 C with continuous gentle agitation.

Question 29: The shelf life of granulocytes is:

A. 4 hours.
B. 6 hours.

C. 12 hours.
D. 24 hours.
E. 5 days.

Question 30: Which of the following patients is a candidate for granulocyte transfusions?

A. An 80-year-old man with widely metastatic adenocarcinoma with extensive marrow replacement. His tumor has failed to respond to chemotherapy and he is currently under hospice care. His absolute neutrophil count is 100/µL. He is septic with positive blood cultures for *Escherichia coli*. He has been treated with appropriate antibiotics but has not responded.
B. A 25-year-old woman with acute leukemia. She is at day 17 after chemotherapy and has responded well to treatment. She is experiencing fevers. Her absolute neutrophil count is 900/µL. Repeated blood cultures have been negative and there is no obvious infection site.
C. A 56-year-old woman with acute leukemia. She is at day 5 after chemotherapy and her leukemia has shown a good response to treatment. She is experiencing fevers and has pulmonary infiltrates on chest radiograph. Her absolute neutrophil count is 200/µL. Bronchoscopy shows evidence of cytomegalovirus (CMV) pneumonitis. No other infection is identified.
D. A 30-year-old man with acute leukemia. He is at day 7 after chemotherapy and his leukemia has shown a good response to treatment. He now has a perirectal abscess. The abscess has been drained and cultured. It grew *E coli* and he has been treated with 3 days of appropriate antibiotics. Despite this, the area of infection appears to be enlarging. His absolute neutrophil count is 50/µL.
E. A 40-year-old man with non-Hodgkin lymphoma. He is at 3 weeks after chemotherapy with a good response. He has developed a lobar pulmonary infiltrate, and sputum cultures grew *Streptococcus pneumoniae*. He was just started on antibiotics. His absolute neutrophil count is 1000/µL.

Question 31: Granulocytes should:

A. Be administered through a microaggregate filter.
B. Be washed.
C. Be ABO-compatible with the intended recipient.
D. Never be transfused to patients with a history of febrile transfusion reactions.
E. Be given within 48 hours of preparation.

Question 32: Which of the follow statements concerning optimizing the collection of granulocytes is *true*?

A. Administration of hydroxyethyl starch (HES) to apheresis donors enhances granulocyte yield.
B. Administration of corticosteroids enhances granulocyte yield.
C. Administration of granulocyte colony-stimulating factor (G-CSF) enhances granulocyte yield.
D. Administration of corticosteroids and G-CSF is superior to the administration of either agent alone.
E. All of the above are true.

Question 33: Which of the following is an adverse reaction caused by the infusion of HES during granulocyte collection?

A. Back pain.
B. Weight gain.
C. Tetany.
D. Paresthesia.
E. Headache.

Question 34: Which of the following statements is *true* concerning the irradiation of granulocytes?

A. It is associated with decreased granulocyte function and should be avoided.
B. It inactivates CMV, which may be present in the granulocytes.
C. It prevents transfusion-associated graft-vs-host disease (GVHD).
D. It changes the shelf life of granulocytes to 1 hour.
E. It prevents alloimmunization to HLA antigens.

ANSWERS

Question 1: C

Explanation:

- Storage temperature: 1 to 6 C.
- Transport temperature: 1 to 10 C.

Question 2: E

Explanation:

- See Table 3-2A for shelf life for RBCs using different anticoagulant/preservative solutions.

Table 3-2A.

Anticoagulant/ Preservative	ACD/CPD/ CP2D	CPDA-1	AS
Storage/shelf life (days)	21	35	42
Hematocrit	≤80%	≤80%	52 to 60%

ACD = acid citrate dextrose; CPD = citrate phosphate dextrose; CP2D = citrate phosphate dextrose (twice the amount); CPDA-1 = citrate phosphate dextrose adenine; AS = additive solution.

- Additive solution is added to the concentrated RBCs after the removal of platelet-rich plasma and provides optimal red cell preservation. The composition of additive solutions varies. See Table 3-2B for the composition.

Table 3-2B.

	AS-1	AS-3	AS-5
Dextrose (mg/mL)	2200	1100	900
Adenine (mg/mL)	27	30	30
Monobasic sodium phosphate (mg/mL)	0	276	0
Mannitol (mg/mL)	750	0	525
Sodium chloride (mg/mL)	900	410	877
Sodium citrate (mg/mL)	0	588	0
Citric acid (mg/mL)	0	42	0

- Shelf life of RBCs in an open system: 24 hours at 1 to 6 C.
- Shelf life of frozen RBCs: 10 years.
- Volume varies according to anticoagulant/preservative with ACD, CPD, CP2D, and CPDA-1 having volumes of 250 to 300 mL and AS having volumes of 350 to 450 mL.

Question 3: A

Explanation:

- Changes in CPDA-1 RBCs stored at 1 to 6 C are described in Table 3-3. Similar changes are seen with other anticoagulant/preservative solutions.

Table 3-3.

Changes	CPDA-1	
	Day 0	Day 35
% viable cells at 24 hours	100	71
pH	7.55	6.71
ATP (% of initial)	100	45 ±12
2,3-DPG (% of initial)	100	<10
Plasma K+ (mmol/L)	5.10	78.50
Plasma hemoglobin	78	658

Question 4: B

Explanation:

- The returned component (whole blood or RBCs) is acceptable for reissue if the temperature is maintained between 1 and 10 C. The rationale behind the 30-minute rule is that a unit of RBCs at 1 to 6 C that is then moved to room temperature will warm to a temperature of 10 C after 30 minutes.
- The conditions for reissuing the component for transfusion are as follows:
  - Intact seal.
  - Maintenance of the temperature between 1 and 10 C.
  - Attachment of at least one sealed segment of the integral donor tubing.
  - Records indicating that the unit was inspected and acceptable before reissuing.

Question 5: E

Explanation:

- The maximal shelf life of irradiated RBCs is 28 days even if the original expiration would exceed this period. If an irradiated unit's shelf life is less than 28 days, then that remains the shelf life of the unit following irradiation. In other words, the shelf life of an irradiated unit is 28 days or its original shelf life, whichever comes first.
- Irradiation is associated with unacceptable 24-hour red cell survival (<75% recovery) after 28 days.
- Irradiation is also associated with an increase in supernatant potassium. At 48 hours after irradiation, the supernatant potassium doubles.
- Irradiation does not affect the shelf life of platelets.

Question 6: B

Explanation:

- Currently available leukocyte reduction filters result in a 4- to 5-log reduction in leukocytes.
- Leukocyte-reduced RBC components (LR-RBCs) must contain less than 5.0×10^6 leukocytes per unit.
- LR-RBCs must contain at least 85% of the original RBCs.
- The shelf life of LR-RBCs is the same as the original RBC unit.
- Irradiation affects the proliferative activity of lymphocytes through DNA damage. Irradiation prevents graft-vs-host disease (GVHD). It does not provide the benefits of leukocyte reduction such as prevention of HLA alloimmunization, avoidance of febrile reactions, and prevention of cytomegalo-virus (CMV) transmission.
- Theoretically, leukocyte reduction could prevent GVHD and has done so in animal models. The minimum number of leukocytes required for the prevention of GVHD is not known. Hence, LR-RBCs cannot be used for prevention of GVHD.
- Inverted spin centrifugation was formerly used for leukocyte reduction. It was a means of isolating and removing leukocytes via centrifugation. It is no longer used.
- Thawing and deglycerolization results in LR-RBCs. However, this is labor intensive and results in significant loss of the red cell component.
- Washing does not result in significant leukocyte reduction.

Question 7: D

Explanation:

- A 20% concentration of glycerol is alternatively used in some component preparation labs.
- Advantages and disadvantages of these methods are described in Table 3-7.

Table 3-7.

Concentration of Glycerol	Speed of Freezing	Freezing Temperature	Storage Temperature	Glycerolization	Deglycerolization
20% (low glycerol method)	Rapid	≤−196 C	≤−120 C	Complex	Simple
40% (high glycerol method)	Slow	≤−80 C	≤−65 C	Simple	Complex

Question 8: C

Explanation:

- Inadequately removed glycerol can cause in-vivo or in-vitro hemolysis. The presence of glycerol in the red cells renders them hypertonic relative to solutions with physiologic osmolalities. If the cells are placed in these solutions, there is movement of water into the cells, resulting in their rupture. During the process of deglycerolization, solutions of progressively lower osmolality are used to wash the red cells. This allows for the removal of the glycerol from the cells without excess hemolysis.
- Glycerol is approved by the FDA.
- It is unknown whether glycerol may cause renal toxicity, anaphylaxis, or thrombocytopenia.
- Following the deglycerolization process, ≥80% of the red cells must be recovered.

Question 9: E

Explanation:

- When thawed and deglycerolized without using additional wash fluid, frozen red cells from a donor with sickle cell trait form a semi-solid dark gel. In some cryopreservation programs, donations are screened for hemoglobin S before freezing is undertaken.
- Inadequate deglycerolization causes in-vivo or in-vitro hemolysis.
- Bacterial contamination changes the color and appearance of the unit and may cause hemolysis.
- Insufficient anticoagulation would result in the presence of clots within the unit.
- Use of hypotonic solutions for washing would result in hemolysis.

Question 10: A

Explanation:

- In order to calculate the percentage of donors who would be compatible with the patient with these six clinically significant antibodies, the following calculations are performed:
  - 15% of people of European ethnicity are Rh-negative (ie, D antigen-negative).
  - >99% of D-negative individuals are C-negative and E-negative.
  - The remaining phenotypes are independent of one another. To calculate the frequency of the combined phenotype, the individual frequencies are multiplied together.
  - The frequency (%) of antigen-negative units is:
    - D−   15
    - C−   99 (of Rh-negative units)
    - E−   99 (of Rh-negative units)
    - K−   91
    - S−   45
    - Jk^b−   28
  - The frequency of the combined phenotype is: $0.15 \times 0.99 \times 0.99 \times 0.91 \times 0.45 \times 0.28 = 0.01685$ or ~1.7%.

- Another way to look at the frequency of finding a unit that meets this patient's needs is to start with an Rh-negative unit, because all units in the blood bank are of known D antigen type. If one begins in this way, then ~11% of all Rh-negative units will also lack the C, E, K, S, and Jk^b antigens (ie, 0.99 × 0.99 × 0.91 × 0.45 × 0.28).
- In this clinical situation, the best choice is to refrigerate the units until the expiration time and discard if not clinically needed. Choice C might also be considered; however, because 11% of Rh-negative units will meet this patient's needs and there is a loss of red cells via hemolysis from deglycerolization, refreezing is not the best option.
- The shelf-life of deglycerolized RBCs stored at 1 to 6 C is 24 hours because the routine process is an open system and there is a danger of bacterial contamination.
- Automated instruments that can wash (deglycerolize) RBCs in a closed system are available. If one of these systems is used, the RBCs can be stored at 1 to 6 C for up to 14 days. After 14 days, there is significant increase in potassium and hemoglobin in the supernatant fluid.
- The laboratory values indicate that the patient likely has an adequate oxygen-carrying capacity. Based upon the laboratory values, transfusion of RBCs is not indicated. However, the decision to transfuse should be based upon a patient's symptoms and clinical situation and not strictly upon laboratory values. Mere availability of a rare unit is not an indication for transfusion.
- Autologous units are not crossed over for allogeneic use.

Question 11: C

Explanation:

- S–, s–, U– units are exceedingly rare. If unused, these units should be refrozen before the 24-hour expiration. After refreezing they can be stored for up to 10 years but when thawed, the amount of time before expiration will be the amount of time left from the original thaw/deglyceralization process (the clock does not start over; it only pauses).
- The cells could also be rejuvenated. Rejuvenation restores the adenosine triphosphate and 2,3 diphosphoglycerate levels of the RBCs. RBCs in a closed system can be rejuvenated up to 3 days after expira-

tion. Such cells can then be frozen. Rejuvenated RBCs must be washed to remove the rejuvenation solution because the inosine in the solution is toxic.
- The units should not be released into general inventory because of their rarity.
- The patient should be encouraged to donate blood in the future (autologous or allogeneic) because of their extremely rare blood type.
- Frozen RBC characteristics:
  - Preparation: within 6 days after collection or 3 days after expiration (with rejuvenation).
  - Shelf life:
    - 10 years (medical director can prolong the shelf life based upon the value of the rare unit).
    - 24 hours after deglycerolization if an open system is used to deglycerolize the cells.
    - 14 days after deglycerolization if an FDA-licensed closed system is used to deglycerolize the cells.
  - Freezing and storage temperatures are given in Table 3-7.

Question 12: D

Explanation:

- The shelf life of platelets without gentle agitation is 24 hours.
- Gentle agitation is necessary to allow for adequate oxygen exchange through the platelet bag. Failure to do so could result in a decrease in pH below acceptable levels and activation of the platelets.
- The shelf life of platelets with gentle agitation is 4 hours (open system, because of the danger of bacterial contamination during pooling/collection with growth during storage) or 5 days (closed system, because of the danger of bacterial contamination during collection with growth during storage).

Question 13: B

Explanation:

- If platelets are to be harvested from whole blood donations, the blood must be maintained at 22 to 24 C.
- The platelet count, leukocyte content, and volume of platelet units is shown in Table 3-13.
- Components containing $<5.0 \times 10^6$ leukocytes per unit are considered CMV-reduced-risk (equivalent to CMV-negative units) and can prevent or delay HLA alloimmunization.
- Components containing $<5.0 \times 10^8$ leukocytes per unit are required for the prevention of febrile nonhemolytic transfusion reactions.

Table 3-13.

Product	Platelet Count	Volume	Leukocytes
Platelets	5.5×10^{10}	~50 mL	$>10^9$
Platelets Leukocytes Reduced	5.5×10^{10}	~50 mL	$<8.3 \times 10^5$
Pooled Platelets Leukocytes Reduced	Depends upon pool size	Depends upon pool size	$<5.0 \times 10^6$
Apheresis Platelets	3.0×10^{11}	~300 mL	$>10^9$
Apheresis Platelets Leukocytes Reduced	3.0×10^{11}	300 mL	$<5.0 \times 10^6$

Question 14: C

Explanation:

- The minimum acceptable pH of platelet units at the end of the storage period is ≥6.2.
- A pH lower than 6.2 could indicate inadequate gas exchange through the bag during storage or bacterial contamination and growth. A pH <6.2 results in platelet activation and loss of function.

Question 15: B

Explanation:

- During storage, platelets activate.
- pH decreases during storage.
- Normal platelet shape is discoid and becomes spherical with activation. During storage, the shape changes to spherical.
- If a platelet product is backlit, a shimmering effect can be seen as the tumbling discoid platelets reflect the light at different angles. When the platelets activate and become spheres, the light is reflected at the same angle, resulting in the loss of the swirling effect.
- Loss of the swirl effect is frequently used as a surrogate marker for bacterial contamination of platelet products. It is important to note it can be lost as a result of anything that causes activation, including pH <6.2, temperature <20 C, and age of the product.
- Platelet glycoprotein levels *decrease* during storage as a result of platelet activation.

BLOOD COMPONENTS 89

Question 16: D

Explanation:

- In a nonalloimmunized, hematologically stable adult, the transfusion of 1 unit of platelet concentrate is expected to increase the platelet count by 5000 to 10,000/µL.
- The transfusion of 1 unit of Apheresis Platelets or 1 unit of Pooled Platelets (usually a pool of six) is expected to increase the platelet count by 30,000 to 40,000/µL.

Question 17: B

Explanation:

- The plasma present in an apheresis platelet component is from a single donor, whereas that present in a pooled component is a mix of the number of donors in the pool. If an HLA or granulocyte antibody is present in a donor, pooling this will reduce the concentration of the antibody. This may result in a greater reduction of the risk of TRALI as compared to using an apheresis unit from one donor.
- Because apheresis platelets are derived from a single donor, the provision of apheresis platelets reduces donor exposure in comparison to pooled platelet concentrates, thereby reducing the risk of disease transmission.
- Apheresis platelets contain HLA antigens only from one donor. In a pool, there are antigens from each contributing donor. Although this may seem to be a significant advantage with regard to alloimmunization to HLA, it is not so important because white cells are more immunogenic than platelets. It is more important that the components be leukocyte reduced.
- The incidence of bacterial contamination in pooled platelet units derived from six whole blood donations has been found to be five times greater than that of apheresis platelets. This is because six venipunctures are performed with the pooled component, with the possibility of contamination with skin flora from each, vs one venipuncture for apheresis components.

Question 18: E

Explanation:

- FFP characteristics:
  - Volume: 200-250 mL/unit.
  - Contents: all coagulation factors at physiologic concentrations.
  - Shelf life: 12 months at ≤–18 C or 7 years at ≤–65 C.
  - Transport temperature: maintain in the frozen state.
  - Thawing temperature: 30 to 37 C.
  - Storage/shelf life after thawing: 24 hours at 1 to 6 C (preserves Factor V and VIII levels).
  - Transport temperature after thawing: 1 to 10 C.
  - Dose: 10-15 mL/kg with further therapy guided by clinical response and prothrombin time (PT)/partial thromboplastin time (PTT) measurements.

Question 19: B

Explanation:

- Several additive solutions containing various combinations of saline, adenine, phosphate, mannitol, glucose, and bicarbonate are available for prolonged storage. See Table 3-2B. The expiration date for RBCs stored at 1 to 6 C in additive solution is 42 days.
- For the preparation of FFP, plasma must be separated from red cells within 8 hours of whole blood collection if the anticoagulant is CPD, CP2D, or CPDA-1. If the anticoagulant is ACD, plasma must be separated from red cells within 6 hours of whole blood collection.
- To prepare Cryoprecipitated AHF, FFP is thawed at 1 to 6 C.
- Platelets derived from a unit of whole blood must contain 5.5×10^{10} platelets in 90% of the units tested. Apheresis Platelets must contain 3×10^{11} platelets in 90% of the units tested.
- The shelf life of frozen RBCs stored at ≤–65 C is 10 years.

Question 20: D

Explanation:

- Group B individuals have B antigen on their RBCs. Group O and group A FFP would contain anti-B that could potentially cause hemolysis. Group AB FFP does not contain isohemagglutinins.
- Cryoprecipitated AHF is not a substitute for FFP. FFP contains physiologic concentrations of *all* coagulation and anticoagulant factors, whereas Cryoprecipitated AHF contains only fibrinogen, Factor VIII, Factor XIII, and von Willebrand factor (vWF).

Question 21: C

Explanation:

- Cryoprecipitated AHF is prepared by thawing FFP at 1 to 6 C. Cryoprecipitated AHF must be frozen within 1 hour.
- CRP (also termed cryosupernatant) is the fraction of plasma remaining after the removal of cryoprecipitable proteins (ie, cryoprecipitate or Cryoprecipitated AHF).
- CRP is not the therapeutic equivalent of FFP because it lacks certain coagulation factors.
- CRP is routinely used as a raw material in manufacturing the following:
  - Albumin solutions.
  - Immunoglobulin preparations.
  - Non-Factor VIII coagulation factor concentrates.
- CRP contains approximately half of the fibrinogen, Factor VIII, and fibronectin present in FFP. CRP is depleted of the largest multimers of vWF.
- CRP is *not* deficient in ADAMTS13, a vWF-cleaving protease, the deficiency of which has been implicated in thrombotic thrombocytopenic purpura (TTP). Refractory TTP is the only FDA-approved indication for CRP.
- Center for Biologics Evaluation and Research regulations do not allow FFP collected by apheresis to be used for the production of Cryoprecipitated AHF, and therefore CRP is not generated from it.

Question 22: A

Explanation:

See Table 3-22.

Table 3-22.

Category	Storage	Transport	Expiration
Cryoprecipitated AHF	≤−18 C	Maintenance of the frozen state	1 year
Cryoprecipitated AHF thawed at 37 C	20 to 24 C	20 to 24 C	Open system or pooled: 4 hours Pooled before freezing: 6 hours Single thawed unit: 6 hours

Question 23: C

Explanation:

See Table 3-22.

Question 24: B

Explanation:

Quality assurance:

- Minimum of 150 mg of fibrinogen per tested unit.
- Minimum of 80 International Units of Factor VIII per tested unit.

BLOOD COMPONENTS 93

Question 25: D

Explanation:

- Contents of Cryoprecipitated AHF are given in Table 3-25.

Table 3-25.

Contents	Quantity in 1 Bag of Cryoprecipitate
Fibrinogen	>150 mg
von Willebrand factor	~50% present in the original unit
Factor VIII	≥80 units
Factor XIII	~20% to 30% present in the original unit
Fibronectin	

Question 26: D

Explanation:

- Preparation:
  - Prepared by thawing FFP between 1 and 6 C and expressing the cryoprecipitate-reduced supernatant after centrifugation, leaving a volume of 5 to 10 mL of cryoprecipitated proteins and plasma.
  - Cryoprecipitate is refrozen at −18 C within 1 hour.
- See Table 3-22.

Question 27: C

Explanation:

- Dosing:
  - Standard empiric dosing consists of 10 units followed by an assessment of effect through coagulation testing.

- If Cryoprecipitated AHF is being used to replace fibrinogen, the number of units necessary to reach this goal can be calculated. Similarly, if it is being used to replace Factor VIII, a dose can be calculated.
- The calculation to determine the dose of Cryoprecipitated AHF to reach a desired fibrinogen level is as follows:
  - Weight (kg) × 70 mL/kg = blood volume (mL)
    71 × 70 = 4970 mL
  - Blood volume (mL) × (1.0 − hematocrit) = plasma volume (mL)
    4970 × (1 − 0.3) = 3479 mL
  - (Desired fibrinogen level in mg/dL − initial level) × plasma volume / 100 mL/dL = mg of fibrinogen needed
    (200 − 90) × 3479/100 = 3827
  - mg fibrinogen needed / 250 mg fibrinogen per bag = number of bags required
    3827/250 = 14

Question 28: C

Explanation:

- Storage: 20 to 24 C without agitation. Agitation results in granulocyte activation and degranulation. Storage below room temperature results in a loss of function.

Question 29: D

Explanation:

- Shelf life: The bactericidal function of granulocytes rapidly decreases after granulocyte collection. Granulocytes should be transfused as soon as possible, but the shelf life of this component according to AABB standards is 24 hours.

Question 30: D

Explanation:

- Indications for granulocyte transfusions in adult patients:
  - Infection unresponsive to appropriate antimicrobial therapy.
  - Transient (reversible) marrow depression.
  - Absolute neutropenia (<500/μL).
- Indications for granulocyte transfusion in neonatal and pediatric patients:
  - Bacterial sepsis.
  - Transient (reversible) marrow depression.
  - Neutropenia with absolute neutrophil count of <3000/μL and decreased marrow neutrophil stores as indicated by less than 7% of marrow nucleated cells being metamyelocytes or more mature forms.
- Controversial indications:
  - Systemic fungal infection.
  - Prophylaxis during cancer chemotherapy.
- Patient A has no hope of marrow recovery and therefore does not fulfill criteria.
- Patient B has no evidence of infection and has an absolute neutrophil count above 500/μL.
- Patient C has a viral infection. This would not respond to granulocyte transfusions.
- Patient E has not had an appropriate course of antibiotics and his absolute neutrophil count is greater than 500/μL.

Question 31: C

Explanation:

- Characteristics of granulocytes collected by leukapheresis are described in Table 3-31.
- Administration:
  - ABO compatibility and crossmatching are required because the red cell content is >2mL.
  - Microaggregate and/or leukocyte-reduction filters are not used during granulocyte transfusion.

Table 3-31.

Characteristic	Quantity
Granulocyte content	$\geq 1 \times 10^{10}$ in 75% units tested
Red cell content	20 to 50 mL (hematocrit 10%)
Platelet content	3×10^{11} (equivalent to 1 platelet pheresis unit)
Total volume	250 to 300 mL

Question 32: E

Explanation:

- HES is a rouleaux-promoting agent that increases the sedimentation of red cells during centrifugation. This allows greater separation of the granulocytes from the red blood cells and enhances collection efficiency.
- There are reports of anaphylactic reactions and persistent localized skin reactions related to the administration of HES.
- Corticosteroids cause the marginated pool of granulocytes to enter the circulation. This increases the circulating pool and decreases the egress of granulocytes from the circulation. It results in a twofold greater collection of granulocytes compared with unstimulated donors. It has been shown that corticosteroid administration does *not* adversely affect granulocyte function. It decreases apoptosis, a beneficial effect that prolongs circulation.
- G-CSF stimulates increased production of granulocytes by the marrow and also decreases apoptosis. It results in a four- to fivefold-greater collection of granulocytes compared with unstimulated donors. It has been shown that G-CSF administration does *not* adversely affect granulocyte function. It decreases apoptosis, a beneficial effect that prolongs circulation and increases bacteriocidal activity.
- The combination of corticosteroids and G-CSF results in a tenfold-greater collection of granulocytes compared with unstimulated donors.

Question 33: B

Explanation:

- Back pain and headache are common side effects of G-CSF administration. They are thought to result from stretching of pain receptors in the marrow space by the active growth and proliferation of the neutrophils and their precursors. G-CSF may also be associated with nausea.
- Citrate is used as an anticoagulant for granulocyte collections. It anticoagulates blood by chelating calcium so that it is not available to participate in the coagulation cascade. Hypocalcemia is a manifestation of citrate toxicity. The effects of hypocalcemia range from minor circumoral paresthesias and muscle tremor to more severe complications such as tetany and cardiac effects.
- Weight gain occurs with HES. As a slowly excreted colloid, it can expand the donor's intravascular volume. It also can leave the intravascular space, resulting in tissue build up with the movement of water into the third space.
- Additional reactions to HES include:
  - Anaphylactoid reactions caused by the generation of complement fragments by the alternate complement pathway.
  - Intractable pruritis caused by skin deposition.
  - Prolongation of the PTT as well as decreases in fibrinogen levels. This is thought to result from the dilutional effects from volume expansion, as well as decreases in Factor VIII activity and Factor VIII antigen levels. HES increases vWF antigen turnover resulting in decreased antigen levels. As Factor VIII is stabilized by vWF, Factor VIII levels decline as well. Bleeding time may also be prolonged because of decreased vWF.
- These dose-dependent risks are usually not of concern in the setting of granulocyte collection where exposure is limited.
- Corticosteroid administration can also complicate underlying diseases in the donor, such as hypertension, diabetes mellitus, and peptic ulcer disease.

Question 34: C

Explanation:

- Complications of granulocyte transfusion:
  - Acute pulmonary insufficiency and distress.
  - Transfusion-associated GVHD.
  - HLA alloimmunization.
- Irradiation does not damage granulocytes with respect to bactericidal function and, therefore, is not contraindicated.
- Irradiation prevents transfusion-associated GVHD, which has a high mortality rate (approximately 95%). Irradiation prevents replication of DNA in lymphocytes in the component and thereby prevents lymphocyte proliferation. Patients receiving granulocytes are usually profoundly immunosuppressed and at risk of GVHD. Numerous cases of transfusion-associated GVHD caused by granulocytes have been reported and therefore *all* granulocyte products should be irradiated.
- Irradiation does *not* inhibit CMV and does *not* prevent HLA alloimmunization.
- Irradiation has no effect on the expiration time of granulocytes. They should not be stored for more than 24 hours and should be transfused as soon as possible after preparation.

REFERENCES

1. Price TH, ed. Standards for blood banks and transfusion services. 26th ed. Bethesda, MD: AABB, 2009.
2. Kakaiya R, Aronson CA, Julleis J. Whole blood collection and component processing. In: Roback JD, Combs MR, Grossman BJ, Hillyer CD, eds. Technical manual. 16th ed. Bethesda, MD: AABB, 2008:189-228.
3. Smith JW, Burgstaler EA. Blood component collection by apheresis. In: Roback JD, Combs MR, Grossman BJ, Hillyer CD, eds. Technical manual. 16th ed. Bethesda, MD: AABB, 2008:229-40.
4. Lockwood WB, Leonard J, Liles SL. Storage, monitoring, pretransfusion processing, and distribution of blood components. In: Roback JD, Combs

MR, Grossman BJ, Hillyer CD, eds. Technical manual. 16th ed. Bethesda, MD: AABB, 2008:283-300.
5. Winters JL, Pineda AA. Hemapheresis. In: McPherson RA, Pincus MR, eds. Henry's clinical diagnosis and management by laboratory methods. 21st ed. Philadelphia: Saunders Elsevier, 2006:685-715.

In: Blackall D, Figueroa P, Winters J
Transfusion Medicine Self-Assessment and Review, 2nd Edition
Bethesda, MD: AABB Press, 2009

4

Carbohydrate Blood Group Antigens

QUESTIONS

Question 1: Which of the following is a carbohydrate blood group antigen?

A. D.
B. Le^b.
C. Jk^a.
D. Lu^a.
E. S.

Question 2: A patient's red cells react with anti-A and the serum reacts with group B red cells. The ABO blood group identification is:

A. A.
B. B.
C. O.
D. O$_h$.
E. AB.

Question 3: Which of the following ABO donor-recipient pairings is most likely to show a compatible crossmatch? Note: Antibody screening revealed the absence of unexpected antibodies in the patient.

A. Donor: group A_1B—Patient: group A_1.
B. Donor: group B—Patient: group O.
C. Donor: group A_2B—Patient: group B.
D. Donor: group O—Patient: group B.
E. Donor: group A—Patient: group B.

Question 4: The enzyme responsible for conferring H activity on the red cell membrane is:

A. D-galactosyltransferase.
B. UDP-glucuronosyltransferase (UGT).
C. L-fucosyltransferase.
D. Glycosyltransferase.
E. N-acetylgalactosaminyltransferase.

Question 5: The terminal sugar molecule that defines blood group A is:

A. N-acetyl-D-neuraminic acid.
B. L-fucose.
C. N-acetyl-D-galactosamine.
D. D-galactose.
E. N-acetyl-D-glucosamine.

Question 6: A bleeding patient is in need of group O blood. From which US ethnic group would one find the most group O donors?

A. European-American.
B. African-American.
C. Asian.

D. Native American.
E. Melanesian.

Question 7: In the ABO blood group, the mating of which two phenotypes can produce offspring with each of the common four blood types (A, B, AB, and O)?

A. AB and O.
B. AB and A.
C. AB and AB.
D. A and B.
E. AB and B.

Question 8: What is the color of the liquid in the bottle that contains commercial anti-B reagent?

A. Blue.
B. Yellow.
C. Brown.
D. Green.
E. Red.

Question 9: Which of the following characterizes the anti-A found in group O individuals?

A. Formed as a result of A antigen exposure in the context of red cells.
B. IgM and IgG isotypes are present.
C. Requires the addition of anti-human globulin to agglutinate group A red cells.
D. Inactive at 37 C.
E. Cannot agglutinate A_1B and A_2B red cells.

Question 10: Which one of the following statements is true?

A. The *ABO* and *Rh* gene loci are present on chromosome 9.
B. Anti-A and anti-B produced by group B and group A individuals are predominantly IgM.
C. A mixed field reaction is typically observed between anti-A and A_2 red cells.
D. The A_1 and A_2 subgroups are distinguished serologically with the *Ulex europaeus* lectin.
E. Serum of Bombay phenotype individuals (O_h) will agglutinate group O red cells but will not agglutinate group A or group B red cells.

Question 11: A blood donor has the genotype *hh, AB*. What is his apparent red cell phenotype?

A. A.
B. B.
C. O.
D. AB.
E. Cannot be determined.

Question 12: Bombay phenotype (O_h) individuals:

A. Have red cells that do not agglutinate with either anti-A or anti-B but do agglutinate with *Ulex europaeus* lectin.
B. Have naturally occurring anti-A, anti-B, and anti-H.
C. Can be transfused safely with blood from donors of any blood group (A, B, AB, O).
D. Have naturally occurring anti-A and anti-B but they are not reactive at 37 C.
E. Inherit *SeSe* and the *Se* locus.

Question 13: A 50-year-old man with adenocarcinoma of the colon is scheduled for colonic resection. His antibody screen is positive, and the antibody identification panel shows reactivity with all cells. The patient's direct antiglobulin test is negative. Crossmatching 50 group O units fails to identify a compatible unit. Because of the presumed presence of an antibody to a high-incidence antigen, family members are asked to make directed donations. The ABO and Rh typings of the family members are as follows:

> Patient's mother: Group A, Rh positive.
> Patient's father: Group O, Rh positive.
> Patient: Group O, Rh positive.
> Patient's wife: Group B, Rh positive.
> Patient's child # 1: Group A, Rh positive.
> Patient's child # 2: Group B, Rh positive.
> Patient's child # 3: Group AB, Rh positive.
> Patient's child # 4: Group O, Rh positive.

The patient is crossmatch-incompatible with his father and child # 4. The problem is referred to you. You advise:

A. Testing a new sample from each family member because either a technical or a clerical error has caused the ABO discrepancy.
B. Testing the patient's cells with *Dolichos biflorus* lectin.
C. Arranging a confidential conference with the patient to inform him of the possibility that he may not be the biologic father of the first and third children; parentage testing should be performed for confirmation.
D. Testing the patient's cells with *Ulex europaeus* lectin.
E. Testing the patient's cells with O_h serum.

Question 14: Which one of the following antibodies strongly agglutinates O cells and A_2 cells, but either does not agglutinate or only weakly agglutinates A_1 and A_1B cells?

A. Anti-Le^a.
B. Anti-A_1.

106   TRANSFUSION MEDICINE SELF-ASSESSMENT AND REVIEW

C. Anti-A.
D. Anti-H.
E. Anti-B.

Question 15: Which of the following red cell types would be best for demonstrating the presence of anti-I in a patient's serum?

A. Adult cells.
B. O_h Bombay cells.
C. Cord cells.
D. Le(a+b+) cells.
E. i adult cells.

Question 16: A 35-year-old woman presents with a compound fracture of her right femur caused by a motor vehicle accident. Her orthopedic surgeon orders 4 units of blood. The patient has a historic blood type of A, Rh positive. Results of the ABO typing, antibody screen, and subsequent work-up are given in Table 4-16A through 4-16C. Which of the following statements is *true* concerning this antibody?

A. The specificity is anti-Pr.
B. This antibody is usually clinically significant.
C. The patient should be transfused with A_1, Rh-positive, I-negative blood.
D. The specificity is anti-I.
E. The specificity is anti-IH.

Table 4-16A.

Forward Typing				Reverse Typing	
Anti-A	Anti-B	Anti-A,B	Anti-A_1 Lectin	A_1 Cells	B Cells
+	−	+	+	1+	4+

Table 4-16B.

Cell	D	C	c	E	e	f	V	C^w	K	k	Kp^a	Kp^b	Js^a	Js^b	Fy^a	Fy^b	Jk^a	Jk^b	Le^a	Le^b	P_1	M	N	S	s	Lu^a	Lu^b	Xg^a	IS	AHG	Ficin
I	+	+	0	0	+	0	0	0	+	+	0	+	0	+	+	+	0	+	0	+	+	+	+	+	+	0	+	0	3+	0	4+
II	+	0	+	+	0	0	0	0	0	+	0	+	0	+	0	+	+	0	+	0	+	+	+	0	+	0	+	+	3+	0	4+
1	+	+	0	0	+	0	0	0	+	+	0	+	0	+	+	+	+	0	+	0	+	+	+	+	+	0	+	+	3+	0	4+
2	+	+	0	0	+	0	0	+	0	+	0	+	0	+	0	+	+	0	+	0	+	+	+	0	+	0	+	0	3+	0	4+
3	+	+	0	0	+	0	0	0	0	+	0	+	0	+	+	0	0	+	+	+	+	0	+	0	+	0	+	+	3+	0	4+
4	+	0	+	+	0	+	+	0	+	+	0	+	0	+	+	+	+	0	0	+	+	+	+	+	0	0	+	0	3+	0	4+
5	0	+	+	0	+	+	0	0	0	+	0	+	0	+	0	0	0	+	+	+	+	+	+	0	+	0	+	+	3+	0	4+
6	0	0	+	0	+	+	+	0	+	+	0	+	0	+	+	+	+	+	+	0	+	0	+	0	+	0	+	0	3+	0	4+
7	0	0	+	0	+	+	0	0	0	+	0	+	0	+	+	0	+	+	+	0	+	0	+	0	+	+	+	+	3+	0	4+
8	0	0	+	+	+	+	0	0	+	+	0	+	0	+	+	+	+	+	+	0	0	+	+	+	+	0	+	0	3+	0	4+
9	0	0	+	0	+	+	0	0	0	+	0	+	0	+	+	0	0	+	+	0	+	+	+	0	0	0	+	+	3+	0	4+
10	0	0	+	0	+	+	0	0	0	+	0	+	0	+	0	0	0	+	0	0	0	0	+	0	+	0	+	0	3+	0	4+
Patient's cells																													1+	0	3+

Table 4-16C.

Red Cell Tested	Results
O I adult	3+
A₁ I adult	1+
A₂ I adult	2+
O_h Bombay	0
O cord	W+
O i adult	0
A₁ i adult	0

Question 17: Which of the following statements is true regarding an acquired B antigen?

A. It can be acquired through multiple transfusions.
B. It is not detected with monoclonal anti-B.
C. It occurs more frequently in lupus.
D. It has been associated with gram-positive bacteria.
E. It is seen more often in patients with colorectal carcinoma.

Question 18: A 65-year-old woman presents with an abdominal mass detected by computed tomography (CT) scan. A type and screen is ordered before scheduling the patient for an invasive diagnostic procedure. Her ABO typing results are shown in Table 4-18.

Her most likely diagnosis is:

A. Hepatocellular carcinoma.
B. Carcinoma of the ovary.
C. Carcinoma of the pancreas.
D. Carcinoma of the rectum.
E. Meig's syndrome.

Table 4-18.

Forward Grouping			Reverse Grouping	
Anti-A	Anti-B	Anti-A,B	A₁ Cells	B Cells
4+	1+	4+	–	4+

Question 19: A 50-year-old man presents with an abdominal mass detected by CT scan. The patient has a previous history of typing as B, Rh positive. A type and screen is ordered before scheduling the patient for an invasive diagnostic procedure. The ABO typing results are shown in Table 4-19.

His most likely diagnosis is:

A. Hepatocellular carcinoma.
B. Testicular carcinoma.
C. Carcinoma of the pancreas.
D. Melanoma.
E. Adrenal adenocarcinoma.

Table 4-19.

Forward Typing			Reverse Typing	
Anti-A	Anti-B	Anti-A,B	A₁ Cells	B Cells
–	–	–	4+	–

Question 20: A type and screen is ordered for a 74-year-old man with chronic lymphocytic leukemia (CLL). The forward and reverse grouping results are shown in Table 4-20A.

Retesting after incubation for 15 minutes at 4 C demonstrates the results shown in Table 4-20B.

Table 4-20A.

Forward Grouping			Reverse Grouping	
Anti-A	Anti-B	Anti-A,B	A$_1$ Cells	B Cells
4+	–	4+	–	–

Table 4-20B.

A$_1$ Cells	B Cells	O Cells	Autocontrol
–	2+	–	–

This ABO discrepancy was most likely caused by:

A. Clerical error.
B. Technical error.
C. Weak or missing isohemagglutinins.
D. Weak or missing antigen.
E. Rouleaux.

Question 21: A 55-year-old man with the gradual onset of confusion and lethargy is admitted for severe back pain. Radiographs demonstrate a vertebral compression fracture as well as multiple osteolytic lesions. The forward and reverse grouping results are shown in Table 4-21A.

Table 4-21A.

Forward Grouping			Reverse Grouping	
Anti-A	Anti-B	Anti-A,B	A₁ Cells	B Cells
4+	2+	4+	2+	4+

A technique that could help to resolve this ABO discrepancy is:

A. Enzyme treatment of the screening cells.
B. Adsorption and elution.
C. Saline replacement.
D. Prewarming the patient's sample.
E. Testing for polyagglutination.

Question 22: A newly-admitted patient has forward and reverse grouping results as shown in Table 4-22.

Table 4-22.

Forward Grouping			Reverse Grouping	
Anti-A	Anti-B	Anti-A,B	A₁ Cells	B Cells
4+	—	4+	2+	4+

The test that would *not* be helpful in solving this discrepancy is:

A. Antibody screening with group O red cells.
B. Direct antiglobulin test (DAT).
C. Red cell phenotyping with anti-A₁ lectin.
D. Red cell testing for polyagglutinability.
E. Autoabsorption of the patient's serum and retesting.

Question 23: The most commonly identified antibody directed against the antigens of the P blood group system and/or globoside collection is:

A. Anti-P_1.
B. Anti-P_2.
C. Anti-P.
D. Anti-p^k.
E. Anti-Tj^a.

Question 24: Which of the following statements concerning the P_1 antigen and anti-P_1 is true?

A. Anti-P_1 is predominantly an IgG antibody.
B. The P_1 antigen is expressed well on cord red cells, equal to that of adult red cells.
C. Antibodies to P_1 demonstrate equal reactivity with all red cells expressing P_1.
D. The P_1 antigen is a member of the P blood group system.
E. Antibodies to P_1 are clinically significant.

Question 25: With regard to neutralization, which of the antibody/neutralizing substance pairs is correct?

A. Anti-I and human urine.
B. Antibodies to Lewis antigens and breast milk.
C. Anti-Chido and plasma.
D. Anti-Sd^a and hydatid cyst fluid.
E. Anti-P_1 and guinea pig urine.

Question 26: An antibody associated with a positive Donath-Landsteiner test is most likely to have specificity for which blood group antigen?

A. E.
B. M.
C. I.
D. P.
E. Lu^a.

Question 27: Which of the following statements is correct?

A. Paroxysmal nocturnal hemoglobinuria (PNH) is associated with a biphasic hemolysin.
B. Paroxysmal cold hemoglobinuria (PCH) is associated with anti-P.
C. *Mycoplasma pneumoniae* infection is associated with anti-P$_1$PP^k (anti-Tj^a).
D. The McLeod phenotype is associated with the Rh$_{null}$ genotype.
E. Anti-I is commonly associated with infectious mononucleosis.

Question 28: A 20-year-old man presents with a dry cough, headache, and fever for the past 7 to 10 days. Starting 3 days ago, he noted worsening malaise and shortness of breath as well as a darkening of his urine. His wife noted that his eyes were yellow. A complete blood count reveals a hematocrit of 15% and a white cell count of 60,000/μL. His platelet count is normal. Peripheral smear examination demonstrates clumping of the red cells. His DAT is positive with a polyspecific antihuman globulin (AHG) reagent, negative with anti-IgG, and positive with anti-C3d. A chest radiograph shows patchy lower lobe infiltrates. Titers for *Mycoplasma pneumoniae* IgM antibodies are positive. Titers for IgG antibodies are negative. The patient's forward and reverse ABO typings are discrepant. The most likely specificity of the antibody causing his anemia is:

A. Anti-Fy^a.
B. Anti-HI.
C. Anti-I.
D. Anti-Pr.
E. Anti-i.

Question 29: Which of the following antibodies is characteristically associated with in-vitro hemolysis?

A. Anti-C.
B. Anti-D.
C. Anti-Fy^a.
D. Anti-K.
E. Anti-Le^a.

Question 30: Which of the following phenotypes can form both Le^a and Le^b antibodies?

A. Le(a+b−).
B. Le(a−b+).
C. Le(a−b−).
D. Le(a+b+).

Question 31: Which of the following antibodies is associated with hemolytic disease of the fetus and newborn (HDFN)?

A. Anti-A,B.
B. Anti-I.
C. Anti-Le^a.
D. Anti-Le^b.
E. Anti-P$_1$.

Question 32: Table 4-32 represents an antibody identification panel from a pregnant woman who is in her 32nd week of gestation. Which of the following statements is *true* concerning the antibody identified?

Table 4-32.

Cell	D	C	c	E	e	f	V	C^w	K	k	Kp^a	Kp^b	Js^a	Js^b	Fy^a	Fy^b	Jk^a	Jk^b	Le^a	Le^b	P$_1$	M	N	S	s	Lu^a	Lu^b	Xg^a	IS	AHG	CC
I	+	+	0	0	+	0	0	0	+	+	0	+	0	+	+	+	0	+	0	+	+	+	+	+	+	0	+	0	1+	0	
II	+	0	+	+	0	0	0	0	0	+	0	+	0	+	0	+	+	0	+	0	+	+	+	0	+	0	+	+	0	0	+
1	+	+	0	0	+	0	0	0	+	+	0	+	0	+	+	+	+	0	+	0	+	+	+	+	+	0	+	+	0	0	+
2	+	+	0	0	+	0	0	+	0	+	0	+	0	+	+	+	+	0	+	0	+	+	0	0	+	0	+	+	0	0	+
3	+	0	+	0	+	+	0	0	+	+	0	+	0	+	0	+	0	+	+	+	+	0	+	0	+	0	+	0	1+	0	
4	+	+	+	+	+	+	0	0	0	+	0	+	0	+	+	0	+	0	0	0	+	+	+	+	0	0	+	+	0	0	+
5	0	0	+	0	+	+	0	0	+	+	0	+	0	+	0	+	0	+	+	+	+	0	+	+	+	0	+	0	1+	0	0
6	0	+	+	+	+	+	0	0	0	+	0	+	0	+	+	0	+	0	+	0	+	0	+	0	+	0	+	+	1+	0	+
7	0	0	+	0	+	+	0	0	+	+	0	+	0	+	+	+	+	+	+	0	0	+	+	0	+	0	+	0	0	0	+
8	0	0	+	0	+	+	0	0	0	+	0	+	0	+	+	0	+	+	+	0	0	+	0	0	+	+	+	+	0	0	+
9	0	0	+	0	+	+	0	0	0	+	0	+	0	+	+	+	0	+	+	0	+	0	+	+	0	0	+	0	0	0	+
10	0	0	+	0	+	+	0	0	0	+	0	+	0	+	0	0	0	+	0	0	+	0	+	0	+	0	+	0	0	0	+
Patient's cells																															

A. The woman must be negative for the antigen to which the antibody is directed.
B. The antigen is destroyed by enzymes.
C. The pregnancy is at risk for severe hemolytic disease of the fetus and newborn.
D. The antigen is passively adsorbed to the red cell membrane.
E. The antibody commonly causes in-vivo hemolysis.

Question 33: A 60-year-old man is scheduled to undergo a three-vessel coronary artery bypass graft (CABG) procedure. His typing is A, Rh positive. His antibody screen is positive, and the antibody identification panel is provided in Table 4-33A. The panel is interpreted as an anti-Le^b. As units are being set up for surgery, the technologist mistakenly crossmatches four Le^b-positive, group A, Rh-positive red cells (RBC) units and four Le^b-positive, group O, Rh-positive RBC units in addition to Le^b-negative RBC units. The results are shown in Table 4-33B.

The antibody causing these reactions is most likely:

A. Anti-Le^{bL}.
B. Anti-H.
C. Anti-Le^a.
D. Anti-Le^{bH}.
E. Anti-Le^3.

Table 4-33A.

Cell	D	C	c	E	e	f	V	Cw	K	k	Kpa	Kpb	Jsa	Jsb	Fya	Fyb	Jka	Jkb	Lea	Leb	P1	M	N	S	s	Lua	Lub	Xga	IS	AHG	CC
I	+	+	0	0	+	0	0	0	+	+	0	+	0	+	+	+	0	+	0	+	+	+	+	+	+	0	+	0	1+	4+	
II	+	0	+	+	0	0	0	0	0	+	0	+	0	+	+	0	+	0	+	0	+	+	+	0	+	0	+	+	0	0	+
1	+	+	+	0	+	0	0	0	+	+	0	+	0	+	+	+	+	0	+	0	+	+	+	+	+	0	+	+	0	0	+
2	+	+	0	0	+	0	0	+	0	+	0	+	0	+	+	+	0	0	+	0	+	0	0	0	+	0	+	0	0	0	+
3	0	0	+	+	0	+	0	0	0	+	0	+	0	+	+	+	0	+	0	+	+	+	+	0	+	0	+	+	1+	4+	
4	+	0	+	0	+	+	0	0	+	+	0	+	0	+	0	0	+	+	0	+	+	+	+	0	+	0	+	0	0	0	+
5	0	+	+	0	+	+	0	0	0	+	0	+	0	+	0	+	0	+	0	+	+	+	+	+	+	0	+	+	1+	4+	
6	0	0	+	+	+	+	0	0	0	+	0	+	0	+	+	0	+	+	0	0	+	+	+	0	+	0	+	0	1+	4+	
7	0	0	+	0	+	+	0	0	+	+	0	+	0	+	+	+	+	0	+	0	0	+	0	+	+	+	+	+	0	0	+
8	0	0	+	+	+	+	0	0	0	+	0	+	0	+	0	0	+	+	+	0	0	+	+	+	0	0	+	0	0	0	+
9	0	0	+	0	+	+	0	0	0	+	0	+	0	+	+	+	+	0	+	0	0	+	0	0	+	0	+	+	0	0	+
10	0	0	+	0	+	+	0	0	0	+	0	+	0	+	0	0	0	+	0	0	+	0	+	0	+	0		0	0	0	+
Patient's cells																															

Table 4-33B.

Red Cell Phenotype	Crossmatch Reaction
Four group A, Rh-positive, Le^b-positive	Crossmatch-compatible
Four group A, Rh-positive, Le^b-negative	Crossmatch-compatible
Four group O, Rh-positive, Le^b-positive	Crossmatch-incompatible
Four group O, Rh-positive, Le^b-negative	Crossmatch-compatible

---

Question 34: Which of the following phenotypes or haplotypes more frequently occurs in African-Americans than in European-Americans?

A. A.
B. I-negative adult.
C. Le(a–b–).
D. p.
E. P$_2$.

ANSWERS

Question 1: B

Explanation:

- Le^b is a carbohydrate blood group antigen that, along with Le^a, results from the interaction of genes at two independent loci, *Le* and *Se*.
- Lewis antigens are not intrinsic to red cells; instead, they are located on type 1 glycosphingolipids in the plasma that adsorb to the surface of cells.
- Le^b is the receptor for *Helicobacter pylori*.
- The other blood group antigens listed are either proteins or glycoproteins.

Question 2: A

Explanation:

- ABO blood group antibodies are predominantly naturally occurring IgM antibodies with optimal reaction temperatures of 4 C. IgG antibodies are also present in varying titers. These antibodies are reactive at 37 C. By 3 to 6 months of age, all healthy normal individuals possess ABO antibodies. These are directed against the ABO antigens that they lack.
- ABO blood groups are detected by the following:
  - Forward grouping or cell typing: testing the patient's or donor's red cells with commercial anti-A (blue bottle) and commercial anti-B (yellow bottle).
  - Reverse grouping or serum typing: testing the patient's or donor's serum with A$_1$ red cells and group B red cells.
- Representative typing reactions of ABO blood groups and the O$_h$ (Bombay) phenotype are shown in Table 4-2.
- O and O$_h$ phenotypes cannot be differentiated by routine forward and reverse grouping reactions.
- O$_h$ individuals have a potent anti-H, which is detected in the indirect antiglobulin test. Since the red cells used in antibody screen and antibody identification panels are all group O, the serum, because of anti-H, would react with all of these cells.

Table 4-2.

	Forward Grouping		Reverse Grouping	
Blood Group	Anti-A	Anti-B	A₁ Cells	B Cells
A	+	−	−	+
B	−	+	+	−
O	−	−	+	+
AB	+	+	−	−
O_h	−	−	+	+

Question 3: D

Explanation:

- The crossmatch is a serologic test in which recipient serum is mixed with donor red cells for the assessment of compatibility.
- Evaluation of possible answers is given in Table 4-3.
- A person with group O is called a universal red cell donor.
- A person with group AB is called a universal red cell recipient.

Table 4-3.

Choice	Antigens on Donor Red Cells	Antibodies in Serum of Patient	Major Crossmatch
A	A1, B	Anti-B	Incompatible
B	B	Anti-A, anti-B, anti-A,B	Incompatible
C	A₂, B	Anti-A	Incompatible
D	−	Anti-A	Compatible
E	A	Anti-A	Incompatible

Question 4: C

Explanation:

- A, B, and H genes encode glycosyltransferase enzymes that transfer immunodominant sugar molecules to specific acceptor substances (substrates). This results in the production of A, B, and H antigens on the erythrocyte membrane.
- The homozygous inheritance of an amorphic O allele results in the blood group O phenotype and H substance on the RBC membrane.
- The homozygous inheritance of an amorphic h allele results in the Bombay phenotype (O_h).
- UGT is a hepatic enzyme that is required for the conjugation of bilirubin with glucuronic acid. UGT = uridine diphosphate-glucuronosyltransferase.
- ABH antigen biochemistry is outlined in Table 4-4.

Table 4-4.

Gene	Glycosyl-transferase	Immunodominant Sugar Molecule	Substrate Acceptor	Antigen Found on the RBC Membrane
H	α-2-L-fucosyltransferase	L-fucose	Precursor chain type II	H
h	—	—	—	Precursor chain type II (unchanged)
A	α-3-N-acetyl-D-galactosaminyltransferase	N-acetylgalactosamine	H (Type I and II)	A
B	α-3-D-galactosyltransferase	D-galactose	H (Type I and II)	B

Question 5: C

Explanation:

- *N*-acetyl-D-glucosamine is present on the oligosaccharide chain of the carbohydrate antigens of the ABO, P, Lewis, and Ii blood group systems.
- *N*-acetylneuraminic acid is a sialic acid present on the glycophorin molecules.
- The terminal sugar molecule that defines blood group A is *N*-acetyl-D-galactosamine.
- The terminal sugar molecule that defines blood group B is D-galactose.
- Blood group O individuals have the H antigen on their red cells. The terminal sugar molecule that defines the H antigen is L-fucose.

Question 6: D

Explanation:

- Approximate frequencies of the O blood group in various populations are given in Table 4-6.
- Blood group O results from an amorphic allele at the *ABO* locus on chromosome 9 that possesses no transferase activity. As a result, the H antigen present on red cells is not modified.
- Most *O* genes represent *A* genes that contain mutations that eliminate N-acetylgalactosamine transferase activity.

Table 4-6.

African-American	Asian-American	European-American	Native American
49%	41%	44%	79%

Question 7: D

Explanation:

- In the ABO blood group system, the mating of two individuals with A and B phenotypes can produce offspring with the A, B, AB, and O phenotypes. However, this can only occur if these individuals have the *AO* and *BO* genotypes, respectively.
- This is depicted in greater detail in Table 4-7.

Table 4-7.

Phenotype of the Mating Pair	Possible Genotypes of the Mating Pair	Possible Genotypes of the Offspring	Possible Phenotypes of the Offspring
AB and O	A/B; O/O	A/O; B/O	A, B
AB and A	A/B; A/O or A/A	A/A; A/B; A/O; B/O	A, AB, B
AB and AB	A/B; A/B	A/A; A/B; B/B	A, AB, B
A and B	A/O or A/A; B/O or B/B	A/O; B/O; A/B; O/O	A, B, AB, O
AB and B	A/B; B/O or B/B	B/B; A/B; A/O; B/O	B, AB, A

Question 8: B

Explanation:

- Anti-A reagent has a blue label and the liquid is blue.
- Anti-B reagent has a yellow label and the liquid is yellow.
- Some antihuman globulin (AHG) reagents have a green label or the liquid is green.
- Anti-D reagent has a gray label and the liquid is colorless.
- There are no red- or brown-colored bottles containing commercial reagents for ABO typing.

Question 9: B

Explanation:

- The isohemagglutinins anti-A and anti-B are produced by environmental exposure to carbohydrates similar to the A and B antigens found on red cells. Because they do not result from exposure to red cells, these antibodies are referred to as naturally occurring. However, the implication that they are formed without an antigenic stimulus is incorrect.
- Full adult expression of isohemagglutinins is reached at about 6 months of postnatal life. The antibodies are not readily identifiable in fetal blood.
- The isohemagglutinins have IgM, IgG, and IgA components, though the IgM component typically predominates.
- The antibodies can activate complement in vivo, are reactive at 37 C, and can cause intravascular hemolysis, resulting in acute hemolytic transfusion reactions.
- An IgG component can cross the placenta and potentially cause ABO hemolytic disease of the fetus and newborn.
- Anti-A can agglutinate A_1, A_2, A_1B, and A_2B red cells.
- Exposure of individuals lacking A and/or B antigens to A and/or B antigens through transfusion of incompatible red cells, transfusion of non-red-cell-containing components containing soluble A and/or B antigens, pregnancy with an ABO-incompatible fetus, and inoculation with vaccines containing A and/or B antigens can result in changes in the isohemagglutinins present in the individual. These changes include increased avidity, increased IgG concentration, increased reactivity at 37 C, increased titer, and a resulting increased chance of hemolysis if transfusion with ABO-incompatible red cells occurs.

Question 10: B

Explanation:

- The *ABO* locus is present on chromosome 9. *Rh* gene loci are present on the short arm of chromosome 1.
- Anti-A and anti-B produced by group B and group A individuals, respectively, are predominantly IgM. Smaller quantities of IgG and IgA are also present.
- A mixed-field agglutination reaction may be observed in the following situations:
  - Between anti-A and weak subgroups of A such as A_3.
  - Between anti-B and some weak subgroups of B.
  - Recent transfusion of group O RBCs to a non-group-O recipient.
  - Blood group chimerism, as in cases of marrow transplantation (if the donor and recipient have different ABO groups) or dizygotic twins of different blood types who have exchanged hematopoietic progenitor cells *in utero*.
  - Between anti-Sd^a and Sd^a-positive red cells in the antiglobulin phase of testing.
  - Between anti-Lu^a or anti-Lu^b and Lu^a- and Lu^b-positive red cells, respectively.
- The lectin *Dolichos biflorus* distinguishes A_1 from other subgroups of A (eg, A_2).
- Serologic tests of the A_1 and A_2 subgroups are described in Table 4-10.
- A_1 and A_2 are the major subgroups of A. Approximately 80% of group A individuals are A_1 and ~20% are A_2.
- Anti-A_1 is present in 1% to 8% of individuals of the A_2 blood group.
- Anti-A_1 is present in 22% to 35% of individuals of the A_2B blood group.
- The serum of Bombay phenotype individuals will agglutinate group O, group A, group B, and group AB red cells.
- A_2 transferase is a mutant form of A_1 transferase that can only add the N-acetyl galactosamine to straight-chain H antigen, while A_1 transferase can add the sugar to both straight-chain and branched-chain H antigen. This accounts for the quantitative and qualitative differences between A_1 and A_2 antigens.

Table 4-10.

Reagent	A$_1$ Cells	A$_2$ Cells
Anti-A	+	+
Anti-A$_1$	+	−
Dolichos biflorus	+	−

Question 11: C

Explanation:

- The genotype *hh, AB* has the O$_h$ Bombay phenotype and types as an apparent O phenotype.
- The *h* gene is a mutated form of the *H* gene.
- Bombay individuals lack the *H* gene and thus lack the substrate to make A or B substances even if the *A* and/or *B* genes are present.
- The H transferase (FUT1), Se (FUT2), and Le (FUT3) are located on chromosome 19. All are derived from a common ancestral gene.

Question 12: B

Explanation:

- O$_h$ Bombay individuals lack A, B, and H substance on their red cells and produce anti-A, anti-B, anti-A,B, and anti-H. All of these may cause intravascular hemolysis.
- *Ulex europaeus* lectin has anti-H specificity. Thus, O$_h$ red cells do not agglutinate with *Ulex europaeus* lectin.
- The concentration of H substance on the RBC membrane is O>>A$_2$>>B>>A$_2$B>>A$_1$>>A$_1$B>>O$_h$.
- Anti-H in O$_h$ Bombay individuals is usually IgM, strongly reactive at 37 C, and fixes complement. Thus, O$_h$ individuals can only be transfused safely with red cells from other O$_h$ individuals.

CARBOHYDRATE BLOOD GROUP ANTIGENS

- Anti-H produced by A_1 or A_1B individuals is usually IgM, reactive at room temperature or colder, and is clinically insignificant.
- At the genotypic level, the O_h phenotype arises from the inheritance of *hh* at the *H* locus and *sese* at the *Se* locus. This is in contrast to individuals of the para-Bombay phenotype who have a normal *Se* gene.

Question 13: D

Explanation:

- The patient has the Bombay phenotype (O_h). The apparent discrepancy will be resolved by testing his cells with anti-H or *Ulex europaeus* lectin. These will *not* agglutinate his cells. A positive reaction will be observed when group O red cells are tested with anti-H or *Ulex europaeus* lectin.
- Reverse grouping reactions of Group O serum and O_h Bombay serum are given in Table 4-13.
- *Ulex europaeus* lectin can differentiate cells with varying concentrations of the H antigen.
- Naturally occurring anti-H is present in the patient's serum. The patient will be crossmatch-incompatible with all group O red cells. He will be crossmatch-compatible with O_h Bombay phenotype red cells only.
- A technical or a clerical error is a common cause of ABO typing discrepancies, which is not applicable in this case.
- *Dolichos biflorus* is used for distinguishing A_1 and A_2 subgroups. A positive reaction is observed with A_1 and A_1B cells. A negative reaction is observed with A_2 and A_2B cells.
- Testing the patient's cells with O_h serum is a reasonable choice; however, O_h serum is not readily available.

Table 4-13.

	O Cells	O_h Cells	A_1 Cells	A_2 Cells	B Cells
Ulex europaeus	4+	−	Weak +	3+	2+
O serum	−	−	4+	4+	4+
Bombay O_h serum	4+	−	4+	4+	4+

- The first and the third children have inherited the unexpressed A allele from their father.
- The deduced genotypes of the family members are:
    - Patient's mother: A/A or A/O; H/h
    - Patient's father: O/O; H/h
    - Patient: O/A; h/h
    - Patient's wife: B/O; H/H or H/h
    - Patient's child # 1:   A/O; H/h
    - Patient's child # 2:   B/O; H/h
    - Patient's child # 3:   A/B; H/h
    - Patient's child # 4:   O/O; H/h

Question 14: D

Explanation:

- The concentration of the H antigen on red cells varies according to the A and/or B transferase genes present. In the presence of an A_1 gene, the majority of the H antigen is converted to the A_1 antigen. In the presence of an A_2 gene, only a portion of the H antigen is converted.
- The relative concentrations of the H antigen on red cells is: $O >> A_2 >> B >> A_2B >> A_1 >> A_1B >> O_h$.
- Reactions with serum containing carbohydrate antibodies are shown in Table 4-14.

Table 4-14.

Serum containing:	Reaction with:				
	A_1 Cells	A_2 Cells	B Cells	A_1B Cells	O Cells
Anti-Le^a	Will agglutinate Le(a+b−) cells and Le(a+b+) cells, irrespective of ABO type of the cells				
Anti-A_1	+	−	−	+	−
Anti-A	+	+	−	+	−
Anti-H	−	2+	1+	−	3+ to 4+
Anti-B	−	−	+	+	−

Question 15: C

Explanation:

- Reactions observed with a patient's serum containing anti-I are shown in Table 4-15.
- O_h Bombay cells have an increased expression of the I antigen because of the absence of the H antigen. The use of these cells would not help to confirm the presence of anti-I. In addition, these cells are rare and are usually not available.
- While i adult cells could be used to identify the presence of anti-I, they are rare and are usually not available.
- i adult is a very rare phenomenon associated with a recessive inheritance.
- Fetal and newborn red cells express a rich concentration of the i antigen and, conversely, have little or no I antigen. These cells are widely available. As a result, they are most frequently used to demonstrate the specificity of anti-I.
- The red cells of most children express an I antigen concentration equivalent to that found in adults by the age of 18 to 24 months.
- Autoanti-I is most commonly a benign, cold-reacting, naturally occurring, IgM, low-titer antibody found in the sera of most healthy individuals.
- Autoanti-I may also be a cause of cold autoimmune hemolytic anemia (cold agglutinin syndrome, CAS). CAS can be associated with certain infectious agents (eg, *Mycoplasma pneumoniae*, Epstein-Barr virus) or with certain malignant conditions (eg, Waldenström's mac-

Table 4-15.

Cells	H	I	i	Reaction with Anti-I
Cord O	+	−	+	−
Adult O	+	+	−	4+
O_h	−	+	−	4+
i adult	+	−	+	−

Antigen Present on Red Cells: H, I, i

roglobulinemia, multiple myeloma, and non-Hodgkin lymphoma). It can also be idiopathic. When autoanti-I is associated with hemolysis, the antibody typically has a high titer and a high thermal amplitude.

Question 16: E

Explanation:

- Anti-IH is a common cold agglutinin. It recognizes the compound antigen composed of I and H. As a result, the antibody does not react with O_h Bombay red cells (lack H) or O_i adult red cells (lack I), and they react only weakly or not at all with cord cells (lack I).
- Because the amount of H antigen varies according to the ABO type, the reactivity of cells with anti-IH also varies. Group O reagent red cells will react strongly (3+ or 4+). Cells with decreasing amounts of H will react more weakly (eg, A_1 patient cells and A_1 typing cells may react 1+).
- Anti-IH is usually clinically insignificant, with rare reports of it causing cold hemagglutinin disease. As a result, there is no need to transfuse I-negative red cells, which are extremely rare.
- Anti-IH, like most cold agglutinins, is enhanced by enzyme treatment. Anti-Pr cannot be the specificity, as enzymes destroy this antigen.
- Anti-I would not show the variation in strength, by ABO blood group, seen with this antibody.

Question 17: E

Explanation:

- An acquired B antigen, in A_1 and A_2 individuals, is caused by a deacetylase enzyme produced by gram-negative bacteria and is associated with intestinal obstruction caused by carcinoma of the colon and rectum. The deacetylase converts N-acetyl-D-galactosamine, the immunodominant sugar molecule of the A antigen, to D-galactosamine, which is similar to D-galactose, the immunodominant sugar of the B antigen.

CARBOHYDRATE BLOOD GROUP ANTIGENS 131

- Bacterial enzymes from *Proteus vulgaris* or *Escherichia coli 086* may act on the red cell membrane and convert an A antigen into an apparent B antigen. As a result, group A cells will appear to be AB.
- Fatal intravascular hemolytic transfusion reactions have occurred in group A individuals who appeared to be AB and received AB RBCs.
- Acquired B is a rare phenomenon. The ABO grouping discrepancy caused by acquired B can be resolved by the following means:
  - Monoclonal anti-B: Some clones do not react with acquired B antigen; some, such as ES-4, do.
  - Adjustment of the pH of anti-B from a group A individual to a pH of 6:
  - This antiserum may not react with acquired B antigen but may react with the normal B antigen.
  - Adjustment of the pH of monoclonal anti-B from clone ES-4 to a pH of 6: This antibody may not react with acquired B antigen but may react with the normal B antigen.
  - Mouse monoclonal antibody directed specifically against an epitope of the acquired B antigen.
  - Reacetylation of the acquired B antigen by treating the red cells with acetic anhydride.
  - Use of lectins *Griffonia simplicifolia* and *Phaseolus lunatus*.
  - Addition of galactosamine will disperse the agglutination induced by the addition of anti-B in acquired B antigen but not that seen with the normal B antigen.
  - Determining the presence of A or B antigens in the saliva of a secretor.
  - Determining the presence of A or B transferase activity in the serum of the individual.
  - Use of DNA technology to identify the presence or absence of the *H*, *A*, and *B* genes.

Question 18: D

Explanation:

- The patient is group A with acquired B antigen. This phenomenon is seen most frequently with colorectal carcinoma.
- Tumors of the ovary (mostly fibromas), ascites, and hydrothorax constitute Meig's syndrome. Carcinomas of the liver, ovary, pancreas,

and Meig's syndrome are usually not associated with acquired B phenomenon.

Question 19: C

Explanation:

- Some tumors—most notably adenocarcinomas of the pancreas, stomach, ovary, and biliary system—can produce large amounts of soluble A and B substances. These can neutralize anti-A and anti-B typing reagents unless the cells are adequately washed before typing. In this case, washing the cells thoroughly should correct the discrepant forward type.

Question 20: C

Explanation:

- ABO discrepancies in reverse groupings, caused by weak or missing isohemagglutinins, are often seen in patients with hypogammaglobulinemia (eg, CLL, Hodgkin disease), neonatal patients, elderly patients, and immunocompromised patients.
- The discrepancy may be resolved by retesting after incubation for 15 to 60 minutes. Reverse grouping reactions can further be enhanced by incubation at colder temperatures (eg, 4 to 18 C). An autocontrol must also be performed, as incubating at lower temperatures may result in agglutination caused by cold-reactive autoantibodies.
- Clerical and technical errors can lead to ABO discrepancies. As part of resolving ABO discrepancies, testing should be repeated with careful attention to standard operating procedures (SOPs).
- Weak or missing antigens can be seen with subgroups of A and B, leukemia, Hodgkin disease, and the presence of soluble blood group substances. Different techniques are required to determine the cause depending on which situation is involved (eg, absorption and elution for weak or missing antigens in leukemia and Hodgkin disease, washing for soluble blood group substances, etc).

CARBOHYDRATE BLOOD GROUP ANTIGENS   133

Question 21: C

Explanation:

- Enzyme treatment destroys some antigens (eg, Fy^a, Fy^b, M, N, S, s), eliminating agglutination caused by alloantibodies. Enzyme treatment enhances the binding of some alloantibodies (eg, Rh system) as well as warm-reactive autoantibodies and most cold autoantibodies.
- Rouleaux is responsible for the ABO discrepancy in this case. Rouleaux appears as a "stack of coins" under the microscope and results from an alteration of the zeta potential of the red cells by elevated levels of plasma protein. It most commonly results from increased plasma protein levels caused by plasma cell dyscrasias (eg, multiple myeloma, Waldenström's macroglobulinemia) or hypergammaglobulinemia. Aggregation (not agglutination) can also occur as a result of plasma expanders (eg, dextran) or Wharton's jelly contamination. Multiple washings of red cells can resolve forward grouping discrepancies in these cases.
- Reverse grouping discrepancies can be resolved by the saline replacement technique. This removes the plasma with its abnormal protein. In this technique, the typing red cells are washed and resuspended in saline after incubation with the patient's serum.
- Spontaneous agglutination of the patient's red cells, as well as typing cells, can occur with cold autoantibodies. If the patient's sample, as well as the screening cells and saline wash solution, are kept at 37 C, binding of the autoantibody can be avoided and false reactions prevented.
- Polyagglutination occurs when antigens are acquired or inherited to which all human sera contain naturally occurring antibodies. These can be identified using panels of lectins, as shown in Table 4-21B.
- Osteoclastic bone resorption, often seen in multiple myeloma, causes pathologic fractures and hypercalcemia manifested by confusion, lethargy, weakness, and polyuria.

Table 4-21B.

	T	Th	Tk	Tn	Cad
Arachis hypogaea	+	+	+	0	0
Dolichos biflorus	0	0	0	+	+
Glycine max	+	0	0	+	+
Salvia sclarea	0	0	0	+	0
Salvia horminum	0	0	0	+	+

Question 22: D

Explanation:

- Forward grouping indicates that the patient is blood group A. Reverse grouping suggests that the patient is blood group O (because of the 2+ reaction with A_1 cells as well as the reaction with B cells).
- Possible explanations for this ABO grouping discrepancy are:
  - The patient is A_2 with anti-A_1 present in the serum.
  - Presence of an unexpected cold-reacting antibody (eg, anti-Le^a, anti-M) in the patient's serum reacting with the corresponding antigen on the A_1 typing cells.
  - Presence of a cold autoantibody in the patient's serum.
- If the patient is group A, with an unexpected antibody in the serum, the antibody will be identified by antibody screening with group O red cells.
- A DAT could identify the presence of a cold autoantibody that is agglutinating the A_1 red cells. This antibody should also be detected by the antibody screen and panel identification. Demonstrating that the antibody is present on the patient's red cells indicates the presence of an autoantibody and not an alloantibody.
- If red cell phenotyping with anti-A_1 lectin (*Dolichos bifloris*) is negative, the patient is presumed to be A_2 and anti-A_1 is a possibility. In this case, the serum should be tested with three more A_1 red cell samples to confirm the identity of the anti-A_1.

CARBOHYDRATE BLOOD GROUP ANTIGENS

- Polyagglutination testing with a lectin panel would not be helpful because there are no inconsistencies in the forward grouping of the patient's red cells.
- By removing an autoantibody through absorption with the patient's own red cells, the resulting absorbate could be used to perform the reverse typing without difficulty.

Question 23: A

Explanation:

- Phenotype frequencies and associated antigens and antibodies in the P system are shown in Table 4-23.
- Anti-P_1 is the most common specificity encountered in the P blood group system. It is produced by individuals with the P_2 phenotype.
- Anti-P_1 is usually a naturally occurring IgM antibody that is reactive at immediate spin with an optimal reaction temperature below 22 C. It may interfere with compatibility testing, specifically ABO typing, but does not cause hemolysis. As a result, it is clinically insignificant. The antibody binds complement and may be detected by polyspecific AHG reagents.
- Anti-P_2 does not exist. P_2 is a phenotype composed of the antigens P and P^k. Individuals with the P_2 phenotype lack P_1 and can make anti-P_1.

Table 4-23.

Phenotype	Antigens	Antibody	Phenotype Frequency (%) Whites	Blacks
P_1	P_1, P, P^k	—	79	94
P_2	P, P^k	Anti-P_1	21	6
P^k	P^k	Anti-P	Very rare	Very rare
p or P_{null}	—	Anti-P_1PP^k (formerly anti-Tj^a)	Very rare	Very rare

- Individuals with a P_2 or P_1 phenotype have the P antigen, which is lacking in 1:100,000 to 1:200,000 individuals.
- Anti-P and anti-P_1PP^k (formerly referred to as anti-Tj^a) are very rare and can cause hemolysis in vivo and in vitro.
- Anti-P_1PP^k is associated with spontaneous abortions occurring early in the pregnancies of p women.
- The P blood group system, and the biochemically related globoside collection, contains the antigens P, P_1, P^k, and LKE (Luke). The biosynthetic pathway of these antigens is represented in Fig 4-23.
- The P antigen is the cell surface receptor for parvovirus B19, which causes erythema infectiosum (Fifth disease). Individuals of the p phenotype, who lack globoside, are naturally resistant to infection with this pathogen.

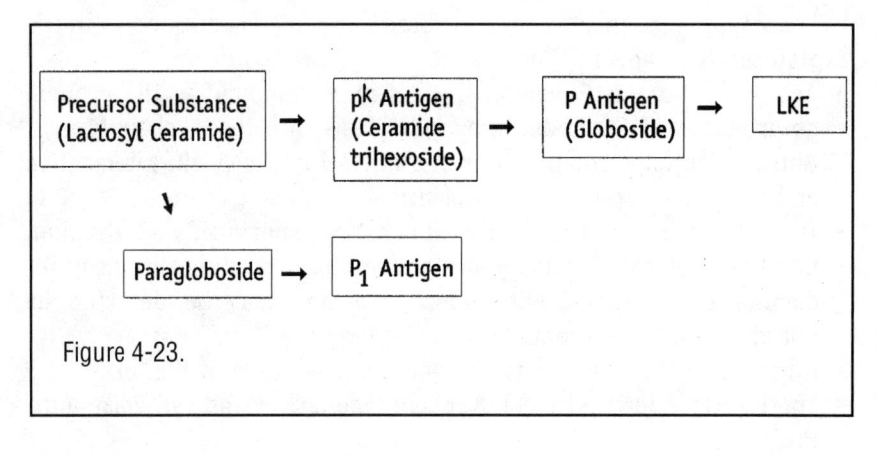

Precursor Substance (Lactosyl Ceramide) → p^k Antigen (Ceramide trihexoside) → P Antigen (Globoside) → LKE

Paragloboside → P_1 Antigen

Figure 4-23.

Question 24: D

Explanation:

- The P_1 antigen is not well developed at birth and does not reach adult levels until the age of 7.
- Antibodies to P_1 show variations in their strength of reactivity with different red cells. This does not represent a dosage effect, however. A true dosage effect depends on the number of copies of the gene for the antigen (the dose) that the individual possesses. With the P_1 antigen, individuals inherit P_1 genes that demonstrate differences in the strength of antigen expression (weak or strong). This is not

dependent upon the number of genes inherited and, therefore, is not a dosage effect.
- Anti-P$_1$ is predominantly an IgM, cold-reactive antibody. As such, it is rarely clinically significant.
- Anti-P$_1$ is sometimes found in people with parasitic infections.
- Earthworms, hydatid cyst fluid, pigeon egg whites, pigeon droppings, turtledove egg whites, turtledove droppings, and *Clonorchis sinensis* contain large amounts of the P$_1$ antigen that can be used to neutralize antibodies to P$_1$.

Question 25: C

Explanation:

- Lewis antigens may be present in the saliva and can be used to neutralize Lewis antibodies. They are not, however, present in breast milk.
- The antigens of the Chido/Rodgers blood group system are located on C4, the fourth component of the complement cascade. Enzymes destroy these antigens. Antibodies to these antigens are frequently of high titer but exhibit low avidity binding and are clinically insignificant. Plasma can neutralize them.
- The I antigen is present in saliva and breast milk but is not present in urine.
- The Sd^a antigen is neutralized by guinea pig urine, and the P$_1$ antigen is neutralized by hydatid cyst fluid, among other substances (see the explanation for Question 24).

Question 26: D

Explanation:

- Paroxysmal cold hemoglobinuria (PCH) is caused by an IgG biphasic hemolysin that most commonly has P blood group specificity. The antibody (autoanti-P) optimally binds red cells at 4 C. However, complement is activated and red cells are lysed at 37 C.

- The Donath-Landsteiner test consists of incubating a patient's serum with P-positive red cells at 4 C alone, at 37 C alone, and at 4 C followed by 37 C.
- Positive Donath-Landsteiner test results are shown in Table 4-26.
- The Donath-Landsteiner test is positive when the degree of hemolysis is greater in test tube 3 than it is in either test tube 1 or test tube 2.
- PCH is an autoimmune hemolytic anemia that, in the past, was characteristically associated with syphilis. This association is now uncommon, with PCH much more commonly occurring secondary to viral infections, particularly in young children.

Table 4-26.

	Test Tube 1	Test Tube 2	Test Tube 3
Incubating temperature	4 C	37 C	4 C followed by 37 C
Hemolysis	+/−	+/−	+++

Question 27: B

Explanation:

- PNH is a progenitor cell disorder characterized by episodic intravascular hemolysis and large vessel thrombosis. A defect in the ability to form glycosylphosphatidylinositol linkages results in a deficiency of decay accelerating factor and membrane inhibitor of reactive lysis on the red cell membrane. These are important regulators of complement activation. The resulting sensitivity to complement causes the hemolysis.
- PCH is a syndrome often seen following viral infections such as mumps, measles, chickenpox, influenza, or mononucleosis as well as *Mycoplasma* infections. The disorder can also be seen with syphilis, the disease classically associated with PCH.
- PCH is most commonly seen in children and is responsible for 40% of autoimmune hemolytic anemia cases in children less than 5 years of age.
- The Donath-Landsteiner test confirms the diagnosis of PCH.

- Therapy for PCH includes treating the underlying infection and avoiding cold temperatures. Steroids are not effective. Because red cells lacking the P antigen are rare (1:100,000 to 1:200,000), transfusion with P-negative red cells is not an option.
- Anti-I is associated with *Mycoplasma pneumoniae* infection but is detected in <50% of cases.
- Anti-P$_1$PP^k is a mixture of IgG antibodies directed against the antigens P$_1$, P, and P^k. It was formerly thought that these antibodies were directed against a single antigen; thus, the alternative antibody designation is anti-Tj^a. Anti-P$_1$PP^k is associated with early habitual abortion.
- The McLeod phenotype is associated with the absence of the Kx antigen and results in a decreased expression of Kell system antigens.
- Autoanti-i is found in the serum of some patients with infectious mononucleosis.

Question 28: C

Explanation:

- The patient is suffering from atypical pneumonia caused by *M. pneumoniae* infection. In addition, he has cold agglutinin syndrome (CAS).
- CAS has a peak incidence at 70 years of age. It may be primary or occur secondary to malignancies including lymphomas, chronic lymphocytic leukemia, and plasma cell dyscrasias (eg, multiple myeloma, Waldenström's macroglobulinemia). CAS is also associated with disease caused by infectious agents including *M. pneumoniae*, Epstein Barr virus (infectious mononucleosis), cytomegalovirus, parvovirus B19, and HIV.
- CAS results when an autoantibody, usually IgM, develops to antigens present on the red cell. These antibodies bind at cooler sites of the body (ie, the periphery) and fix complement. The antibody then disassociates at the warmer temperatures of the body, leaving complement fixed to the red cell membrane. The complement-coated cells are then removed by macrophages, predominantly those of the liver, through an interaction with their C3b receptors.
- In *M. pneumoniae* pneumonia, cold agglutinins are increased in 30% to 50% of patients; however, CAS occurs in a much smaller percent-

age. When hemolysis occurs, it is usually self-limited and mild, occurring during the second week of infection.
- The most common specificity of the autoantibody in *M. pneumoniae* pneumonia is anti-I, but other specificities can occur, including anti-Pr.
- Pr antigens are found on all red cells. These antigens are destroyed by enzyme treatment. The name Pr is derived from protease, recognizing the fact that these antigens are sensitive to proteases.
- The antigens toward which other cold-reacting autoantibodies are directed (eg, I, i, HI) are *not* destroyed by enzymes. With these antibodies, reactivity may be enhanced with enzyme treatment.
- Fy^a antibodies have not been implicated in cases of post-infectious CAS.
- CAS from causes other than infections (eg, malignancies) are usually chronic conditions that are difficult to treat. As an example, steroid therapy is usually not successful in the treatment of CAS, which contrasts to its high rate of success in the treatment of warm autoimmune hemolytic anemia.

Question 29: E

Explanation:

- With rare exceptions, the in-vitro hemolysis of reagent red cells indicates the presence of antibodies directed against I, Le^a, Le^b, Jk^a, Jk^b, P_1PP^k (Tj^a), or Vel antigens.
- IgM antibodies are responsible for the direct agglutination of cells at room temperature. Antibodies of this type include Le^a, Le^b, P_1, M, N, and Lu^a.
- The majority of antibodies are detected in the antiglobulin phase of testing.

Question 30: C

Explanation:

- The serum of individuals with the various Lewis phenotypes may contain the Lewis antibodies shown in Table 4-30A.
- Individuals with the Le(a–b+) phenotype do not make anti-Le^a because they possess the *Le* gene. A small amount of the type I chain is not converted to the H antigen by the *Se* gene but, instead, is converted to Le^a in these individuals. The amount is too small to detect by routine serologic methods but is sufficient to induce tolerance towards the Le^a antigen.
- Inheritance of the *Le* and the *Se* genes results in different Lewis phenotypes, as shown in Table 4-30B.
- The biosynthetic pathway of Lewis antigens is shown in Fig 4-30.
- The Le (a+b+) phenotype is rare in whites and blacks but is found in 3% of Asians. Individuals with this phenotype have an abnormal *Se* gene that cannot efficiently convert a type I precursor chain to a type I H antigen. This allows for the conversion of some of the type I chain to the Le^a antigen.

Table 4-30A.

Phenotypes	Anti-Le^a	Anti-Le^b
Le (a+b+)	–	–
Le (a+b–)	–	+
Le (a–b–)	+	+
Le (a–b+)	–	–

Table 4-30B.

Gene	Antigen	Phenotype
Le and *Se*	Le^b	Le (a–b+)
Le	Le^a	Le (a+b–)
le/le	—	Le (a–b–)

Figure 4-30.

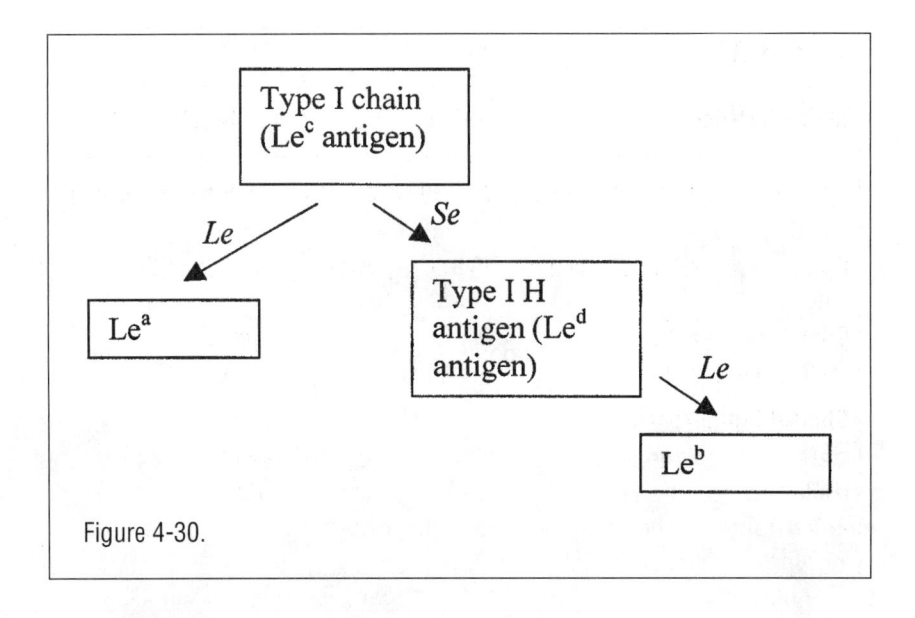

Question 31: A

Explanation:

- Anti-A and anti-B antibodies are predominantly IgM antibodies found in the plasma of group B and A individuals, respectively. They are rarely associated with HDFN.
- Anti-A,B, along with anti-A and anti-B, is found in the plasma of group O individuals. This antibody, which reacts with group A and B red cells, has both IgG and IgM components. As such, anti-A,B can cross the placenta and bind to the A and/or B antigens on fetal red cells, which may lead to hemolysis. For this reason, HDFN is almost always seen in neonates born to a group O mother.
- Anti-Le^a, Anti-Le^b, anti-I, and anti-P$_1$ are IgM, cold-reactive antibodies that are not associated with HDFN and are only rarely associated with hemolytic transfusion reactions, if ever. Aside from the fact that they are IgM antibodies, these antibodies are not associated with HDFN because their corresponding antigens are found on tissues other than red cells or in soluble form. In addition, the antigens are not expressed fully on cord red cells.
- Table 4-31 lists the characteristics and clinical significance of Lewis blood system antibodies.

Table 4-31.

Characteristics	Anti-Le^a	Anti-Le^b
Naturally occurring or immune	Naturally occurring	Naturally occurring
Class	IgM/IgG	IgM
Optimal temperature of reactivity	≤RT (24 C), may react up to 37 C	≤RT (24 C)
Complement fixation	Yes	Yes
In-vitro hemolysis	Sometimes	Rare
Clinical Significance:		
HDN	No	No
HTR	Few	No

RT = Room Temperature

Question 32: D

Explanation:

- The antibody is anti-Le^b. Lewis antigens frequently disappear during pregnancy, with the subsequent development of Lewis antibodies—most frequently, Le^b. This is called the Brendemoen phenomenon.
- Lewis antigens are extrinsic to the red cell membrane being adsorbed from the plasma. Changes in plasma characteristics during pregnancy may explain the Brendemoen phenomenon.
- Lewis antibodies are usually IgM and are not capable of crossing the placenta. This, and the fact that Lewis antigens are poorly expressed at birth, explain why they do not cause HDFN.
- The enzymatic treatment of red cells enhances the reactivity of antibodies to Lewis antigens.
- Lewis antibodies can cause hemolysis in vitro, as can the following antibodies: anti-A, -B, -A,B, -I, -Jk^a, -Jk^b, -P$_1$PP^k (Tj^a), and -Vel. The presence of hemolysis during antibody screening or identification suggests that one of these antibodies is present. Nevertheless, Lewis antibodies are clinically insignificant.
- Le^b is the receptor for *Helicobacter pylori*.

Question 33: D

Explanation:

- Anti-Le^b exists in two forms. Anti-Le^{bL} reacts with all Le^b-positive cells, regardless of their ABO type. Anti-Le^{bH} reacts only with group O and A$_2$ red cells expressing the Le^b antigen. This antibody recognizes a compound antigen of Le^b and H. Anti-Le^{bH} can be neutralized by either Le^b substance or H substance, whereas anti-Le^{bL} is neutralized only by Le^b substance.
- Anti-H would react with all of the cells found on an antibody identification panel because all of these cells are group O and have large amounts of H substance. All of the O cells crossmatched would have been incompatible. Some of the A cells, depending on their A subtype (A$_1$ vs A$_2$), may also have been incompatible.
- The antigen Le^3 does not exist.

Question 34: C

Explanation:

- Certain phenotypes are present at a higher frequency in African-Americans as compared to European-Americans.
- The phenotype/haplotype frequency (%) in African-Americans and European-Americans are compared in Table 4-34.

Table 4-34.

Phenotype/Haplotype	Frequency (%) African-Americans	European-Americans
A	27	40
I-negative adult	Very rare	Very rare
Le(a–b–)	22	6
p	Very rare	Very rare
P$_2$	6	21

REFERENCES

1. Cooling L. ABO, H, and Lewis blood groups and structurally related antigens. In: Roback JD, Combs MR, Grossman BJ, Hillyer CD, eds. Technical manual. 16th ed. Bethesda, MD: AABB, 2008:361-85.
2. Klein HG, Anstee DJ. ABO, Lewis and P groups and Ii antigens. In: Klein HG, Anstee DJ, Blood transfusion in clinical medicine. 11th ed. Malden, MA: Blackwell Scientific, 2005:114-62.
3. Reid ME, Lomas-Francis C. The blood group antigens factsbook. 2nd ed. San Diego, CA: Elsevier, 2004.
4. Reid ME, Westhoff CM. Human blood group antigens and antibodies. In: Hoffman R, Benz E, Shattil S, Furie B, eds. Hematology: Basic principles and practices. 5th ed. Philadelphia: Elsevier. 2009: 2163-78.
5. Kowalski M. ABO and Rh typing discrepancies. In: Rudmann SV, ed. Serologic problem solving: A systematic approach for improved practice. Bethesda, MD: AABB Press, 2005:153-81.

5

Protein-Based Blood Group Antigens

QUESTIONS

Question 1: Which of the following statements is *true*?

A. The Colton blood group antigens, Co^a and Co^b, are located on the red cell membrane protein CHIP-1 (channel-forming integral protein-1).
B. The Kidd blood group antigens, Jk^a and Jk^b, are located on erythrocyte chemokine receptors.
C. The Cartwright antigens, Yt^a and Yt^b, are located on decay accelerating factor (DAF)/CD55 of erythrocytes.
D. The Cromer antigens are located on erythrocyte acetylcholinesterase (AChE).
E. The Duffy antigens are located on the urea transport proteins of the kidney.

Question 2: Which of the following Rh antigens is *most* common in people of African ethnicity (Blacks) and people of European ethnicity (Whites)?

A. D.
B. C.
C. E.

D. c.
E. e.

Question 3: Which of the following Rh antigens is *least* common in Black and White populations?

A. D.
B. C.
C. E.
D. c.
E. e.

Question 4: The *most* common Rh haplotype in Whites is:

A. R^1.
B. R^2.
C. R^z.
D. r.
E. R^0.

Question 5: A 27-year-old African-American man with sickle cell disease (hemoglobin SS) presents to a hospital for the first time and requires a blood transfusion. He tells his physicians that he has been transfused heavily in the past but he can't recall when or where that occurred. In order to avoid exposure to blood group antigens to which the patient may have formed alloantibodies, the transfusion medicine specialist chooses to give blood of the Rh phenotype most likely to match the patient's own Rh phenotype. Statistically speaking, which of the following Rh phenotypes is most likely the best match?

A. R^0.
B. R^1.
C. R^2.
D. R^z.
E. r'.

Question 6: A 19-year-old woman of European ethnicity presents to a mobile blood drive at her college. She fulfills all eligibility criteria and donates a unit of whole blood. The results of her ABO and Rh typings are shown in Table 5-6.

Table 5-6.

	Forward Typing					Reverse Typing	
Anti-A	Anti-B	Anti-A,B	Anti-D	Weak D Test	Weak D Control	A$_1$ Cells	B Cells
0	0	0	0	2+	0	4+	4+

Components generated from the donation should be labeled as:

A. Group A, Rh negative.
B. Group O, Rh positive.
C. Group O, weak D.
D. Group A, Rh positive.
E. Group O, Rh negative.

Question 7: The same individual described in Question 6 is involved in an automobile accident 3 months later. Three units of red cells are ordered. The safest red cell component to transfuse would be:

A. Group A, Rh negative.
B. Group O, Rh positive.
C. Group A, weak D.
D. Group A, Rh positive.
E. Group O, Rh negative.

Question 8: Three years later, the patient in Question 6 is pregnant. At 3 months of gestation, her antibody screen is positive. The antibody identification panel identifies anti-D. The most likely explanation for this finding is that the patient is:

A. Weak D phenotype because of weak D mutation, and now she has alloanti-D.
B. Partial D genotype, and now she has alloanti-D.
C. Rh-negative genotype, and now she has alloanti-D.
D. Weak D phenotype because of a C gene in the *trans* position to the D gene, and now she has alloanti-D.
E. Rh-positive phenotype with an autoanti-D.

Question 9: Granulocyte function is impaired in chronic granulomatous disease (CGD). An association exists between this clinical condition and a depression of which of the following antigen systems?

A. Rh.
B. P.
C. Kell.
D. Duffy.
E. Kidd.

Question 10: Which of the following statements is *true* regarding the McLeod phenotype?

A. The red cells have enhanced expression of Kell system antigens and the Kx antigen.
B. Anti-K is detected in the serum.
C. Levels of serum creatine phosphokinase are depressed.
D. It is associated with impaired red cell urea transport.
E. Acanthocytes are seen on the peripheral blood smear.

Question 11: Antibodies with high titer and low avidity have which of the following characteristics?

A. They have strong reactivity with reagent red cells.
B. They are strongly reactive with even high dilutions of patient serum.
C. They may interfere with the detection of clinically significant alloantibodies.
D. They are implicated frequently in hemolytic transfusion reactions.
E. They are IgM antibodies best detected with an antiglobulin reagent.

Question 12: Which of the following antibodies exhibits high titer and low avidity behavior?

A. Anti-Chido (Ch).
B. Anti-Lu[b].
C. Anti-M.
D. Anti-S.
E. Anti-Wr[b].

Question 13: A patient's serum reacts weakly with 16 of 16 group O panel cells only at the antihuman globulin (AHG) phase of testing. No reaction was noted in the autocontrol. Further testing with ficin-treated panel cells demonstrated no reactivity at the AHG phase. Which of the following antibodies is most likely responsible for these results?

A. Anti-Js[a].
B. Anti-k.
C. Anti-e.
D. Anti-Ch.
E. Anti-Kp[a].

152 TRANSFUSION MEDICINE SELF-ASSESSMENT AND REVIEW

Question 14: A 75-year-old man is to undergo right total knee arthroplasty for degenerative joint disease. On presurgical testing, his antibody screen is found to be positive. An antibody identification panel is shown in Table 5-14A and additional test results are given in Table 5-14B. The most likely specificity of the antibody is:

A. Anti-e.
B. Anti-JMH.
C. Anti-Kn^a.
D. Anti-Fy^b.
E. Autoantibody.

Question 15: What is the titer of anti-K in the serum being examined in Table 5-15?

A. 8.
B. 1:8.
C. 16.
D. 1:16.
E. 1:32.

Table 5-15.

Dilution	1:1	1:2	1:4	1:8	1:16	1:32	1:64	1:128
Anti-K	4+	3+	2+	1+	m+	0	0	0

m = microscopically positive

Table 5-14A.

Cell	D	C	c	E	e	f	V	C^w	K	k	Kp^a	Kp^b	Js^a	Js^b	Fy^a	Fy^b	Jk^a	Jk^b	Le^a	Le^b	P$_1$	M	N	S	s	Lu^a	Lu^b	Xg^a	IS	AHG	Ficin
I	+	+	0	0	+	0	0	0	+	+	0	+	0	+	+	+	+	0	0	+	+	+	+	+	+	0	+	0	0	1+	0
II	+	0	+	+	+	0	0	0	0	+	0	+	0	+	0	+	+	+	+	0	+	+	0	0	+	0	+	+	0	1+	0
1	+	+	0	0	+	0	0	0	+	+	0	+	0	+	+	+	+	0	+	0	+	+	+	+	+	0	+	+	0	1+	0
2	+	+	+	0	+	0	0	+	0	+	0	+	0	+	0	+	0	+	0	0	+	0	+	0	+	0	+	0	0	1+	0
3	+	0	+	+	+	+	0	0	0	+	0	+	0	+	+	0	+	+	0	+	+	+	+	0	+	0	+	+	0	1+	0
4	+	0	+	0	+	+	+	0	+	+	0	+	0	+	0	0	+	0	+	0	+	+	+	0	+	0	+	0	0	1+	0
5	0	0	+	+	+	+	0	0	0	+	0	+	0	+	+	+	+	+	+	+	+	0	+	+	0	0	+	+	0	1+	0
6	0	0	+	0	+	+	0	0	+	+	0	+	0	+	0	0	0	+	0	0	0	+	+	0	+	+	+	0	0	1+	0
7	0	0	+	0	+	+	0	0	0	+	0	+	0	+	+	+	+	+	+	+	+	0	+	0	+	0	+	+	0	1+	0
8	+	+	0	+	0	0	+	0	0	+	0	+	0	+	+	0	+	0	+	0	0	+	+	+	0	+	+	0	0	1+	0
9	0	0	+	0	+	+	0	0	0	+	0	+	0	+	+	+	0	+	0	0	0	+	0	0	+	0	+	+	0	1+	0
10	0	0	+	0	+	+	0	0	0	+	0	+	+	+	0	0	0	+	0	0	+	0	+	+	+	0	+	0	0	1+	0
Patient's cells																															

Table 5-14B.

Titer	1	2	4	8	16	32	64	128	256	512	1024
Cell I	1+	1+	1+	1+	1+	1+	1+	1+	1+	1+	w+

Question 16: Which of the following is true concerning the Sd^a antigen and the antibodies that recognize it?

A. The Sd^a antigen is expressed on 10% of red cell samples.
B. Sd^a is located on the C4 component of complement.
C. Anti-Sd^a is neutralized by human plasma.
D. The presence of anti-Sd^a is suggested by refractile orange agglutinates on microscopy.
E. Anti-Sd^a has been associated with hemolytic disease of the fetus and newborn (HDFN).

Question 17: Which of the following statements is true of the antigens of the Lutheran blood group system and the antibodies that recognize them?

A. Lu^a is a high-incidence antigen.
B. Anti-Lu^a causes hemolytic transfusion reactions.
C. The Lu(a–b–) phenotype is common in individuals of African ethnicity.
D. The Lu(a–b–) phenotype results only from an autosomal recessive gene.
E. Antibodies to Lu^a produce a mixed-field pattern of reactivity with Lu^a positive cells.

Question 18: A 35-year-old woman presents with a lacerated liver following an automobile accident. Four Red Blood Cell (RBC) units are ordered. The patient has no history of transfusion but does have a history of five pregnancies. She types as group A, Rh positive. Her antibody screen is positive with the antibody identification panel given in Table 5-18A. Additional testing is also performed, as shown in Table 5-18B.

Table 5-18A.

Cell	D	C	c	E	e	f	V	C^w	K	k	Kp^a	Kp^b	Js^a	Js^b	Fy^a	Fy^b	Jk^a	Jk^b	Le^a	Le^b	P_1	M	N	S	s	Lu^a	Lu^b	Xg^a	IS	AHG	CC
I	+	+	0	0	+	0	0	0	+	+	0	+	0	+	+	+	0	+	0	+	+	+	+	+	+	0	+	0	0	1+	
II	+	0	+	+	0	0	0	0	0	+	0	+	0	+	0	+	+	0	+	0	+	+	+	0	+	0	+	+	0	1+	
1	+	+	0	0	+	0	0	0	+	+	0	+	0	+	+	+	+	0	+	0	+	+	+	+	+	0	+	+	0	1+	
2	+	+	0	0	+	0	0	+	0	+	0	+	0	+	+	+	+	0	0	0	+	+	0	0	+	0	+	0	0	1+	
3	+	+	0	+	0	0	0	0	+	+	0	+	0	+	0	0	0	+	+	+	+	0	+	0	+	0	+	+	0	1+	
4	+	0	+	0	+	+	0	0	0	+	0	+	0	+	+	0	+	+	0	0	+	+	+	+	0	0	+	0	0	1+	
5	0	0	+	0	+	+	0	0	+	+	0	+	0	+	+	0	0	+	+	+	+	0	+	0	+	0	+	+	0	0	+
6	0	0	+	0	+	+	0	0	0	+	0	+	0	+	+	+	+	+	0	+	+	0	+	0	+	0	+	0	0	0	+
7	0	0	+	0	+	+	0	0	0	+	0	+	0	+	0	+	+	+	+	0	+	0	+	0	+	+	+	+	0	0	+
8	0	0	+	0	+	+	0	0	0	+	0	+	0	+	+	0	0	+	+	0	0	+	0	+	0	0	+	0	0	0	+
9	0	0	+	0	+	+	0	0	0	+	0	+	0	+	+	+	0	+	+	0	+	+	+	+	+	0	+	+	0	0	+
10	0	0	+	0	+	+	0	0	0	+	0	+	0	+	0	0	+	+	0	0	0	0	+	0	+	0	+	0	0	0	+
Patient's cells																															

Table 5-18B.

Cell	IS	AHG	Check Cell
Rh-negative fetal red cells	0	3+	
Rh-positive fetal red cells	0	3+	

Which of the following statements about this antibody and the antigen to which it is directed is *true*?

A. The antigen is named after its discoverers, Levine and Stetson.
B. The antibody was originally produced by immunizing guinea pigs with red cells from rhesus monkeys.
C. The antigen is destroyed by enzyme treatment.
D. The antibody is capable of fixing complement and causing intravascular hemolysis.
E. The antigen is poorly expressed on fetal red cells.

Question 19: The most common red cell typing in Blacks is:

A. Lu(a–b–).
B. Jk(a–b–).
C. Fy(a–b–).
D. O_h.
E. Js(a–b–).

Question 20: Which blood group protein acts as a receptor for the malaria parasite *Plasmodium vivax*?

A. Duffy.
B. MN.
C. Kidd.
D. Kell.
E. Lutheran.

Question 21: The S and s blood group antigens are carried on which molecule?

A. Glycophorin A.
B. Glycophorin B.
C. Glycophorin C.
D. Glycophorin D.
E. Glycophorin E.

Question 22: The human blood group glycophorin molecules are heavily glycosylated and carry the vast majority of which membrane-associated carbohydrate?

A. N-acetylglucosamine.
B. N-acetylgalactosamine.
C. Fucose.
D. Galactose.
E. Sialic acid.

Question 23: A patient with an anti-U requires transfusion. Blood from a donor of which ethnic background is most likely to lack the U blood group antigen?

A. African.
B. Asian.
C. European.
D. Native American.
E. All donors are equally likely to lack the U antigen.

Question 24: A 30-year-old pregnant woman delivers a full-term female neonate who is noted to be jaundiced at birth. Laboratory evaluation reveals that the baby has an elevated bilirubin level, is anemic, and has an elevated reticulocyte count. Her direct antiglobulin test (DAT) is strongly reactive, but both she and her mother have negative antibody screens. The antibody that is most likely responsible for these findings is:

A. Anti-C^w.
B. Anti-Lu^a.
C. Anti-Le^a.
D. Anti-M.
E. Anti-S.

Question 25: The baby described in Question 24 requires an exchange transfusion for severe hyperbilirubinemia. Blood from which of the following donors would be most appropriate for transfusion?

A. The baby's mother.
B. The baby's father.
C. The baby's 18-year-old brother.
D. Any random blood donor.
E. Blood from a rare donor inventory.

ANSWERS

Question 1: A

Explanation:

- The water transporter Aquaporin-1 is located on the erythrocyte membrane protein CHIP-1 and carries the Colton blood group antigens, Co^a and Co^b.
- The Kidd blood group antigens, Jk^a and Jk^b, are carried by the human erythroid urea transport protein HUT11.
- Red cells with the rare null phenotype in the Kidd system, Jk(a–b–), resist lysis in 2M urea.
- The Cartwright antigens, Yt^a and Yt^b, are located on AChE. Acetylcholinesterase is important in neural transmission by degrading acetylcholine within synapses. Its function on erythrocytes is unknown. AChE is linked to the red cell membrane through a glycosylphosphatidylinositol (GPI) linkage.
- The Cromer antigens are located on DAF/CD55 and are linked to the plasma membrane of erythrocytes through a GPI linkage.
- Erythrocytes of patients with paroxysmal nocturnal hemoglobinuria (PNH) exhibit a deficiency of GPI-linked proteins. This results in a lack of Cromer, Cartwright, and Dombrock blood group antigens as well as the John Milton Hagen (JMH) antigen.
- Cromer-negative individuals have a mildly increased sensitivity to complement-mediated lysis. This led to the discovery of another GPI-linked molecule, CD59 or membrane inhibitor of reactive lysis, which also plays a key role in inactivating complement.
- The Duffy (Fy) protein is the receptor for the chemokines interleukin-8 (IL-8), RANTES (regulated on activation, normal T expressed and secreted), MGSA (melanoma growth secreting activity), and MCP-1 (monocyte chemoattractant protein-1). This receptor may allow the red cells to act as scavengers of excess chemokines in the circulation.
- The biologic function or significance of selected blood-group-carrying surface proteins are shown in Table 5-1.

Table 5-1.

Function or Significance	Specific Function	Blood Group Antigens
Receptor	Receptor for chemokines	Duffy
	Complement component C3b/C4b receptor type I (CR1)	Knops
	Lymphocyte homing receptor/ hyaluronan receptor	Indian
Transport protein	Human erythroid urea transporter proteins	Kidd
	Human erythroid water transporter proteins	Colton
	Band 3 protein–Anion exchange	Diego and Wright
Complement pathway	Complement component 4 (C4)	Chido/Rodgers
	Decay accelerating factor (DAF)/CD55	Cromer
Adhesion molecule	CD44 adhesion molecule	Indian
Structural integrity	Glycophorin C and D	Gerbich
	Band 3 protein	Diego
Microbial receptor	Plasmodium sp.	Duffy, Cad, MNSs
	Parvovirus B19	P
	Polio virus	Indian
	E. coli, coxsackie virus, and echovirus	Cromer
	Haemophilus influenzae	Anton (AnWj)

Question 2: E

Explanation:

See Explanation for Question 3.

Question 3: C

Explanation for Questions 2 and 3:

The frequency of the Rh system antigens (D, C, E, c, and e) in Blacks and Whites is shown in Table 5-3.

Table 5-3.

Frequency (%)		
Blacks	**Whites**	**Fisher-Race Terminology**
92	86	D
33	70	C
21	30	E
97	80	c
99	98	e

Question 4: A

Explanation:

- The observed frequency of Rh haplotypes in Whites is R^1 (42%) $\gg$ r (37%) $\gg R^2$ (14%) $\gg R^0$ (4%).
- The observed frequency of Rh haplotypes in Blacks is R^0 (44%) $\gg$ r (26%) $\gg R^1$ (17%) $\gg R^2$ (11%).
- The frequency of the R^z, r', r", and r^y haplotypes in Blacks and Whites is very rare.
- The principal Rh gene complexes and the antigens encoded are shown in Table 5-4.

Table 5-4.

Haplotype	Genes Present	Antigens Present	Phenotype
R^1	RHD, RHCe	D, C, e	R_1
R^2	RHD, RHcE	D, c, E	R_2
R^0	RHD, RHce	D, c, e	R_0
R^Z	RHD, RHCE	D, C, E	R_Z
r'	RHCe	C, e	r'
r"	RHcE	c, E	r"
r	RHce	c, e	r
r^y	RHCE	C, E	r^y

Question 5: A

Explanation:

- Alloimmunization is a significant problem among sickle cell patients, with up to 30% of sickle cell patients being alloimmunized depending on the population of patients being studied. This is particularly problematic among the chronically transfused.
- Although incompletely understood, the major cause for the high rate of alloimmunization among sickle cell patients appears to be the fact that sickle cell patients (predominantly of African ethnicity) are more likely to lack certain blood group antigens in comparison to a blood donor population that is predominantly of European ethnicity (eg, see Table 5-3). This means that they are more likely to be exposed to foreign blood group antigens.
- The most common blood group antibodies detected in sickle cell patients are anti-C, anti-E, and anti-K. This results from the fact that 1) these are among the most immunogenic of all blood group antigens and 2) the corresponding antigens (ie, C, E, and K) are more frequently found in blood donors of European ethnicity.

- Although neither universally accepted nor applied, a means to avoid alloimmunization among sickle cell patients is to establish a baseline blood group antigen phenotype and then selectively match for the Rh antigens and K antigen. From the standpoint of the Rh antigens, this then means that blood lacking the C and E antigens (ie, c- and e-positive) would be provided.
- Among donors of European ethnicity, the r phenotype (cde) is most likely to lack the C and E antigens. Among donors of African ethnicity, the R^0 phenotype (cDe) is most likely to lack the C and E antigens.
- See Table 5-5 for the frequencies of the Rh phenotypes found in donor groups of various ethnicities in the United States.

Table 5-5.

Phenotype	Frequency %			
	African-American	Asian-American	European-American	Native American
R^1	17	70	42	44
R^2	11	03	14	34
R^0	44	03	04	02
R^Z	00	01	00	06
r'	02	02	02	02
r"	00	00	01	06
r	26	03	37	11
r^y	0	0	0	0

Question 6: B

Explanation:

See Question 8.

Question 7: E

Explanation:

See Question 8.

Question 8: B

Explanation for Questions 5 through 8:

- A weak D phenotype can be caused by the following:
  - Inheritance of a D gene that codes for decreased expression (referred to as inherited weak D).
  - Inheritance of a C gene on the chromosome opposite the D gene (referred to as weak D caused by gene interaction or C trans). Examples include CDe/Ce (R^1/r') and cDE/Ce (R^2/r').
- These weak D phenotypes are caused by a decreased number of D antigens per red cell (200 to 10,000) compared with the normal Rh phenotype (10,000 to 33,000). Thus, there is a *quantitative* difference in the D antigen. These individuals have the D antigen on their red cells; therefore, they should be considered Rh positive when donating and receiving blood. These individuals do not form anti-D.
- A partial D phenotype occurs when an individual inherits a D gene that does not encode all of the epitopes present on the D antigen. Thus, there is qualitative difference in the D antigen.
  - Ideally, these individuals would be considered Rh negative when receiving transfusions because they can form antibodies to the epitopes of the D antigen that they lack. However, it is not possible, in routine Rh typing, to distinguish weakened D antigen expression due to either quantitative or qualitative differences in the D antigen.
  - These individuals should be considered Rh positive when donating blood because Rh-negative individuals may recognize the epitopes of the D antigen present on transfused red cells and form antibodies.
- Inherited weak D phenotypes and weak D phenotypes caused by gene interactions are more common than partial D phenotypes. Together, these three phenotypes occur in 1% of all Rh-positive individuals.

- The partial D phenotypes may type like an individual who has one of the weak D phenotypes; that is, they type as Rh negative with anti-D reagents in direct agglutination testing and positive in the weak D test.
- Because it is impossible to distinguish the weak D phenotypes from the partial D phenotypes without special reagents, it is safest to treat individuals with a positive weak D as Rh negative for the purpose of transfusion. However, when using sensitive gel and solid-phase-based testing methods, the majority of these individuals may go undetected and are therefore treated as Rh positive.
- The weak D test is performed as follows:
  - Following a negative typing with anti-D, the red cells are incubated for 30 minutes at 37 C. A weak D negative control is also incubated and consists of the patient's red cells to which the diluent of the anti-D reagent has been added but to which anti-D has *not* been added.
  - After incubation, the cells are washed.
  - Antihuman globulin (AHG) is added, and the cells are centrifuged and examined for agglutination.
- The presence of agglutination in the weak D test with no agglutination in the control indicates that the D antigen is present, anti-D has bound, and the AHG has produced agglutination.
- Agglutination in the negative control indicates that IgG other than anti-D is present on the patient's red cells (eg, a warm autoantibody) and the results of the weak D test cannot be interpreted (ie, they may be positive because anti-D has bound or some other IgG antibody is present).
- Anti-D can be seen in Rh-positive individuals who have autoantibodies that mimic anti-D. Anti-D can also be seen in the passenger lymphocyte syndrome. If Rh-positive individuals receive an organ from an Rh-negative individual, donor lymphocytes in the transplanted organ may become sensitized with resultant production of anti-D.

Question 9: C

Explanation:

- CGD is a primary immunodeficiency disorder in which phagocytes can ingest bacteria but are unable to kill them because of a defective oxidative burst. This results from abnormalities in nicotinamide adenine dinucleotide phosphate oxidase. This abnormality leads to the formation of granulomas and recurrent infections. CGD is often associated with a depression of Kell blood group system antigens, a component of the McLeod phenotype.
- The McLeod phenotype is characterized by the following:
  - Acanthocytes.
  - Compensated hemolytic anemia with increased reticulocytes, increased lactate dehydrogenase, decreased haptoglobin, and hypersplenism.
  - Decreased red cell permeability to water.
  - Increased phosphorylation of spectrin.
  - Increased red cell carbonic anhydrase.
  - Decreased expression of Kell system antigens.
  - Increased creatine kinase MM isoenzymes.
  - Progressive neurologic changes including areflexia, choreiform movements, dysarthria, wasting of muscles, and cardiomyopathy.
- Kell antigens are produced at the KEL locus on chromosome 7 at 7q33-7q35. The expression of Kell antigens also depends on the presence of the Kx protein encoded by the XK gene on chromosome X at Xp21 (locus XK).
- Molecular biologic investigations have demonstrated a 50-kb deletion in a critical region of the XK gene in individuals with the McLeod phenotype.
- The mutated gene either does not transcribe the Kx protein or it encodes a defective protein, which does not get incorporated into the erythrocyte membrane. This results in a decreased expression of Kell system antigens.
- The genes for Duchenne muscular dystrophy, retinitis pigmentosa, and CGD are closely associated with the XK locus.
- The K_0 (Kell null) phenotype is associated with a complete lack of Kell system antigens, but the Kx protein has markedly increased

expression on the red cell membrane. These rare individuals do not have the features associated with the McLeod phenotype.

Question 10: E

Explanation:

- Patients with chronic granulomatous disease and the McLeod phenotype can produce a combination of anti-Kx and anti-Km (formerly referred to as anti-KL). Km is a basic structural antigen of the Kell system. Individuals with anti-Kx and anti-Km are compatible only with red cells from other patients with the McLeod phenotype. Individuals with the McLeod phenotype without CGD may form anti-Km. In these individuals, red cells from those with either the K_0 or the McLeod phenotype are compatible.
- Red cells of the rare Jk(a–b–) phenotype have impaired urea transport and resist lysis in 2M urea.
- Also see the explanation for Question 9.

Question 11: C

Explanation:

See Question 12.

Question 12: A

Explanation for Questions 11 and 12:

- Characteristics of antibodies that exhibit high titer and low avidity behavior include the following:
  - Most react with high-frequency antigens.
  - They demonstrate weak reactivity that persists despite serial dilution of the serum. This reactivity is caused by a very high titer (does not dilute) in the presence of a low avidity (weak strength

of reaction). The weak reactivity has been found to result from low numbers of antigens on the red cell surface rather than an intrinsically low avidity of the antibody.
  - The pattern of reactivity is not always reproducible.
  - These are IgG antibodies that react at the AHG phase of testing.
- These antibodies may cause problems in antibody identification and compatibility testing. Finding crossmatch-compatible units may be difficult or impossible because many of the antigens are high frequency. For this reason, crossmatch-incompatible units may need to be transfused.
- These antibodies are not clinically significant. They do not cause hemolytic transfusion reactions or hemolytic disease of the fetus and newborn.
- Antigens with corresponding antibodies exhibiting high titer and low avidity behavior are listed in Table 5-12.
- Lu^b is a high-frequency member of the Lutheran blood group system and the antithetical partner of Lu^a. Although anti-Lu^b is a rare antibody, it is considered to be clinically significant.
- Anti-M and anti-S are directed against antigens carried by glycophorin A and glycophorin B, respectively. They do not exhibit high titer and low avidity behavior.
- Anti-Wr^b is a very rare alloantibody. The frequency of the Wr^b antigen is 99.99%. It does not have the weak reactivity that persists despite serial dilution of the serum.
- See the explanation for Question 13 for information on the Chido/Rodgers blood group system and anti-Ch antibodies.

Table 5-12.

Antigens	Formal Names
Ch	Chido
Rg	Rodgers
Csa	Cost Sterling
Yka	York
Kna	Knops
McCa	McCoy
JMH	John Milton Hagen
MPD	Minnie Pearl Davis

Question 13: D

Explanation:

- The relative frequency of blood group antigens can help to determine the likelihood that the identified immune response represents the corresponding antibody.
- It is important to note that the frequency of antigens on an antibody identification panel may not represent the frequency of antigens in the population. The frequency is determined by the following:
  - The cells available to the manufacturer.
  - The requirement that a sufficient number of antigen-positive and -negative cells be present to rule in or rule out clinically significant antibodies.
- The reactivity of selected antibodies with panel cells is shown in Table 5-13.
- Anti-Ch is the most likely specificity responsible for the results described in this Question.
- The Chido/Rodgers (Ch/Rg) blood group system is comprised of 9 antigens found on the C4A and C4B complement components:
  - Ch/Rg antigens are generally high frequency and the antibodies exhibit high titer and low avidity behavior.

Table 5-13.

Antibody	Antigen % Whites	Antigen % Blacks	Expected Reactivity with Group O Panel Cells (of 16)	AHG Reactivity	Reactivity with Enzyme-Treated Cells
Anti-Ch	98	98	16/16 (100%)	w+	0 or ↓
Anti-k	99.8	>99.9	16/16 (100%)	1 to 4+	Equivalent
Anti-e	98	98	15/16 (95%)	1 to 4+	↑
Anti-Js[a]	0.01	20	0/16 to 1/16 (0 to 5%)	1 to 4+	Equivalent
Anti-Kp[a]	2	2	0/16 to 1/16 (0 to 5%)	1 to 4+	Equivalent

- ○ Chido, Rodgers, and Lewis antigens are adsorbed onto the red cell membrane from surrounding plasma.
- ○ Antibodies to these antigens can be neutralized by plasma.
- Two tests can confirm the specificity of anti-Ch and anti-Rg:
  - ○ Plasma or serum neutralization technique (inhibits antibody reactivity).
  - ○ Testing against C4d-coated red cells (enhances antibody reactivity).
- The lack of C4B (Ch−) is associated with an increased susceptibility to bacterial meningitis in children. The lack of C4A (Rg−) is associated with a much greater disposition for systemic lupus erythematosus.
- Anti-Js^a and anti-Kp^a are directed against low-frequency members of the Kell blood group system. These antibodies do not exhibit the serologic behavior described in the Question.
- Anti-k and anti-e are directed against high-frequency members of the Kell and Rh blood group systems. However, their reactivity is not decreased with the use of ficin-treated red cells and may even be enhanced.

Question 14: B

Explanation:

- The titer results (Table 5-14B) are consistent with an antibody exhibiting high titer and low avidity behavior. In contrast, Table 5-14C compares this type of antibody with that of antibodies (anti-Fy^b and anti-e) that do not exhibit this type of behavior.
- The JMH antigen is a high-incidence antigen. The antigen can be transiently depressed after disease and can be lost after age 50. Antibodies to JMH can develop in these settings. Older individuals who have anti-JMH in their serum will frequently have positive autocontrols and direct antiglobulin tests (DAT) as in the patient described.
- Antibodies that do not exhibit high titer and low avidity behavior, such as anti-e and anti-Fy^b, should demonstrate a weakening of the antibody with serial dilutions.

Table 5-14C.

Titer	1	2	4	8	16	32	64	128	256	512	1024
HTLA	1+	1+	1+	1+	1+	1+	1+	1+	1+	1+	w+
Anti-Fy^b, Anti-e	4+	3+	2+	1+	w+	0	0	0	0	0	0

- While anti-Kn^a frequently behaves as an antibody with high titer and low avidity, it is not destroyed by enzymes and does not cause a positive DAT.
- Autoantibodies, warm- and cold-reacting, are enhanced with enzyme treatment, not destroyed. The exception is anti-Pr. The Pr antigen is destroyed by enzyme treatment. Anti-Pr is usually a cold-reacting antibody that would not fit with the reactivity seen in this patient.

Question 15: A

Explanation:

- The titer is the reciprocal of the highest serum dilution causing visible (macroscopic) agglutination. In this case, the highest serum dilution is 1:8. The reciprocal of this is 8.
- Titration is a semiquantitative technique to measure the amount of antibody in the serum or the strength of an antigen on the red cell.

Question 16: D

Explanation:

- Anti-Sd^a has not been associated with HDFN and is not present on fetal red cells.
- 91% of the population is positive for the Sd^a antigen.
- The Sd^a antigen is present on the Tamm-Horsfall glycoprotein in urine and is excreted by renal tubular epithelial cells.
- The urine from Sd^a-positive individuals can neutralize anti-Sd^a. All guinea pigs are Sd^a positive, so their urine can be used to neutralize these antibodies as well. As guinea pigs are not always available, pooled urine from 10 individuals is frequently used to ensure that at least one Sd^a-positive urine sample is in the pool.
- A characteristic finding of anti-Sd^a is the microscopic presence of orange refractile agglutinates in a field of unagglutinated red cells.
- Sd^a-antigen expression may decrease during pregnancy. The Sd(a−) phenotype is observed in 30% to 75% of all pregnancies.

- The reduced expression of LW and Lewis antigens may also be seen in pregnancy.

Question 17: E

Explanation:

- The Lu(a–b–) phenotype is very rare in all populations. It may result from the following:
  - An autosomal amorphic recessive gene (Lu).
  - An autosomal dominant suppressor gene (InLu).
  - An X-linked recessive suppressor gene (XS2).
- With the autosomal dominant suppressor, other red cell antigens have reduced expression, including P1, AnWj, Indian, Knops, and MER2.
- Two major antigens belong to the Lutheran blood group system: Lu^a (8% of Whites and 5% of Blacks) and Lu^b (>99% of all populations).
- Lutheran antigens are poorly developed at birth, and the corresponding antibodies generally do not cause HDFN. There are no reports of intravascular hemolysis associated with Lutheran antibodies. However, anti-Lu^b (but not anti-Lu^a) is associated with decreased red cell survival and extravascular hemolysis.
- Antibodies to Lu^a and Lu^b cause a mixed-field appearance on antibody screening.
- The Lu(a–b–) phenotype is associated with red cell morphologic abnormalities, as noted in Table 5-17.
- The Lutheran gene is linked to the C3 and secretor genes on chromosome 19.

Table 5-17.

Phenotype	Antigens Missing	Morphology
Rh_{null}	Lacks Rh, Duffy, and LW antigens	Stomatocytes
McLeod	Lacks Kx and Kell system antigens	Acanthocytes
Lu(a–b–)	Lacks Lu^a, Lu^b, and Lu^3 (Depending upon the genetic cause, other antigens may also be absent)	Poikilocytosis

- Lutheran antigens are located on a single-pass membrane-spanning protein that may function as an adhesion molecule and may mediate intracellular signaling.

Question 18: B

Explanation:

- The antibody is anti-LW^a.
- The LW blood group system is named after Landsteiner and Weiner, the discoverers of the system. Levine and Stetson first described anti-D.
- Anti-LW^a was produced by inoculating guinea pigs with rhesus monkey red cells. Originally, these antibodies were thought to be the same as the anti-D described by Stetson and Levine because both antibodies reacted with 85% of Whites and appeared to recognize the same antigen. As a result, the system that contains the D antigen was mistakenly called the Rh (Rhesus) system. It was subsequently discovered that LW antigens are not the same as the D antigen. LW antigens are strongly expressed on all Rh-positive red cells, but they are more weakly expressed on Rh-negative red cells, which explains the apparent 85% frequency of the LW^a antigen. The actual frequency of LW^a in Whites is almost 100%.
- LW antigens are not destroyed by enzymes, but they are destroyed by dithiothreitol treatment.
- Antibodies to LW system antigens do not fix complement and do not cause intravascular hemolysis. They are IgG antibodies that do not cause clinically significant hemolytic transfusion reactions or HDFN.
- LW system antigens are strongly expressed on fetal red cells, including Rh-negative red cells. These reagents can be used to distinguish anti-LW from anti-D, as shown in Table 5-18C.
- The LW antigen system contains three antigens: LW^a (100% of all populations), LW^b (<1% of Europeans, except for Estonians–8%, Finns–6%, and Poles–4%), and LW^{ab} (100% of all populations).
- The LW gene encodes a glycoprotein of 241 amino acids that functions as an intercellular adhesion molecule. The LW glycoprotein binds to the leukocyte integrins CD11 and CD18.
- Autoantibodies to LW antigens have been reported with some malignancies.

Table 5-18C.

Antibody	Cell	IS	AHG	Check Cell
Anti-D	Rh+ adult	0	4+	
	Rh– adult	0	0	+
	Rh+ cord	0	4+	
	Rh– cord	0	0	+
Anti-LW	Rh+ adult	0	4+	
	Rh– adult	0	1+	
	Rh+ cord	0	4+	
	Rh– cord	0	4+	

Question 19: C

Explanation:

- Duffy system phenotypes and antigen frequencies are listed in Table 5-19.
- Lu(a–b–), Jk(a–b–), Js(a–b–), and O_h (Bombay) phenotypes are very rare in all populations.
- Fy(a–b–) is not a true null phenotype. Duffy mRNA is not detected in the marrow of Fy(a–b–) individuals; however, it is detected in other tissues including the lung, spleen, and colon.

Table 5-19.

Reaction with			Phenotype Frequency (%)	
Anti-Fy^a	Anti-Fy^b	Phenotype	Blacks	Whites
+	0	Fy(a+b–)	9	17
0	+	Fy(a–b+)	22	34
+	+	Fy(a+b+)	1	49
0	0	Fy(a–b–)	68	Very rare

- The Fy(a−b−) phenotype in Blacks is caused by a single amino acid substitution at position −46 in the Duffy (Fy^b) gene. This mutation impairs the promoter activity in erythroid cells by disrupting the binding site for the GATA1 erythroid transcription factor.
- Blacks with the Fy(a−b−) phenotype are homozygous for an apparently normal Fy^b allele (found in other tissues). These individuals may make anti-Fy^a but rarely produce anti-Fy^b.

Question 20: A

Explanation:

- The Duffy protein plays an important role in malaria transmission. The invasion site depends on the presence of the Fy^6 epitope, which is the receptor site for the malaria parasite *Plasmodium vivax*.
- Fy^6 is present on all red cells with an Fy(a+) or Fy(b+) phenotype. It is absent on red cells with the Fy(a−b−) phenotype. This favors the natural selection of individuals with the Fy(a−b−) phenotype in areas where *P. vivax* would be endemic by providing resistance to malaria. In West Africa, individuals with the Fy(a−b−) phenotype are found in greater frequency than in areas where P. vivax is absent.
- The protective effect of the Fy(a−b−) phenotype does not extend to the malaria parasite *P. falciparum*, which infects cells of all Duffy phenotypes.
- As many as 30% of Blacks in Africa are heterozygous for hemoglobin S (Hb S) in areas where malaria is endemic. This frequency is likely related to the protection against *P. falciparum* that Hb S affords. About 8% of Blacks in Africa are heterozygous for Hb S in areas where malaria is not endemic. *P. falciparum* malaria is milder and seldom lethal in Hb AS individuals in comparison to Hb AA individuals.
- Certain inherited abnormalities of red cells offer protection against malaria, as shown in Table 5-20.

Table 5-20.

Geographic Location	Increased Incidence of	Red Cell Abnormalities	Protection Against
Melanesia	Stomatocytic elliptocytes and α-thalassemia minor	Membrane; hemoglobin synthesis	*P. falciparum*
West Africa	Fy(a–b–)	Absent Duffy protein	*P. vivax*
Central Africa	Hb AS	Hemoglobinopathy	*P. falciparum*
South Asia	Hb ES	Hemoglobinopathy	*P. falciparum*
Sardinia	G6PD deficiency and β-thalassemia	Glycolytic pathway; hemoglobin synthesis	*P. falciparum*
Africa, Southeast Asia	S–s–U– phenotype and glycophorin A/B variants (eg, He and St[a] antigens)	Abnormalities of glycophorin B	*P. falciparum*
Papua New Guinea	Leach phenotype (Gerbich –2, –3, –4)	Absence of glycophorins C/D	*P. falciparum*

Question 21: B

Explanation:

See Question 23.

Question 22: E

Explanation:

See Question 23.

Question 23: A

Explanation for Questions 21 through 23:

- The human glycophorin molecules are single-pass integral membrane proteins that are heavily glycosylated and carry numerous blood group antigens.
- There are four glycophorin molecules—glycophorins A, B, C, and D. The glycophorin E gene (*GYPE*) is adjacent to *GYPB* but does not appear to encode a membrane glycoprotein.
- Glycophorins A and B are highly homologous and carry the M/N and S/s antigens, respectively. The first 26 amino acids of glycophorins A and B are identical, with glycophorin B carrying a domain with the same structure as the N blood group antigen. This antigen is referred to as "N" [ie, N-like or 'N' (N in quotes)].
- Glycophorins C and D, like A and B, are homologous and carry antigens of the Gerbich blood group system.
- The glycophorin molecules carry the vast majority (>90%) of the red cell-associated sialic acid. This is the primary reason why the red cell has a heavy negative charge, a feature that may be responsible for the repulsive force that keeps adjacent red cells apart.
- The physiologic function of glycophorin A and glycophorin B is unknown but, like the Duffy blood group antigens, they may play a role in malaria invasion. Glycophorins A and B are putative red cell receptors for *P. falciparum* malaria.
- Glycophorin C and glycophorin D appear to be involved in red cell membrane integrity through an interaction with cytoskeletal protein 4.1. Glycophorins C and D are markedly reduced in protein 4.1-deficient red cells, which is a cause of hereditary elliptocytosis.
- The immune response to the M and N antigens is predominantly IgM and naturally occurring. There are only scattered case reports of hemolysis caused by antibodies directed against these antigens. In contrast, the immune response to S/s and the Gerbich antigens is IgG and generally requires red cell exposure. These antibodies are considered to be clinically significant with respect to hemolysis.
- Glycophorin B carries the U blood group antigen, a very high-frequency antigen in all populations studied. However, donors of African ancestry are most likely to lack U (1%). Therefore, they should be sought out if a patient with anti-U requires transfusion.

Question 24: A

Explanation:

- The neonate described in this case vignette has findings consistent with HDFN. Hyperbilirubinemia, anemia, and a reticulocytosis are indicative of hemolysis, whereas the reactive DAT indicates that this is an immune-mediated process.
- HDFN results from a maternal IgG blood group antibody that crosses the placenta and binds to fetal/neonatal red cells expressing the cognate antigen.
- Even with Rh Immune Globulin prophylaxis, anti-D remains the most common cause of HDFN.
- In this case, anti-C^w is the most likely responsible antibody because it is an IgG immune response that has been implicated in cases of HDFN. It is important, however, that although it can cause hemolysis, this antibody would not commonly be detected in the context of an antibody screen because the C^w antigen is a low-frequency member of the Rh blood group system present on only 2% of donor red cells.
- The anti-S immune response is IgG, but since the S antigen is of relatively high frequency (55% of Whites and 30% of Blacks), anti-S should be detected in the context of an antibody screen.
- Le^a antibodies are predominantly IgM, cold-reacting antibodies that have not been implicated in cases of HDFN. They may or may not be detected in the antibody screen, depending on the antibody identification system that is used.
- Although anti-Lu^a may be an IgG antibody and it is of relatively low frequency (8% of Whites and 5% of Blacks), anti-Lu^a has been implicated in only mild cases of HDFN, and this is very rare.
- Anti-M is typically a complex mixture of IgG and IgM isotypes, but the IgM component predominates in most individuals, and the antibody is cold-reactive. Although these antibodies may be detected in the context of the antibody screen, it is extremely rare for them to be clinically significant.

Question 25: D

Explanation:

- The baby in this case has severe HDFN caused by anti-C^w. As such, the most appropriate unit for transfusion would be from an ABO- and Rh-compatible donor who is C^w-negative.
- The baby's father would not be an acceptable candidate for blood donation as he is almost certainly C^w-positive. This is based on the fact that HDFN results from an immune response in the mother directed against an antigen on fetal/neonatal red cells that is paternally derived.
- The baby's brother would not be the most suitable blood donor because there is a high likelihood (at least 50%) that he too will be C^w-positive.
- Obtaining blood from a rare donor inventory would not be appropriate because C^w-negative units are easily obtained from standard blood donors. Units from rare donor inventories should be reserved for patients who have antibodies for which it will be exceedingly difficult to identify antigen-negative units of blood.
- Based on the pathogenesis of HDFN, it is axiomatic that the mother of this neonate will be C^w-negative. She is not, however, the most appropriate blood donor because she is in the immediate postpartum period, and the identification of C^w-negative units from the standard donor population will not be difficult.
- C^w-negative blood is readily and most appropriately obtained from random blood donors because approximately 98% of all such donors will be C^w-negative. Although expensive, reagent anti-C^w is available to ensure that the donor unit lacks the C^w antigen. Alternatively, plasma samples from either mother or baby could be used for cross-matching purposes because they will both contain the C^w antibody.

REFERENCES

1. Westhoff CM. The Rh system. In: Roback JD, Combs MR, Grossman BJ, Hillyer CD, eds. Technical manual. 16th ed. Bethesda, MD: AABB, 2008:387-409.
2. Daniels G. Other blood groups. In: Roback JD, Combs MR, Grossman BJ, Hillyer CD, eds. Technical manual. 16th ed. Bethesda, MD: AABB, 2008:411-36.
3. Klein HG, Anstee DJ. The Rh blood group system (and LW). In: Klein HG, Anstee DJ. Blood transfusion in clinical medicine. 11th ed. Malden, MA: Blackwell Publishing, 2005:163-208.
4. Klein HG, Anstee DJ. Other red cell antigens. In: Klein HG, Anstee DJ. Blood transfusion in clinical medicine. 11th ed. Malden, MA: Blackwell Publishing, 2005:209-52.
5. Reid ME, Lomas-Francis C. The blood group antigens factsbook. 2nd ed. San Diego, CA: Academic Press, 2004.
6. Reid ME, Westhoff CM. Human blood group antigens and antibodies. In: Hoffman R, Benz E, Shattil S, et al, eds. Hematology: basic principles and practices. 5th ed. Philadelphia: Churchill-Livingstone, 2008:2163-78.

6

Pretransfusion Testing and Antibody Identification

QUESTIONS

Question 1: Which of the following is *not* required on a physician's order for blood components?

A. Patient's first name.
B. Patient's last name.
C. Unique patient identification number.
D. Patient's birth date.
E. Component(s) requested.

Question 2: Which of the following would *not* be adequate for patient identification when drawing samples for pretransfusion testing?

A. Hospital identification band.
B. Identification by a third party if the patient is unresponsive.
C. The patient's stating and spelling his or her name.
D. Blood bank or emergency room identification band.
E. Hospital chart at the foot of the patient's bed.

Question 3: Which of the following sample/patient pairs is acceptable to crossmatch a unit of Red Blood Cells (RBCs)?

A. Sample drawn 5 days before anticipated transfusion; patient delivered an infant 1 month ago.
B. Sample drawn 2 days before anticipated transfusion; patient received RBCs 5 days ago.
C. Sample drawn 4 days before anticipated transfusion; transfusion history is unknown.
D. Sample drawn 7 days before anticipated transfusion; pregnancy history is unknown.
E. Sample drawn 4 days before anticipated transfusion; patient transfused 2 months ago.

Question 4: Which of the following samples is acceptable for pretransfusion testing?

A. Sample labeled at the patient's bedside. Label contains the patient's full name and hospital number.
B. Sample labeled at the nursing station. Label contains the date, the patient's full name, the hospital number, and the initials of the phlebotomist.
C. Sample labeled at the patient's bedside. Label contains the date, the patient's full name, and the phlebotomist's initials.
D. Sample labeled in the hallway outside of the patient's room. Label contains the date, the patient's full name, the hospital number, and the initials of the phlebotomist.
E. Sample labeled at the patient's bedside. Label contains the date, the patient's full name, and the hospital number.

Question 5: According to AABB *Standards for Blood Banks and Transfusion Services (Standards)*, which of the following tests must be performed on every unit of donated blood intended for allogeneic use?

A. Antibodies to hepatitis A virus (HAV).

B. Antibodies to cytomegalovirus (CMV).
C. Parvovirus RNA.
D. Hepatitis C virus (HCV) RNA.
E. Antibodies to hepatitis B surface antigen (HBs).

Question 6: How many days must a recipient's blood specimen be retained following transfusion?

A. 3 days.
B. 7 days.
C. 14 days.
D. 21 days.
E. 35 days.

Question 7: A type-and-crossmatch order is indicated with which of the following surgical procedures?

A. Cholecystectomy.
B. Excision of a facial seborrheic keratosis.
C. Inguinal hernia repair.
D. Splenectomy.
E. Routine Caesarian section.

Question 8: In which of the following cases is weak-D testing required?

A. Pregnant woman types as Rh negative.
B. Blood donor types as Rh negative.
C. Pregnant woman types as Rh positive.
D. Male surgery patient types as Rh negative.
E. Female surgery patient types as Rh positive.

Question 9: Which of the following antibodies is least likely to be a naturally occurring antibody?

A. Anti-D.
B. Anti-M.
C. Anti-I.
D. Anti-Le^b.
E. Anti-N.

Question 10: Which of the following antibodies is most likely to be a naturally occurring antibody?

A. Anti-K.
B. Anti-M.
C. Anti-e.
D. Anti-Jk^a.
E. Anti-Fy^a.

Question 11: The reactivity of which of the following antibodies is usually enhanced by the enzyme treatment of red cells?

A. Anti-M.
B. Anti-Fy^b.
C. Anti-S.
D. Anti-D.
E. Anti-JMH.

Question 12: Which of the following antigens is resistant to denaturation when red cells undergo enzyme treatment?

A. Fy^a.
B. M.
C. N.
D. S.
E. Jk^a.

PRETRANSFUSION TESTING AND ANTIBODY IDENTIFICATION 187

Question 13: A 20-year-old male of African ethnicity with a history of sickle cell disease presents with a painful episode. He is treated with intravenous fluids, oxygen, and analgesics. His hemoglobin is 6 g/dL. Three RBC units are ordered. The patient is group O, Rh-positive. His antibody workup is given in Table 6-13. What is the frequency of compatible donors of European ethnicity?

A. 2.2%.
B. 3.4%.
C. 4.0%.
D. 5.7%.
E. 10%.

Question 14: Which of the following can be used to destroy the antigen to which the antibody identified by the panel in Table 6-14 is directed?

A. Papain.
B. Ficin.
C. Bromelin.
D. Dithiothreitol.
E. *Ulex europaeus*.

Table 6-13.

Cell	D	C	E	c	e	f	V	Cw	K	k	Kpa	Kpb	Jsa	Jsb	Fya	Fyb	Jka	Jkb	Lea	Leb	P	M	N	S	s	Lua	Lub	Xga	IS	AHG	Ficin IS	Ficin
1	+	+	0	+	0	0	0	0	+	0	0	+	0	+	+	+	+	0	0	+	+	+	+	0	+	0	+	0	1+	3+	1+	3+
2	+	0	+	0	+	0	0	0	0	+	0	+	0	+	0	+	0	+	+	0	+	0	+	0	+	0	+	+	0	0	0	0
3	+	0	0	+	+	0	0	0	+	+	0	+	0	+	+	0	0	+	+	+	+	+	0	+	+	0	+	+	1+	1+	1+	0
4	0	0	0	+	+	+	0	0	0	+	0	+	0	+	+	0	+	+	+	+	+	0	+	0	+	0	+	0	0	3+	0	3+
5	0	0	0	+	+	+	0	0	+	+	0	+	0	+	0	+	+	0	0	+	+	+	+	+	0	0	+	0	1+	2+	1+	0
6	+	0	0	+	+	0	0	0	+	+	0	+	0	+	+	+	+	0	0	+	+	0	+	0	+	0	+	0	0	3+	0	3+
7	+	+	0	0	+	0	0	0	+	+	0	+	0	+	+	+	+	+	+	+	+	+	0	+	0	0	+	0	1+	3+	1+	0
8	+	0	+	+	+	0	0	0	0	+	0	+	0	+	0	+	+	0	0	0	0	0	+	+	+	+	+	+	0	0	0	0
9	0	0	+	+	0	0	0	0	0	+	0	+	0	+	+	+	0	+	+	0	+	+	+	0	+	0	+	0	0	3+	0	3+
10	0	0	+	+	0	0	0	0	0	+	0	+	0	+	0	+	0	+	+	+	+	+	+	0	+	0	+	0	0	3+	0	0
Patient's cells																																

Table 6-14.

Cell	D	C	c	E	e	f	V	C^w	K	k	Kp^a	Kp^b	Js^a	Js^b	Fy^a	Fy^b	Jk^a	Jk^b	Le^a	Le^b	P_1	M	N	S	s	Lu^a	Lu^b	Xg^a	IS	AHG	cc
I	+	+	0	0	+	0	0	0	+	+	0	+	0	+	+	+	0	+	0	+	+	+	+	+	+	0	+	0	0	4+	0
II	+	0	+	+	0	0	0	0	0	+	0	+	0	+	0	+	+	0	+	0	+	+	+	0	+	0	+	+	0	0	+
1	+	+	0	0	+	0	0	0	+	+	0	+	0	+	+	+	0	+	0	+	+	+	0	+	+	0	+	+	0	4+	0
2	+	0	+	0	+	+	0	0	0	+	0	+	0	+	+	+	+	0	0	0	+	+	0	0	+	0	+	+	0	0	+
3	+	+	+	0	+	0	0	+	0	+	0	+	0	+	0	+	+	0	0	0	+	+	+	0	+	0	+	+	0	4+	0
4	+	0	+	+	0	+	0	0	+	+	0	+	0	+	0	0	0	+	+	+	+	0	+	0	+	0	+	0	0	0	+
5	0	+	+	0	+	+	0	0	0	+	0	+	0	+	+	0	+	0	0	0	+	+	+	0	+	0	+	+	0	4+	0
6	0	0	+	+	+	+	0	0	+	+	0	+	0	+	+	0	0	+	0	+	+	+	+	+	+	0	+	0	0	0	+
7	0	0	+	0	+	+	0	0	0	+	0	+	0	+	0	+	+	+	+	0	+	0	+	0	+	0	+	+	0	0	+
8	0	0	+	+	0	+	0	0	+	+	0	+	0	+	+	0	+	+	+	0	0	+	+	+	+	+	+	0	0	4+	+
9	0	+	+	0	+	+	0	0	0	+	0	+	0	+	+	+	0	+	0	0	0	0	+	+	0	0	+	+	0	0	+
10	0	0	+	0	+	+	0	0	0	+	0	+	0	+	0	0	0	+	0	0	+	0	+	0	+	0	+	0	0	0	+
Patient's cells																															

Question 15: Which of the following statements about enhancement media and potentiators is correct?

A. Polyethylene glycol (PEG) enhances agglutination by decreasing the negative charge (zeta potential) around red cells.
B. Low ionic strength saline (LISS) enhances antibody uptake by reducing the zeta potential and allows increased attraction between positively charged antibodies and negatively charged red cells.
C. Polybrene (Sigma-Aldrich, St Louis, MO) enhances the uptake of antibodies by neutralizing the negative charges of the sialic acid residues on red cells.
D. Albumin enhances antibody uptake by reducing the net negative charge of the red cell.
E. Enzyme treatment enhances antibody uptake by decreasing the net negative charge of the red cell by removing sialic acid residues.

Question 16: Who first described the antihuman globulin (AHG) test?

A. Coombs.
B. Moreschi.
C. Landsteiner.
D. Levine.
E. von Descatello.

Question 17: The specificity of the anticomplement activity in broad-spectrum AHG is:

A. C1.
B. C2.
C. C3d.
D. C4.
E. C5.

PRETRANSFUSION TESTING AND ANTIBODY IDENTIFICATION

Question 18: Polyspecific or broad-spectrum AHG must contain:

A. Anti-IgA.
B. Anti-IgD.
C. Anti-IgE.
D. Anti-IgG.
E. Anti-IgM.

Question 19: Which of the following represents an appropriate use of the direct antiglobulin test (DAT)?

A. Forward-typing a patient to determine the ABO type.
B. Reverse-typing a patient to determine the ABO type.
C. Performing an antibody screen.
D. Performing a crossmatch.
E. Looking for bound immunoglobulin in a patient with drug-induced hemolysis.

Question 20: Which of the following could cause a false-positive DAT?

A. Use of an EDTA specimen for testing.
B. Saline contaminated with colloidal silica.
C. IgA coating of the red cells.
D. IgM coating of the red cells.
E. Incubating the cells after the addition of the antiglobulin reagent.

Question 21: All of the following are examples of indirect antiglobulin tests (IATs) *except*:

A. Weak-D testing.
B. Antibody identification panel.
C. AHG crossmatch.

D. Antibody elution.
E. Antibody titration.

Question 22: Which of the following is associated with a false-negative IAT?

A. Failure to wash the red cells adequately.
B. Overcentrifugation.
C. Saline contaminated with colloidal silica.
D. AHG reagent containing anti-species antibodies.
E. Sensitized red cells.

Question 23: Which of the following statements concerning the repeat testing of RBC units before transfusion is *true*?

A. The ABO typing must be confirmed from an attached segment.
B. The Rh typing of Rh-positive units must be confirmed from an attached segment.
C. Confirmatory testing must be performed before the original ABO and Rh labels are affixed to the unit.
D. Confirmation of the Rh typing of Rh-negative units is not required.
E. Confirmatory testing for weak D is required.

Question 24: Which of the following patients is eligible for a computer crossmatch?

A. Patient has a history of anti-Fy^a. Historic blood type is A, Rh positive. Typing of current sample is A, Rh positive. Anti-Fy^a is not seen.
B. Patient has no previous blood type or antibody screen results. Current antibody screen is negative. Patient types as O, Rh negative.
C. Patient has a history of a negative antibody screen. Historic blood type is AB, Rh positive. Current antibody screen is positive for anti-c. Current blood type is AB, Rh positive.

D. Patient has no previous blood type or antibody screen results. Current antibody screen is negative. Patient types as B, Rh negative. Repeat typing on the same sample is B, Rh negative.
E. Patient has a history of a negative antibody screen. There is no history of a previous ABO or Rh type. Current antibody screen is negative. Patient types as A, Rh positive.

Question 25: Which of the following blood components does not need to be crossmatched with a patient's serum sample?

A. Leukocyte-reduced RBCs.
B. Apheresis platelet product containing 3 mL of red cells.
C. Granulocyte product collected by apheresis.
D. Pooled platelet product containing 1.5 mL of red cells.
E. Granulocyte product collected by centrifugation of a whole blood donation.

Question 26: Which of the following crossmatch techniques would most likely detect the combination of anti-Wr^a in the recipient and the Wr^a antigen on red cells from a donor?

A. Complete crossmatch.
B. Minor crossmatch.
C. Immediate-spin crossmatch.
D. Computer crossmatch.
E. Platelet crossmatch.

Question 27: A patient with an antibody to a high-incidence antigen has an emergency need for blood. The only available antigen-negative compatible units are ones for which testing for transfusion-transmitted diseases has not been completed. Which of the following statements is *true*?

A. The units should not be labeled to indicate the tests that are pending because this might alarm the patient.

B. The pending testing need not be completed if the units are transfused because the harm has already been done if the units are infected.
C. If the units were apheresis units, additional testing would not be necessary if these represented units of the same component from the same donor transfused into the same recipient within 30 days of the original unit that was fully tested.
D. It is not required that the physician requesting the transfusion be notified of reactive test results because the units have already been transfused.
E. A statement signed by the ordering physician is not needed to document emergency release because this will increase legal liability.

Question 28: Which of the following statements concerning the testing of autologous blood is *true*?

A. If the unit is to be shipped outside the collecting facility, anti-hepatitis B core (HBc) testing need not be performed.
B. If the unit is to be used within the collecting facility, anti-human immunodeficiency virus (HIV)-1/2 testing need not be performed.
C. If the unit is to be shipped outside the collecting facility, anti-HIV-1/2 testing need not be performed.
D. If the unit is to be shipped outside the collecting facility, anti-hepatitis B surface antigen (HBsAg) testing must be performed.
E. If the unit is to be used within the collecting facility, anti-HBs testing must be performed.

Question 29: A 50-year-old man presents for surgical resection of a colonic adenocarcinoma. The patient's history is notable for the transfusion of 6 RBC units approximately 20 years ago following a motor vehicle accident. Preoperative testing reveals a positive antibody screen. The antibody identification panel is provided in Table 6-29. The most likely explanation for these findings is:

A. An alloantibody to e.
B. An alloantibody to k.

Table 6-29.

Cell	D	C	c	E	e	f	V	C^w	K	k	Kp^a	Kp^b	Js^a	Js^b	Fy^a	Fy^b	Jk^a	Jk^b	Le^a	Le^b	P₁	M	N	S	s	Lu^a	Lu^b	Xg^a	IS	AHG	CC
I	+	+	0	0	+	0	0	0	+	+	0	+	0	+	+	+	0	+	0	+	+	+	+	+	+	0	+	0	0	3+	
II	+	0	+	+	0	0	0	0	0	+	0	+	0	+	0	+	+	0	+	0	+	+	+	0	+	0	+	+	0	3+	
1	+	+	0	0	+	0	0	0	+	+	0	+	0	+	+	+	+	0	+	0	+	+	0	+	+	0	+	+	0	3+	
2	+	0	+	0	+	0	0	+	0	+	0	+	0	+	+	+	0	0	0	0	+	0	+	0	+	0	+	0	0	3+	
3	+	0	+	+	0	+	0	0	0	+	0	+	0	+	0	0	+	+	+	+	+	+	+	0	+	0	+	+	0	3+	
4	+	0	+	0	+	+	0	0	+	+	0	+	0	+	+	0	0	0	0	0	+	+	+	+	0	0	+	0	0	3+	
5	0	0	+	+	+	+	0	0	0	+	0	+	0	+	+	0	+	+	+	+	+	0	+	0	+	0	+	+	0	3+	
6	0	0	+	0	+	+	0	0	0	+	0	+	0	+	0	+	+	+	0	0	+	+	+	0	+	0	+	0	0	3+	
7	0	0	+	+	+	+	0	0	+	+	0	+	0	+	+	0	+	+	+	0	+	0	0	0	+	0	+	+	0	3+	
8	0	0	+	0	+	+	0	0	0	+	0	+	0	+	+	+	0	+	+	0	0	+	+	+	+	+	+	+	0	3+	
9	0	0	+	+	+	+	0	0	0	+	0	+	0	+	+	0	0	+	0	0	0	+	0	+	0	0	+	+	0	3+	
10	0	0	+	0	+	+	0	0	0	+	0	+	0	+	0	0	0	+	+	0	+	0	+	0	+	0	0	0	0	3+	
Patient's cells																															

C. An autoantibody.
D. An alloantibody to Wr^a.
E. An alloantibody to Lu^b.

Question 30: A variation of reaction strength is observed with 8 out of 10 panel cells tested in the AHG phase of antibody identification. The autocontrol is negative. These findings are most likely associated with which of the following?

A. Anti-Co^a.
B. Anti-E.
C. Anti-k.
D. Multiple alloantibodies.
E. Warm-reactive autoantibodies.

Question 31: Which of the following is *true* concerning the antigens belonging to the blood group system to which the antibody in Table 6-31 is directed?

A. The antigens are located on a creatinine transporter.
B. Antibodies to these antigens are not associated with hemolysis.
C. Red cells lacking both the "a" allele and the "b" allele are common in people of African ethnicity.
D. The antibodies frequently fall to undetectable levels.
E. The antibodies are the most common cause of HDFN.

Question 32: A type and screen is ordered for a 63-year-old man scheduled for hip replacement surgery. The patient received 2 units of compatible blood 3 years ago as a result of a car accident. His antibody screen is now positive. The problem is referred to you for further evaluation. The results of a 10-cell panel are given in Table 6-32. Which of the following characteristics of the antibody identified is *true*?

A. The antibody is not associated with a dosage effect.

Table 6-31.

Cell	D	C	c	E	e	f	V	Cw	K	k	Kpa	Kpb	Jsa	Jsb	Fya	Fyb	Jka	Jkb	Lea	Leb	P1	M	N	S	s	Lua	Lub	Xga	IS	AHG	CC
I	+	+	0	0	+	0	0	0	+	+	0	+	0	+	+	+	0	+	0	+	+	+	+	+	+	0	+	0	0	0	+
II	+	0	+	+	0	0	0	0	0	+	0	+	0	+	0	+	+	0	+	0	+	+	+	0	+	0	+	+	0	3+	
1	+	+	0	0	+	0	0	+	+	+	0	+	0	+	+	+	+	0	+	0	+	+	0	+	+	0	+	0	0	3+	
2	+	+	+	0	+	+	0	0	0	+	0	+	0	+	+	+	0	0	0	0	+	0	+	0	+	0	+	+	0	3+	+
3	+	0	+	+	+	+	0	0	+	+	0	+	0	+	0	0	0	+	0	+	+	+	+	0	+	0	+	0	0	0	
4	+	0	+	0	+	+	0	0	0	+	0	+	0	+	+	0	+	0	+	0	+	+	+	0	0	0	+	+	0	3+	+
5	0	0	+	+	+	+	0	0	+	+	0	+	0	+	0	0	+	+	0	+	+	+	+	0	+	0	+	0	0	0	
6	0	0	+	0	+	+	+	0	0	+	0	+	0	+	+	+	+	+	+	+	+	+	+	+	+	0	+	+	0	1+	
7	0	0	+	0	+	+	0	0	0	+	0	+	0	+	0	+	+	+	+	0	+	0	+	0	+	0	+	0	0	1+	+
8	+	0	+	+	+	+	0	0	0	+	0	+	0	+	+	+	+	+	+	0	0	0	0	0	+	+	+	+	0	1+	+
9	0	0	+	0	+	+	0	0	0	+	0	+	0	+	+	0	0	+	0	0	0	+	+	+	0	0	+	+	0	0	
10	0	0	+	0	+	+	+	0	0	+	0	+	0	+	0	0	+	0	0	0	+	0	+	0	+	0	+	0	0	0	
Patient's cells																													0		

Table 6-32.

Cell	D	C	c	E	e	f	V	C^w	K	k	Kp^a	Kp^b	Js^a	Js^b	Fy^a	Fy^b	Jk^a	Jk^b	Le^a	Le^b	P_1	M	N	S	s	Lu^a	Lu^b	Xg^a	IS	AhG	CC
I	+	+	0	0	+	0	0	0	+	+	0	+	0	+	+	+	0	+	0	+	+	+	+	+	+	0	+	0	0	0	+
II	+	0	+	+	0	0	0	0	0	+	0	+	0	+	0	+	+	0	+	0	+	+	+	0	+	0	+	+	0	2+	
1	+	+	0	0	+	0	0	0	+	+	0	+	0	+	+	+	+	0	+	0	+	+	+	+	+	0	+	+	0	0	+
2	+	+	+	0	+	0	0	+	0	+	0	+	0	+	0	+	+	0	+	0	+	0	0	0	+	0	+	0	0	0	+
3	+	0	+	+	0	0	0	0	0	+	0	+	0	+	+	0	0	+	0	+	+	+	+	0	0	0	+	+	0	2+	+
4	+	0	+	0	+	+	0	0	0	+	0	+	0	+	0	0	+	0	+	0	+	0	+	0	+	0	+	0	0	0	
5	0	0	+	+	+	+	0	0	+	+	0	+	0	+	+	0	0	+	+	+	+	+	+	+	+	0	+	+	0	0	+
6	0	+	+	0	+	+	0	0	0	+	0	+	0	+	+	+	+	+	0	0	+	0	+	0	+	0	+	0	0	2+	+
7	0	0	+	+	+	+	0	0	0	+	0	+	0	+	0	+	+	+	+	0	+	0	+	0	+	0	+	+	0	0	+
8	0	0	+	0	+	+	0	0	+	+	0	+	0	+	+	0	+	+	+	0	0	+	0	+	+	+	+	0	0	0	+
9	0	0	+	0	+	+	0	0	0	+	0	+	0	+	+	+	0	+	+	0	0	+	+	+	0	0	+	+	0	0	+
10	0	0	+	0	+	+	0	0	0	+	0	+	0	+	0	0	0	+	+	0	+	0	+	0	+	0	+	0	0	0	+
Patient's cells																															

B. The antibody is an IgG immune antibody implicated in HDFN and hemolytic transfusion reactions.
C. Thirty percent of people of European ethnicity can form the antibody on exposure to an immunizing event.
D. The antibody typically shows decreased reactivity with proteolytic enzyme-treated reagent red cells.
E. Between 20% and 30% of donor units will be crossmatch compatible with the patient.

Question 33: Which of the following antigens is associated with polyagglutinability?

A. C antigen.
B. K antigen.
C. Kx antigen.
D. T antigen.
E. V antigen.

Question 34: Which of the following statements is *true* concerning the antibody identified in the panel shown in Table 6-34?

A. It is usually an IgM antibody.
B. Reactivity is enhanced by adjusting the pH to 8.0.
C. It is not associated with a dosage effect.
D. The frequency of the antigen is much lower in people of African ethnicity than in people of European ethnicity.
E. Reactivity is enhanced with enzyme-treated red cells.

Table 6-34.

Cell	D	C	c	E	e	f	V	C^w	K	k	Kp^a	Kp^b	Js^a	Js^b	Fy^a	Fy^b	Jk^a	Jk^b	Le^a	Le^b	P_1	M	N	S	s	Lu^a	Lu^b	Xg^a	IS	AHG	CC
I	+	+	0	0	+	0	0	0	+	+	0	+	0	+	+	+	0	+	0	+	+	+	+	+	+	0	+	0	1+	2+	
II	+	0	+	+	0	0	0	0	0	+	0	+	0	+	0	+	+	0	+	0	+	+	+	0	+	0	+	+	1+	2+	
1	+	+	+	0	+	0	0	+	+	+	0	+	0	+	+	+	+	0	+	0	+	+	+	+	+	0	+	+	1+	2+	
2	+	+	0	0	+	0	0	0	0	+	0	+	0	+	+	+	0	0	+	+	+	+	0	0	+	0	+	0	2+	3+	+
3	+	0	+	+	+	0	0	0	0	+	0	+	0	+	0	+	+	+	0	0	+	+	+	0	+	0	+	+	0	0	
4	+	0	+	0	+	+	0	0	+	+	0	+	0	+	+	0	+	0	+	+	+	+	+	0	0	0	+	0	1+	2+	
5	0	0	+	0	+	+	0	0	0	+	0	+	0	+	+	0	0	+	0	+	+	0	+	0	+	0	+	+	1+	2+	+
6	0	0	+	+	+	+	0	0	+	+	0	+	0	+	0	+	+	+	0	+	+	0	+	0	+	0	+	0	0	0	+
7	0	0	+	0	+	+	0	0	0	+	0	+	0	+	+	+	+	+	+	0	+	+	+	0	+	0	+	+	0	0	
8	0	0	+	0	+	+	0	0	+	+	0	+	0	+	0	0	0	+	+	0	0	0	0	+	0	+	+	0	2+	3+	
9	0	0	+	0	+	+	0	0	0	+	0	+	0	+	+	+	0	+	+	0	0	+	+	+	+	0	+	+	1+	2+	+
10	0	0	+	0	+	+	0	0	0	+	0	+	0	+	0	0	0	+	0	0	+	0	+	0	+	0	+	0	0	0	+
Patient's cells																															

Question 35: Which of the following lectin-antigen pairs is correct?

A. *Vicia graminea* and the B antigen.
B. *Bandeiraea simplicifolia* and the N antigen.
C. *Dolichos biflorus* and the A_1 antigen.
D. *Salvia horminum* and the T antigen.
E. *Arachis hypogaea* and the Cad antigen.

ANSWERS

Question 1: D

Explanation:

- AABB *Standards for Blood Banks and Transfusion Services (Standards)* requires that an order be legible and list two independent identifiers, which may include the following information:
  - First and last names.
  - Unique patient identification number.
- The type of component requested is needed in order to know what to provide the patient.
- Additional information that is frequently collected, but not required, includes the gender of the patient, the age of the patient, the patient's diagnosis, previous transfusion history, pregnancy history, and the requesting physician's name. This information may be useful for problem-solving.

Question 2: E

Explanation:

- The most common cause of ABO-incompatible transfusion reactions is a clerical error. At least two-thirds of these errors occur outside of the laboratory, at the time of pretransfusion sample collection or at the time of transfusion.
- When collecting blood samples, positive identification is required. This consists of one or more of the following:
  - A hospital wristband and/or unique identification band such as a blood bank or emergency room identification band.
  - Identification by a third party (if the patient is unresponsive).
  - The patient's stating his or her name.
- The patient's chart or name on the outside of the hospital room does not represent adequate identification.

Question 3: B

Explanation:

- AABB *Standards* requires that samples be drawn within 3 days of transfusion if the patient has been transfused or pregnant within the past 3 months or if the transfusion and/or pregnancy history is unknown.
- Many institutions, because of difficulties obtaining this information, will use a 3-day rule for all patients.
- The goal of this regulation is to prevent delayed hemolytic transfusion reactions. Individuals with recent transfusions or pregnancies may be forming blood group antibodies that would not be detectable if samples are drawn too far in advance of the anticipated time of transfusion.

Question 4: E

Explanation:

- In order to minimize clerical errors and the risk of ABO-incompatible transfusions, AABB *Standards* requires the following:
  - The intended recipient shall be identified positively at the time of sample collection.
  - Labels shall bear sufficient information for the unique identification of the recipient and include two independent identifiers and the date that the sample was collected.
  - Labels shall be attached to the sample before leaving the side of the intended recipient.
  - There shall be a mechanism to identify the individual who drew the blood from the patient. This may involve the phlebotomist's initialing the sample, signing paperwork, or entering an identifier into the computer. It does *not* have to be initialing of the sample.
  - Before testing is performed, the identifying information on the specimen label must be in agreement with all identifying information on the request form.
- Answer A is incorrect in that the required date is lacking.

- Answer B is incorrect because the sample was not labeled at the patient's bedside.
- Answer C is incorrect in that a second unique identifier such as a hospital number is lacking.
- Answer D is incorrect because the sample was not labeled at the patient's bedside.

Question 5: D

Explanation:

- The following tests are performed on all units of blood intended for allogeneic transfusion and all autologous blood or components that will be transfused outside the collection facility:
  - Serologic test for syphilis.
  - Antibodies to human immunodeficiency virus (HIV)-1/2.
  - Antibodies to human T-cell lymphotropic virus (HTLV)-I/II.
  - Anti-HCV.
  - Antibodies to hepatitis B core antigen (HBc).
  - HBsAg.
  - HIV-1 RNA.
  - HCV RNA.
  - West Nile virus (WNV) RNA (seasonal criteria apply).
- Testing for the HIV p24 antigen is no longer required by the Food and Drug Administration.
- In the US, the alanine aminotransferase (ALT) test (a surrogate test for hepatitis B and hepatitis C) was no longer required as of 1995. However, ALT testing remains a requirement for commercial source plasma in plasmapheresis centers and is frequently performed in blood centers that sell recovered plasma to fractionators.
- No specific donor testing is required for either HAV or parvovirus at this time.
- Although CMV serologic testing is not required of any blood donors, it may be performed in selected donors to aid in the prevention of transfusion-transmitted CMV infection.
- Although positive anti-HBs testing would aid in the identification of those with past hepatitis B virus (HBV) infections, this test would not discriminate between these individuals and those individuals

who have been vaccinated against HBV. As such, it would not be a useful donor test and is not required.

Question 6: B

Explanation:

- The segments from transfused RBC units and the recipient's blood specimen must be sealed and stored at 1 to 6 C for at least 7 days following transfusion (see AABB *Standards*).
- Retention of samples makes it possible to do repeat testing in the setting of transfusion reactions or if additional testing is required.

Question 7: D

Explanation:

- With a type-and-screen order, the recipient's ABO and D antigen type are determined and the serum is screened for clinically significant antibodies. The screen is performed by testing the potential recipient's serum against two or three commercially prepared group O red cell samples with a known antigenic makeup.
- A type-and-crossmatch order includes all of the elements of a type-and-screen order (see above); in addition, however, one or more RBC units are crossmatched so that they may be available immediately for those situations that are more likely to require transfusion.
- A type-and-screen order is appropriate for procedures that may require a transfusion but for which transfusion is not likely (eg, cholecystectomy and routine Caesarian section). In those procedures for which a significant blood loss is not expected (eg, excision of a facial seborrheic keratosis and inguinal herniorrhaphy), a type and screen is not indicated.
- If the antibody screen is negative and a transfusion is required, compatible RBCs can be provided very quickly, generally within 10 to 15 minutes, depending on the method of crossmatching used. This is predicated on having a blood sample in the blood bank for which the

type and screen has been performed and the sample is still suitable for crossmatching.
- If the antibody screen is positive, an antibody identification panel is performed. In such a case, crossmatch-compatible, antigen-negative units can be placed on hold in case they are needed urgently.

Question 8: B

Explanation:

- Weak-D testing is performed by incubating (at 37°C) the patient's red cell sample with anti-D for 15 to 30 minutes. The sample is then washed, antihuman IgG is added, and the sample is centrifuged and examined for agglutination.
- Weak-D testing is required only for Rh-negative blood donors. If weak-D testing was not performed, a weak-D individual could be falsely classified as Rh-negative. The transfusion of their blood to Rh-negative individuals would put them at risk for the development of anti-D.
- Weak-D testing is not indicated for transfusion recipients because the failure to identify a weak-D transfusion recipient has no clinical consequences (ie, they would be falsely classified as Rh-negative even though they are Rh-positive; they would thus receive Rh-negative red cells but this would have no adverse consequences).
- Some institutions perform weak-D testing on all Rh-negative patients because they feel that the administration of Rh-negative red cells to an individual with a weak-D phenotype is a waste of a scarce resource, as these patients are unlikely to form anti-D.
- Other institutions will perform the testing but will still administer Rh-negative red cells to weak-D individuals because those with the partial-D phenotype, a minority of those presenting as weak D, can form anti-D to the components of the D antigen they lack.
- The same logic applies to weak-D typing in Rh-negative pregnant women and the administration of Rh Immune Globulin (RhIG):
  ○ Some institutions perform weak-D typing on all Rh-negative pregnant women and provide RhIG accordingly.
  ○ Some institutions perform weak-D typing on all Rh-negative pregnant women and provide RhIG irrespective of the weak-D type (out

PRETRANSFUSION TESTING AND ANTIBODY IDENTIFICATION

of concern that even a weak-D patient is at increased risk for anti-D development).
- Some institutions do not perform weak-D typing on any Rh-negative patients, pregnant or otherwise.
- If a pregnant woman is Rh negative and a candidate for RhIG therapy, fetal/neonatal weak-D testing is required when the initial test for D is negative.

Question 9: A

Explanation:

See Question 10.

Question 10: B

Explanation for Questions 9 and 10:

- Naturally occurring antibodies are usually IgM, cold-reactive, and present in the serum of individuals who have had no known exposure to red cells expressing the antigen (eg, no previous transfusions or pregnancies).
- Naturally occurring antibodies result from exposure to antigens within the environment, which are also present on red cells. For example, anti-A results from exposure to the same antigen present on microbes within the gastrointestinal tract or antigens present on pollen.
- Immune IgG antibodies are produced by exposure to red cells expressing the foreign antigens. Sources of exposure include pregnancy, transfusion, and organ or hematopoietic progenitor cell transplantation.
- As a rule of thumb, naturally occurring IgM antibodies are directed against carbohydrate epitopes, whereas immune IgG antibodies are directed against peptide epitopes.
- The most common naturally occurring and immune antibodies are listed in Table 6-10.
- Mnemonic for naturally occurring antibodies: LIPMAN (Lewis, Ii, P, M, ABH, N).

Table 6-10.

Naturally Occurring Antibodies	Immune Antibodies
Anti-A, anti-B, anti-A,B, anti-H	Antibodies to Rh system antigens
Anti-I	Antibodies to Kell system antigens
Anti-Le^a, anti-Le^b	Antibodies to Duffy system antigens
Anti-M, anti-N	Anti-S, anti-s
Anti-P$_1$	Antibodies to Kidd system antigens

Question 11: D

Explanation:

See Question 12.

Question 12: E

Explanation for Questions 11 and 12:

- Enzymes that either enhance or destroy antigen-antibody reactions can be very useful in identifying the specificity of alloantibodies, particularly in situations in which there are complex mixtures of multiple alloantibodies.
- Enzymes cleave membrane glycoproteins and sialic acid residues. This removes a steric barrier that may enhance the reactivity of certain antibodies for their corresponding antigens. However, glycoproteins and sialic acid residues are critical components of some blood group antigens, and their removal results in the destruction of these antigens.
- The effects of enzyme treatment on blood group antigen-antibody interactions are described in Table 6-12A.
- Enzymes do not readily destroy s and U antigens of the MNSs blood group system.
- Enzymes have no effect on Kell, Lutheran, and Gerbich 3.
- Commonly used enzymes and their sources are listed in Table 6-12B.

PRETRANSFUSION TESTING AND ANTIBODY IDENTIFICATION 209

Table 6-12A.

Antibodies Enhanced by Enzyme Treatment	Antigens Denatured by Enzyme Treatment
P$_1$ Rh system Le^a, Le^b Jk^a, Jk^b I, i ABH	M, N, S Fy^a, Fy^b, Fy6 Ch^a, Rg^a, JMH In^b Yt^a Pr Tn Xg^a Gerbich 2 and 4 Cromer

Table 6-12B.

Enzyme	Source
Ficin	Figs
Papain	Papaya
Trypsin	Pig stomach
Bromelin	Pineapple

Question 13: C

Explanation:

- Three antibodies are present:
  - Anti-K reacting at immediate spin only.
  - Anti-Fy^a demonstrating dosage (cells 1 and 2 are heterozygous and are 1+, whereas cell 4 is homozygous and is 2+) and destroyed by enzymes.
  - Anti-Jk^b.

- In order to calculate the frequency of compatible donors, the frequency of antigen-negative donors for each antigen must be multiplied together and then multiplied by 100. In this case, the equation is as follows:
  - Frequency of compatible donors = 0.45 (frequency of group O) × 1 (frequency of Rh-positive and -negative donors) × 0.35 (frequency of Fy^a-negative donors) × 0.91 (frequency of K-negative donors) × 0.28 (frequency of Jk^b-negative donors) × 100% = 4.0%.

Question 14: D

Explanation:

- The antibody identified in the panel is anti-K.
- Dithiothreitol (DTT) is a sulfhydryl-reducing agent that can be used to destroy Kell system antigens. Other such agents, including 2-mercaptoethanol (2ME), β-mercaptoethylamine, and 2-aminoethylisothiouronium bromide (AET), also denature Kell system antigens.
- Kell system antigens are not affected by treatment with papain, ficin, or bromelin.
- Trypsin and chymotrypsin, when used in combination, can denature Kell system antigens but do not do so separately.
- Sulfhydryl-reducing agents also denature other antigens, including LW^a, Do^a, Do^b, and Yt.
- DTT also denatures IgM antibodies by reducing the disulfide bond present in the joining chain of the IgM molecule.
- *Ulex europaeus* is a lectin that binds to and causes the agglutination of red cells expressing the H antigen.

Question 15: B

Explanation:

- The process of agglutination can be divided into two phases:
  - The binding of the antibody to its target antigen.
  - Formation of a linked lattice between red cells.

- Numerous enhancing media and potentiators are used to facilitate this process.
- LISS enhances antibody uptake by reducing the zeta potential and allows increased attraction between positively charged antibodies and negatively charged red cells.
- PEG enhances antibody-antigen binding by excluding water from around the red cells, effectively concentrating the antibody and favoring binding to its target. IgM antibodies, such as ABO and Lewis, are weaker or not detected with PEG. Warm autoantibodies are greatly enhanced by PEG.
- Overall, PEG is more sensitive than LISS with respect to alloantibody detection.
- The false-positive rate is higher for PEG in comparison to LISS: 1.3% vs 0.1%.
- Polybrene enhances formation of the linked lattice by neutralizing the negative charges of the sialic acid residues on the red cell, allowing red cells to come closer together. The addition of sodium citrate can disperse the spontaneous agglutination induced by Polybrene. If an antibody is present, the red cells will be crosslinked and will not disperse. If no antibody is present, the red cells will disperse. Polybrene detects ABO antibodies as well as clinically significant alloantibodies.
- Albumin enhances linked lattice formation by reducing the net negative charge of the red cells, allowing the cells to come closer together.
- Enzyme treatment enhances linked lattice formation by decreasing the net negative charge of the red cells by removing sialic acid residues. This allows the red cells to come closer together.

Question 16: B

Explanation:

- Coombs described the antiglobulin test in 1945, but it was subsequently recognized that Moreschi had described the test earlier.
- Landsteiner described the ABO system in 1901.
- Levine and Stetson described the first human example of anti-D in 1939.
- Von Descatello and Sturli described the AB blood type in 1902.

Question 17: C

Explanation:

See Question 18.

Question 18: D

Explanation for Questions 17 and 18:

- Polyspecific or broad-spectrum AHG must contain antihuman IgG and anti-C3d.
- Broad-spectrum AHG may also contain anti-C3b, anti-C4b, anti-C4d, anti-IgM, and anti-IgA specificities, depending on the source. Reactivity with these reagents may be weak and require special manipulation to demonstrate red cell coating with these globulins. This is especially true with regard to anti-IgA and anti-IgM reactivity.
- Polyspecific AHG reagent is used predominantly in the direct antiglobulin test (DAT). Polyspecific AHG is not routinely used in antibody screening or crossmatching because antibodies that are detectable only by their ability to fix complement are rare. In these tests, monospecific AHG, containing only anti-IgG activity, is used.

Question 19: E

Explanation:

- The DAT is used to demonstrate the in-vivo coating of red cells with antibody or complement.
- All of the choices except E involve antibody coating of red cells in vitro (ie, in the test tube).
- The DAT is appropriately used in clinical situations associated with immune-mediated hemolysis, which include the following:
  - HDFN.
  - Autoimmune hemolytic anemia.

- Transfusion reactions.
- Drug-induced hemolysis.

Question 20: B

Explanation:

- The DAT demonstrates in-vivo coating of red cells by antibody or complement. Red cells from the patient are washed, AHG reagent is added, and the cells are immediately centrifuged and examined for agglutination.
- Causes of false-positive DATs include the following:
  - Coating of the red cells by complement in vitro (eg, complement being fixed at cold temperatures during specimen storage).
  - Aggregation of red cells by the gel present in serum separator tubes.
  - Complement fixation by 5% or 10% dextrose in intravenous solutions.
  - Septicemia or bacterial contamination of stored blood samples leading to T activation.
  - Contamination of the saline with materials that can cause spontaneous aggregation of red cells (eg, colloidal silica from glass bottles).
  - Contamination through improperly cleaned glassware.
  - Overcentrifugation.
  - Improperly prepared AHG reagent (eg, containing anti-species antibodies).
- Causes of false-negative DATs include the following:
  - IgA or IgM coating the red cells, not IgG or complement (most AHG reagents do not detect IgA or IgM).
  - Incubating the red cells after addition of the AHG reagent, because this may cause the antibodies in the AHG reagent to disassociate.

Question 21: D

Explanation:

- An IAT demonstrates in-vitro reactions between red cells and antibodies. In other words, the antibody and its target antigen are incubated together in the test tube. The two bind, and this is detected through the addition of an AHG reagent.
- Examples of IATs include the following:
  - Weak-D testing.
  - Antibody screens.
  - Antibody identification.
  - Compatibility testing.
  - Some antigen typings.
  - Antibody titration.
- Antibody elution involves the removal of antibodies bound to red cells either in the patient or in the test tube. In itself, it does *not* involve the detection of antibodies using an antiglobulin reagent.

Question 22: A

Explanation:

- The IAT procedure is performed as follows: Patient serum or a reagent is incubated with either donor or patient red cells, depending upon the type of IAT performed (see Question 21). The cells are then washed and an AHG reagent is added. The cells are centrifuged and examined for agglutination. The presence of agglutination indicates that antibody has bound to the red cells.
- Causes of false-negative tests include the following:
  - Failure to remove unbound globulin such that it neutralizes the AHG reagent (ie, improper or inadequate red cell washing).
  - Loss of bound antibody with time due to delayed testing.
  - Loss of AHG reagent activity due to improper storage (extreme temperature), bacterial contamination, or contamination with human serum.
  - Failure to add the AHG reagent.

PRETRANSFUSION TESTING AND ANTIBODY IDENTIFICATION 215

- Undercentrifugation.
- Too many or too few red cells used.
- Prozone reactions.
- Loss of reactivity of the antigens on the red cells (eg, out-of-date reagent red cells).
- No active complement present to detect IgM antibodies (eg, use of plasma instead of serum).
- Improper incubation temperature or time.
- Too little serum added (too little antibody present on the red cells to be detected by the AHG reagent).
- Causes of false-positive tests include the following:
  - Sensitized red cells (red cells coated with antibody before incubation).
  - Contamination of saline with materials that can cause spontaneous aggregation of the red cells (eg, colloidal silica from glass bottles).
  - Contamination through improperly cleaned glassware.
  - Overcentrifugation.
  - Improperly prepared AHG reagent (containing anti-species antibodies).

Question 23: A

Explanation:

- In order to detect errors in typing and errors in labeling, all RBC or Whole Blood units must be retested to:
  - Confirm the ABO typing.
  - Confirm the Rh typing of Rh-negative units.
- Weak-D testing is not required for Rh-negative units during retesting. (However, it is required for the initial testing; see Question 8.)
- Confirmatory testing of the Rh type of Rh-positive units is not required. If an Rh-negative unit was erroneously labeled as Rh positive, no consequences would occur to an Rh-positive patient who received that unit. This cannot be said for an Rh-negative patient receiving an Rh-positive unit erroneously labeled as Rh negative.
- Confirmatory testing must be performed *after* the ABO and Rh labels are affixed in order to detect errors in labeling.
- Computer confirmation of ABO and Rh can be performed if:

- The computer is validated to prevent the release of ABO- and Rh-mislabeled components.
- There is a method to detect ABO and Rh discrepancies between the current donation and previous donations by the same donor.
- There is a method to identify first-time donors or donors lacking valid ABO or Rh typings such that confirmatory testing can be performed and these results are entered into the computer.
- There is a method to confirm that the ABO and Rh label on the unit agrees with the ABO and Rh typings in the computer.
- The confirmation process is completed before releasing the component.

Question 24: D

Explanation:

- AABB *Standards* requires that if there is no record of previous detection of an antibody, at minimum, testing to detect ABO incompatibility must be performed. This requirement could be fulfilled through a complete crossmatch, an immediate-spin crossmatch, or a computer crossmatch.
- If an antibody is detected or if there is a history of an antibody, then a complete crossmatch must be performed.
- In order to perform a computer crossmatch:
  - The computer system must be validated on-site to ensure that only ABO-compatible red-cell-containing components can be selected for transfusion.
  - Two determinations of the recipient's ABO group must have been made. This requirement may be fulfilled by:
    - Retesting the current sample.
    - Testing a second current sample.
    - Comparison of current testing with previous records.
  - The computer system must contain the following information for the component to be transfused:
    - Donor unit number.
    - Component name.
    - ABO group.
    - The confirmed ABO group.
    - Rh type.

- The computer system must contain the following information for the recipient of the component:
  - Two unique recipient identifiers.
  - ABO group.
  - Rh type.
  - Antibody screen results.
- A method must exist to verify correct entry of the data before the component is released.
- The computer system must contain logic to alert the user to discrepancies between the recipient's and the component's ABO and Rh types (ie, incompatibilities).

Question 25: D

Explanation:

- AABB *Standards* requires that components containing more than 2 mL of red cells must be crossmatched.
- Granulocyte products typically have a significant red cell content and therefore must be crossmatched.
- Components with less than 2 mL of red cells (eg, Fresh Frozen Plasma, Cryoprecipitated AHF, most apheresis platelet products, and most whole-blood-derived platelet pools) do not need to be crossmatched.

Question 26: A

Explanation:

- Anti-Wr^a is almost always an IgG antibody. The antigen is expressed on red cells but *not* platelets, so a platelet crossmatch would not make sense.
- A complete crossmatch consists of testing at immediate spin followed by testing using an AHG reagent. This is also referred to commonly as the AHG crossmatch. The complete crossmatch will detect IgM antibodies as well as IgG antibodies.

- In a minor crossmatch, the donor's plasma is tested with the recipient's red cells to identify antibodies in the donor that could react with recipient red cells. This form of testing was used before the advent of component therapy, when whole blood, containing large amounts of plasma, was transfused. This type of crossmatching is not frequently performed today and would not detect the situation described.
- The immediate-spin crossmatch (also called an incomplete crossmatch) detects IgM antibodies, most importantly ABO antibodies. It is a rapid test. In patients with negative antibody screens, this crossmatch actually represents a final confirmation of ABO compatibility. As a result, most institutions use only the immediate-spin crossmatch when the antibody screen is negative.
- A computer crossmatch uses an appropriately validated computer to compare the ABO and Rh types of a patient with the ABO and Rh types of a red cell component to determine compatibility. It does not detect incompatibility for other antigen systems.
- The platelet crossmatch detects incompatibilities between antibodies in patient serum (anti-HLA and anti-HPA) and antigens on donor platelets. It would not detect incompatibility caused by anti-Wr^a.

Question 27: C

Explanation:

- AABB *Standards* requires that units of blood released before the completion of testing designed to prevent disease transmission must:
  - Be conspicuously labeled with the testing that is not complete.
  - Have the testing completed as soon as possible.
  - Be accompanied by a statement signed by the requesting physician indicating that the clinical situation was urgent enough to require release before the completion of testing.
- In the event that a unit must be released before the completion of all required infectious disease testing, if a test proves to be reactive, the transfusion service and the ordering physician must be notified as soon as possible.
- For a cytapheresis donor dedicated to support a specific patient, testing must be performed before the first apheresis component is released for transfusion and at least every 30 days thereafter.

Question 28: B

Explanation:

- AABB *Standards* notes that all required infectious disease tests, including anti-HIV-1/2, be performed if the unit will be transfused outside the collecting institution.
- If the unit is to be transfused within the collecting facility, these required tests need not be performed.
- The patient's physician must be notified of any abnormal results obtained when autologous units are tested.
- If a unit to be shipped to another facility has abnormal infectious disease test results, the receiving facility must be notified by the shipping facility.

Question 29: C

Explanation:

- The autocontrol (patient red cells incubated with patient serum) is reactive and all of the panel cells are reactive at the AHG phase. The most likely explanation for these findings is a warm-reactive autoantibody.
- The autocontrol is roughly equivalent to the DAT; this suggests the presence of an autoantibody in the patient's serum.
- Another diagnostic possibility in this case is an antibody with high titer and low avidity characteristics; however, this is less likely because:
  ○ The autocontrol may or may not be reactive.
  ○ The autocontrol is usually only reactive if the antibody is anti-JMH.
  ○ The reactivity of all panel cells at the AHG phase will be w+ to 1+. In this case, the reactivity is 3+.
- Lu^b and k are high-incidence antigens. Antibodies directed against these antigens could give a similar pattern on the antibody identification panel. However, the autocontrol would be negative. The same

holds for anti-e, but in the case of this antibody, one cell on the panel will always be e-negative (and, therefore, nonreactive).
- Wr^a is a low-incidence antigen. Antibodies to this antigen would react with few, if any, of the cells on an antibody identification panel.

Question 30: D

Explanation:

- A variation of reaction strength may be observed, in the AHG phase of testing, when multiple blood group alloantibodies are present. Variations can also be seen with P_1 antibodies (because of the variable strength of P_1 antigen expression on red cells) and antibodies exhibiting a dosage effect.
- If anti-Co^a is present, 1 out of 10 panel cells (not 8 out of 10) should show reactivity at the AHG phase of testing during antibody identification. See Table 6-30 for a listing of the frequency of Colton system antigens.
- A dosage effect may be seen with anti-E, but only 2 or 3 out of 10 panel cells should show reactivity at the AHG phase of testing.
- The k antigen is a high-frequency member of the Kell blood group system. Anti-k would be expected to react with all panel cells with an equal strength of reactivity.
- Warm-reactive autoantibodies typically react with all panel cells with an equal strength of reactivity. In addition, the autocontrol would also be reactive.

Table 6-30.

Colton System Antigens	Frequency (%)
Co^a	10.7
Co^b	99.9

PRETRANSFUSION TESTING AND ANTIBODY IDENTIFICATION

Question 31: D

Explanation:

- The antibody is anti-Jk^a, and it demonstrates a dosage effect.
- The Kidd blood group antigens, Jk^a and Jk^b, are located on the human erythroid urea transporter protein HUT1. This is supported by the fact that Jk(a–b–) red cells resist lysis when placed in 2M urea.
- The blood group system associated with a lack of both the "a" and "b" alleles in people of African ethnicity is the Duffy system (Fy), not the Kidd system.
- Kidd antibodies are associated with hemolysis. Most are IgG3, and the Kidd antigens are clustered on the red cell membrane. This could account for the complement activation and intravascular hemolysis sometimes seen with Kidd antibodies.
- Kidd antibodies have a tendency to fall to undetectable levels over time. Because of this, Kidd antibodies are the most commonly implicated antibodies in delayed hemolytic transfusion reactions.
- Because these antibodies are IgG and the antigens are expressed on fetal red cells, Kidd antibodies can cause HDFN. However, this is uncommon. The antibody most frequently implicated in this disease process is anti-D.

Question 32: B

Explanation:

- Anti-E is the confirmed specificity in the patient's serum.
- Screening cell II and panel cells 3 and 6 are positive for the E antigen. A positive reaction is observed between the patient's serum and these three reagent cells at the antiglobulin phase of testing. A negative reaction is observed between the patient's serum and the nine reagent cells negative for the E antigen.
- E antibodies are typically IgG antibodies that are always considered to be clinically significant with respect to hemolysis.
- E antibodies frequently demonstrate a dosage effect when comparing the relative strengths of reactivity of red cells homozygous for E anti-

gen expression (ie, EE) with those heterozygous for expression (ie, Ee). This effect may be more obvious with weakly reactive antibodies.
- Rh antigens are not denatured by enzyme treatment. In fact, the reactivity of Rh system antibodies may be enhanced when they are tested against enzyme-treated red cells.
- E-negative blood components are indicated for this patient. The red cells of approximately 70% of people of European ethnicity and almost 80% of people of African ethnicity type negative for the E antigen.
- Between 70% and 80% of all donor units will be crossmatch compatible with the patient's serum.

Question 33: D

Explanation:

- Polyagglutinability occurs when most human sera agglutinate a red cell. This results from the presence of naturally occurring antibodies directed against antigens present on red cells. In the majority of instances, these are acquired antigens that represent the exposure of cryptic antigens (eg, T, Tk, Tn, Tx).
- C, K, Kx, and V are inherited red cell antigens that are not associated with polyagglutination.
- Antigens associated with polyagglutination are shown in Table 6-33.

Table 6-33.

Antigen	Inherited/ Acquired	Association
T	Acquired	Infection with *Pneumococci, Clostridium perfringens, Vibrio cholerae*, or influenza virus
Tn	Acquired	Infection with *Clostridia, Bacteroides, E. coli*, or *Proteus*; in addition, mutations in hematopoietic progenitor cells
Tk	Acquired	Infection with *Bacteroides fragilis* and *Serretia marcescens*
Tx	Acquired	Infection with *Pneumococci*
Cad	Inherited	
Hemoglobin M- Hyde Park	Inherited	
HEMPAS	Inherited	Congenital dyserythropoietic anemia type II (CDAII), also called HEMPAS (Hereditary Erythrocyte Multinuclearity with Positive Acidified Serum test)
NOR	Inherited	

Question 34: A

Explanation:

- The antibody is anti-M, and it demonstrates a dosage effect.
- Characteristics of anti-M and the M antigen include the following:
  - The antigen is destroyed by enzymes.
  - Antibody reactivity is enhanced by lowering the pH to 6.2.
  - Anti-M is most commonly IgM and naturally occurring.
  - The antibody may be glucose dependent (ie, the presence of glucose in the preservative of the screening cells may inhibit activity).
  - Anti-M can be clinically significant if there is an IgG component, but this is very rare.

- Most antibodies to the M antigen are IgM and react best at room temperature.
- The M antigen is present in 78% of people of European ethnicity and 74% of people of African ethnicity.

Question 35: C

Explanation:

- Lectins are proteins extracted from plants that bind to specific carbohydrate antigens. They are sometimes used as an alternative to reagent antibodies.
- The specificity of the lectin can depend on the dilution of the lectin.
- Examples of lectins and the antigens that they bind include the following:
  - *Arachis hypogaea*, the peanut lectin, which binds to the T, Th, and Tk antigens but not to the Tn and Cad antigens.
  - *Salvia horminum* recognizes the Tn and Cad antigens but not the T, Th, and Tk antigens.
  - *Dolichos biflorus* recognizes either the A_1 antigen or Cad antigen, depending on the dilution.
  - *Vicia graminae* has specificity for the N antigen.
  - *Ulex europaeus* binds to and causes the agglutination of red cells expressing the H antigen.
  - *Bandeiraea simplicifolia* recognizes the B antigen.

REFERENCES

1. Downes K, Shulman I. Pretransfusion testing. In: Roback JD, Combs MR, Grossman BJ, Hillyer CD, eds. Technical manual. 16th ed. Bethesda, MD: AABB, 2008:437-63.
2. Walker P. Identification of antibodies to red cell antigens. In: Roback JD, Combs MR, Grossman BJ, Hillyer CD, eds. Technical manual. 16th ed. Bethesda, MD: AABB, 2008:465-98.

3. Leger R. The positive direct antiglobulin test and immune-mediated hemolysis. In: Roback JD, Combs MR, Grossman BJ, Hillyer CD, eds. Technical manual. 16th ed. Bethesda, MD: AABB, 2008:499-521.
4. Harris T. Antibody identification. In: Rudmann SV, ed. Serologic problem-solving. Bethesda, MD: AABB Press, 2005:17-80.
5. Lieb M. Direct antiglobulin testing: Systematic problem-solving. In: Rudmann SV, ed. Serologic problem-solving. Bethesda, MD: AABB Press, 2005:81-152.

7

Clinical Transfusion Practice and Effective Use of Blood Components

QUESTIONS

Question 1: A 40-year-old male patient with a new diagnosis of acute leukemia is admitted to the hospital for induction chemotherapy. Two weeks later, he is experiencing pancytopenia secondary to myeloablation. In addition, he is febrile, possibly septic, and possibly has disseminated intravascular coagulation (DIC). He has received multiple platelet products but no longer seems to be responding, as evidenced by minimal elevations in posttransfusion platelet counts obtained 1 hour after transfusion. The most likely cause for the patient's apparent platelet refractoriness is:

A. Neutropenic fever.
B. Sepsis.
C. DIC.
D. HLA alloimmunization.
E. Splenomegaly (secondary to leukemic process).

Question 2: Referring back to the case presentation in Question 1, what is the best approach to provide platelet support for the patient with immune-mediated platelet refractoriness?

A. Provide random (ie, non-HLA-matched) apheresis platelets.
B. Provide HLA-matched apheresis platelets.
C. Provide a pool of platelet concentrates.
D. Provide leukocyte-reduced platelets.
E. Provide irradiated platelets.

Question 3: A 68-year-old male patient underwent coronary artery bypass surgery. Preoperative laboratory results included the following:

- Hematocrit = 45%.
- Platelet count = 275,000.
- Prothrombin time (PT) = 12 seconds (normal = 10-13).
- Partial thromboplastin time (PTT) = 30 (normal = 26-36).
- Fibrinogen = 250 mg/dL (normal = 200-400 mg/dL).

Postoperatively, the patient exhibited increased chest tube drainage, 200 mL in the first 2 hours after surgery and 400 mL in the following 2 hours. There was no bleeding at other sites. Postoperative laboratory results included the following:

- Hematocrit = 24%.
- Platelet count = 130,000.
- PT = 14 seconds.
- PTT = 38 seconds.
- Fibrinogen = 150 mg/dL.
- Fibrin degradation products = mildly elevated.

The most likely primary cause for the patient's excessive bleeding is:

A. Decreased platelet count.
B. Platelet dysfunction related to cardiac bypass.
C. Disseminated intravascular coagulation.
D. Coagulation factor deficiency.
E. Surgically correctable lesion.

Question 4: A 62-year-old male patient with a history of alcohol abuse presents to an emergency department vomiting large volumes of blood.

He is tachycardic and his systolic blood pressure is 60 mm Hg. Based on these data alone, which one of the following components is *least* appropriate to give?

A. Fresh Frozen Plasma (FFP).
B. Normal saline.
C. 5% albumin.
D. Whole Blood.
E. Red Blood Cells (RBCs).

Question 5: A 28-year-old male patient presents to an emergency department complaining of a nosebleed. He is otherwise asymptomatic. The following laboratory results are obtained:

- Hemoglobin = 8.0 g/dL.
- White cell count = 7500/µL with a normal differential.
- Platelet count = 7000/µL.

A blood specimen is sent to the blood bank for type and screen determination. A panreactive antibody is identified, and the patient is also found to have a positive direct antiglobulin test (DAT). The most likely diagnosis is:

A. Immune thrombocytopenic purpura (ITP).
B. Thrombotic thrombocytopenic purpura (TTP).
C. Acute leukemia.
D. Evans syndrome.
E. Warm autoimmune hemolytic anemia.

Question 6: Referring back to the case presentation in Question 5, what treatment should the patient receive?

A. No transfusion at this time.
B. Platelet transfusion alone.
C. Red cell transfusion alone.
D. Platelet and red cell transfusion.
E. Therapeutic plasmapheresis.

Question 7: A 65-year-old male patient with pancreatitis is admitted to the hospital with evidence of severe gastrointestinal bleeding and purpuric skin lesions. Laboratory examination reveals the following:

- Hemoglobin = 6.0 g/dL.
- White cell count = 8000/µL with a normal differential.
- Platelet count = 30,000/µL.
- PT = 18 seconds (normal = 10-13).
- PTT = 38 (normal = 26-36).
- Fibrinogen = 120 mg/dL (normal = 200-400 mg/dL).

Fibrin degradation products are detectable and a peripheral blood smear reveals rare schistocytes. The most likely diagnosis is:

A. ITP.
B. TTP.
C. Posttransfusion purpura (PTP).
D. Henoch-Schonlein purpura (HSP).
E. DIC.

Question 8: Referring back to the case presentation in Question 7, what treatment should the patient receive?

A. No transfusion at this time.
B. Platelet transfusion only.
C. FFP transfusion only.
D. Red cell transfusion only.
E. Transfusion of a combination of blood components.

Question 9: A 65-year-old man with chronic lymphocytic leukemia (CLL) presents with a history of fatigue, jaundice, and dark-colored urine. Three weeks ago, he received a transfusion of 2 RBC units at an outside hospital for anemia. His hemoglobin is 7 g/dL. His DAT is 3+ with polyspecific reagent, 3+ with anti-IgG, and negative with anti-

C3d. His antibody identification panel is shown in Table 7-9. Which of the following tests is indicated in order to help identify compatible RBC units for transfusion?

A. Absorb the patient's serum with rabbit erythrocyte stroma.
B. Prewarm the patient's sample and reagents when doing the testing.
C. Absorb the patient's serum with his own enzyme-treated red cells.
D. Absorb the patient's serum with three enzyme-treated screening cells of complementary phenotype.
E. Elute the patient's red cells and use the eluate to identify compatible red cells.

Question 10: Warm-reactive autoantibodies are most commonly directed at which blood group system?

A. Rh.
B. ABO.
C. MNSs.
D. Ii.
E. LW.

Question 11: Which of the following statements regarding warm autoimmune hemolytic anemia is *true*?

A. The autoantibodies generally react with a specific antigen.
B. The DAT is positive and IgG is identified on the red cells.
C. Crossmatches are compatible.
D. Transfusion should be avoided as it exacerbates hemolysis.
E. Initial treatment includes therapeutic plasma exchange.

Question 12: A 65-year-old male patient presents to the emergency department with new-onset jaundice. He is easily fatigued and breathless on exertion. His pulse rate is 120 bpm, and his hematocrit is 16%. The patient states that he has never been transfused. Blood bank evalu-

Table 7-9.

Cell	D	C	c	E	e	f	V	C^w	K	k	Kp^a	Kp^b	Js^a	Js^b	Fy^a	Fy^b	Jk^a	Jk^b	Le^a	Le^b	P_1	M	N	S	s	Lu^a	Lu^b	Xg^a	IS	AHG	CC
I	+	+	0	0	+	0	0	0	+	+	0	+	0	+	+	+	+	+	0	+	+	+	+	+	+	0	+	0	0	3+	
II	+	0	+	+	0	0	0	0	0	+	0	+	0	+	0	+	+	0	+	0	+	+	+	0	+	0	+	+	0	3+	
1	+	+	0	0	+	0	0	0	+	+	0	+	0	+	+	+	+	0	+	0	+	+	+	+	+	0	+	+	0	3+	
2	+	+	+	0	+	0	0	+	0	+	0	+	0	+	+	+	+	0	+	0	+	+	0	0	+	0	+	0	0	3+	
3	+	0	+	+	0	0	0	0	+	+	0	+	0	+	0	+	0	+	0	+	+	+	+	0	0	0	+	+	0	3+	
4	+	0	+	0	+	+	0	0	0	+	0	+	0	+	+	0	+	+	0	0	+	0	+	0	0	0	+	0	0	3+	
5	0	0	+	+	+	+	0	0	+	+	0	+	0	+	+	0	+	+	0	+	+	+	+	+	+	0	+	+	0	3+	
6	0	0	+	0	+	+	0	0	0	+	0	+	0	+	+	+	+	+	0	+	+	0	+	0	+	0	+	0	0	3+	
7	0	0	+	0	+	+	0	0	+	+	0	+	0	+	0	+	0	+	+	0	+	+	+	+	+	0	+	+	0	3+	
8	0	0	+	0	+	+	0	0	0	+	0	+	0	+	+	0	+	+	+	0	0	+	0	0	+	+	+	0	0	3+	
9	0	0	+	0	+	+	0	0	0	+	0	+	0	+	+	+	+	+	+	0	0	+	+	+	0	0	+	+	0	3+	
10	0	0	+	0	+	+	0	0	0	+	0	+	0	+	0	0	+	0	0	0	+	0	+	0	+	0	+	0	0	3+	
Patient's cells																															

ation indicates that the patient has a serum antibody that reacts with all reagent red cells and that his DAT is reactive. Two RBC units are ordered for urgent transfusion. You recommend:

A. Infusion of a crystalloid or colloid because a crossmatch-compatible unit will not be available.
B. The transfusion of 2 units of crossmatch-incompatible blood.
C. Withholding transfusion unless absolutely necessary.
D. That a new sample be obtained for repeat testing.
E. That the blood bank continue to crossmatch units until compatible units are identified.

Question 13: A 75-year-old male patient is scheduled for surgical removal of a colon tumor. His hematocrit is 22%. A 2-unit red cell transfusion is ordered. Each unit should be:

A. Irradiated to prevent transfusion-associated graft-vs-host disease (TA-GVHD).
B. Transfused over 2 to 4 hours.
C. Infused through a blood warmer.
D. Leukocyte-reduced to prevent cytomegalovirus transmission.
E. Washed to prevent an allergic reaction.

Question 14: A 20-year-old male patient has an inherited bleeding disorder characterized by a prolonged bleeding time, a normal platelet count, a variably prolonged PTT, and a normal PT. The most likely diagnosis is:

A. Factor VII deficiency.
B. Factor VIII deficiency.
C. Factor IX deficiency.
D. von Willebrand disease (vWD).
E. Glanzmann's thrombasthenia.

Question 15: The patient presented in Question 14 requires wisdom tooth extraction. Which one of the following is the most appropriate approach?

A. Transfuse a Factor IX concentrate.
B. Transfuse recombinant Factor VIII.
C. Transfuse 2 units of FFP.
D. Transfuse 10 units of Cryoprecipitated AHF.
E. Confirm responsiveness to desmopressin (DDAVP) and treat just before the procedure.

Question 16: A 60-year-old male patient with esophageal cancer is admitted for a chemotherapy treatment. The patient has not been drinking adequate fluids and appears dehydrated. His physician ordered a 4-unit FFP transfusion. No laboratory tests are ordered. The FFP request is brought to you for evaluation. The best approach is to:

A. Release the FFP as ordered.
B. Cancel the order as inappropriate.
C. Order PT/PTT testing to determine the propriety of the order.
D. Release the FFP if it is determined that the patient is bleeding.
E. Consult with the physician and recommend crystalloid infusion.

Question 17: A 3-year-old Rh-negative female patient with a new diagnosis of acute lymphoblastic leukemia is admitted to the hospital for induction chemotherapy. As a consequence of her treatment, she is pancytopenic and requires red cell and platelet transfusions. Two days after an apheresis platelet transfusion, the blood bank realizes that the patient received an aliquot of platelets from an Rh-positive donor. The recommended course of action is to:

A. Do nothing; it is highly unlikely that the patient will mount an anti-D immune response.
B. Administer a single vial of Rh Immune Globulin (RhIG) by the intramuscular route.

C. Administer an appropriate dose of RhIG by the intravenous route.
D. Closely monitor the patient in order to detect the development of anti-D.
E. Continue to provide Rh-positive platelet products.

Question 18: A 20-year-old male trauma victim is admitted to the emergency department following a gunshot wound to the abdomen. He is alert but anxious. In addition, he is tachycardic and hypotensive and has cool, clammy skin. He is only transiently responsive to the infusion of 2 L of normal saline. Blood samples are drawn, including a sample for full serologic evaluation in the blood bank. The most appropriate course of action is to:

A. Order group O-negative, uncrossmatched red cells and begin transfusion.
B. Order group O-negative whole blood and begin transfusion.
C. Wait for the provision of group-specific, crossmatch-compatible blood and begin transfusion.
D. Infuse 2 additional liters of normal saline and assess his response, but hold transfusion.
E. Wait for the results of hemoglobin and hematocrit testing before proceeding with any red cell transfusions.

Question 19: The patient in Question 18 ultimately received 2 units of O-negative uncrossed blood. His genotype is CDe/CDe. The antibody that is most likely to develop is:

A. Anti-d.
B. Anti-c.
C. Anti-E.
D. Anti-e.
E. Anti-Wr^a.

Question 20: With regard to transfusion of patients with sickle cell disease (SCD) which is *true*?

A. Unlike patients transfused for thalassemia, SCD patients are not at risk of developing iron overload.
B. Formation of rare antibodies is common in this patient group.
C. Extravascular hemolytic transfusion reactions are more common than intravascular hemolysis.
D. Units for transfusion should be irradiated.
E. Development of autoantibodies is rare.

Question 21: All of the following are indications for the use of leukocyte-reduced (LR) blood components *except*:

A. To prevent and/or decrease the incidence of alloimmunization to HLA antigens in chronically transfused patients.
B. To prevent febrile nonhemolytic transfusion reactions.
C. To prevent reactivation of endogenous viral infections such as human immunodeficiency virus (HIV) and cytomegalovirus (CMV).
D. To prevent/and or decrease the incidence of transfusion-associated CMV transmission.
E. To prevent and/or decrease the incidence of alloimmunization to HLA antigens in nonhepatic solid-organ transplantation.

Question 22: Which of the following is an established indication for the use of LR blood components?

A. To guard against the immunomodulatory effect of transfusion.
B. To prevent TA-GVHD.
C. To prevent transmission of variant Creutzfeldt-Jakob disease (vCJD) or other prion diseases.
D. To prevent transfusion-related acute lung injury (TRALI).
E. To prevent CMV transmission.

Question 23: Mucosal bleeding is a characteristic of all of the following *except*:

A. Decreased platelet count.

B. A defect in platelet function.
C. vWD.
D. Hemophilia A.
E. Uremia.

Question 24: The most effective component for treating a patient with fibrinogen deficiency is:

A. FFP.
B. Platelets.
C. Fresh Whole Blood.
D. Cryoprecipitated AHF (cryo).
E. Plasma Frozen Within 24 Hours After Phlebotomy.

Question 25: A granulocyte transfusion may be indicated if the patient has:

A. Leukemia.
B. An absolute granulocyte count of 500/µL or less.
C. CMV infection.
D. A localized fungal infection.
E. A leukocyte count of 1000/µL.

Question 26: Which of the following patients is the most appropriate candidate for granulocyte transfusion?

A. 10-year-old child with erythema infectiosum caused by parvovirus B19 and a granulocyte count of 1500/µL.
B. A patient with sepsis on intravenous tobramycin therapy whose granulocyte count has increased from 500/µL to 1400/µL.
C. Persistent fever and a granulocyte count of 450/µL following a 2-day treatment with intravenous gentamicin.
D. Progenitor cell transplant recipient with a granulocyte count of 200/µL.

E. A 25-year-old male patient with fluctuating high fever and a granulocyte count of 4500/µL.

Question 27: Granulocyte transfusions are most effective against which type of infections?

A. Bacterial.
B. Viral.
C. Parasitic.
D. Prion.
E. Fungal.

Question 28: All of the following are indications for the transfusion of washed RBCs *except*:

A. Paroxysmal nocturnal hemoglobinuria (PNH).
B. Maternal red cells required for an infant with hemolytic disease of the fetus and newborn (HDFN) due to a high-incidence antibody.
C. A patient with IgG anti-IgA.
D. The only unit of blood available for large volume transfusion of a neonate is a 21-day-old, irradiated unit.
E. The patient has multiple serious allergic reactions despite premedication with steroids and an antihistamine.

Question 29: A 62-year-old female patient is admitted to the hospital with chief complaints of fatigue, easy bruising of 2 weeks duration, and a sharp localized headache in the left temporal region. A complete blood count shows a hematocrit of 29%, a white cell count of 28,000/µL with 74% blast cells, and a platelet count of 6000/µL. A marrow biopsy is significant for hypercellularity, 95% myeloblasts, and a marked reduction of megakaryocytes. The patient has no history of blood transfusions or pregnancies. The physical examination is significant for several fresh hemorrhages noted on fundoscopic examination. While waiting for the results of definitive diagnostic studies, the most appropriate approach is to transfuse the patient with:

A. Cryoprecipitated AHF.
B. HLA-matched single-donor platelets (Apheresis Platelets).
C. Randomly chosen single-donor platelets (Apheresis Platelets) or pooled platelet concentrates.
D. Granulocyte concentrates.
E. Two units of compatible RBCs.

Question 30: A 17-year-old male Olympic-grade swimmer with newly diagnosed acute lymphoblastic leukemia is receiving prophylactic platelet transfusion for a platelet count of 9000/µL. Approximately 10 minutes after the start of the transfusion, the patient's oxygen saturation drops from 98% to 65%, and the blood pressure drops from 120/60 mm Hg to 80/40 mm Hg. The patient is visibly struggling for breath and rapidly deteriorating. Emergency intubation is required upon which copious amounts of frothy edema fluid are seen to exit from the endotracheal tube. The most likely explanation for the patient's symptoms is:

A. Transfusion-associated circulatory overload.
B. Anaphylactic transfusion reaction.
C. Transfusion-related sepsis.
D. Symptoms related to underlying disease.
E. TRALI.

ANSWERS

Question 1: D

Explanation:

- All of the answers listed are associated with less than optimal platelet transfusion increments. Neutropenic fever and sepsis are associated with platelet activation and utilization. They may also result in myelosuppression, blunting the marrow's ability to compensate for ongoing thrombocytopenia. In contrast, DIC is associated with platelet consumption and splenomegaly is associated with platelet sequestration. Both may result in apparent nonresponsiveness to platelets. Of note, however, all of these processes are associated with much slower kinetics of platelet loss in comparison to immune-mediated clearance.
- When transfusion recipients fail to respond to platelets, as evidenced by a platelet count obtained in close proximity to transfusion (10 minutes to 1 hour), the most likely cause of the nonresponsiveness is immune-mediated destruction.
- Nonimmune causes of platelet refractoriness are typically associated with an initial increase in platelet count followed by inadequate 24-hour posttransfusion platelet counts.
- The antibodies most commonly implicated in immune-mediated platelet refractoriness are directed against Class I HLA antigens (*A* and *B* loci). Antibodies of this type are responsible for nearly all cases of verified immune-mediated refractoriness, with rare cases attributable to antibodies directed against platelet-specific glycoprotein antigens.
- Platelet refractoriness most commonly occurs in those patients who are chronically transfused with cellular blood components (platelets, RBCs), secondary to HLA antigen exposure. Oncology patients who receive myeloablative chemotherapy, with or without hematopoietic progenitor cell transplantation, are among the most common platelet refractory patients.

Question 2: B

Explanation:

- The best way to determine if a patient is likely to have immune-mediated platelet refractoriness is to closely follow posttransfusion platelet counts. As previously mentioned, platelet counts obtained 10 minutes to 1 hour after transfusion are of greatest utility, as immune-mediated platelet destruction will be demonstrable in this time frame. A screen for platelet-reactive antibodies, or a specific test for HLA antibodies, may then be performed on those patients who exhibit poor 10-minute to 1-hour platelet count increments.
- In the management of platelet refractoriness, randomly selected apheresis platelets do not offer any advantage over randomly selected pooled whole blood-derived platelet concentrates, and neither is recommended as a choice for patient management. When no other suitable product is available, pooled platelets may offer the advantage of providing greater opportunity for donor-recipient compatibility.
- HLA-matched platelets:
    - Apheresis platelets that have been HLA-typed and matched to the recipient's HLA type have been the classic approach to provide platelet support for the refractory patient. However, the ability to provide closely matched platelets depends on the relative prevalence of a patient's HLA type in any particular donor population. Because the HLA antigen system is highly polymorphic, it may be difficult to identify and procure an appropriately HLA antigen-matched apheresis platelet product.
- Crossmatched platelets:
    - An alternative to HLA matching is platelet crossmatching. This technique, similar to standard red cell crossmatching, attempts to identify apheresis platelet products that fail to react with a patient's serum antibodies. A variety of different immunoassays have been used to detect these HLA antigen-antibody interactions. Platelet crossmatching provides benefits to patients similar to those achieved through the provision of HLA-matched platelets. In some respects, crossmatching is superior to HLA matching, as it provides HLA- and human-platelet-antigen-compatible platelets, and suitable products may be more readily available than when HLA matching is used.

- Antigen-negative platelets:
  ○ Recently, some centers are identifying the exact HLA specificities of a refractory patient's HLA antibodies (using bead-based assays). Once specificity is determined, apheresis platelets can be identified that lack the antigen(s) recognized by the identified antibodies. Platelets selected by this method provide at least as good a response as most HLA-matched platelets. An additional benefit is that "antigen-negative" platelets may be more readily available than HLA-matched platelets, as the units are chosen from a larger available stock of platelets.
- Leukocyte reduction may prevent or forestall the platelet refractory state but would not be expected to have any effect on managing the platelet refractory state.
- Cellular blood component irradiation prevents transfusion-associated graft-vs-host disease (TA-GVHD) but is not an important means to either prevent or manage the platelet refractory state.

Question 3: E

Explanation:

- A variety of hemostatic abnormalities can occur in association with complex surgical procedures, but in those patients with drain outputs exceeding 200 mL/hour, a surgically correctable lesion is the most likely cause of excess bleeding.
- Other choices:
  ○ Although the patient's postoperative platelet count is low and these platelets may be functionally abnormal (secondary to bypass pump activation), it is unlikely that these factors would account for the volume of bleeding experienced by the patient. In addition, it is likely that the patient would also bleed from sites other than the primary surgical site (eg, mucosal bleeding, oozing from venipuncture sites).
  ○ Patients who suffer extensive tissue injury, including those accompanying elective surgical procedures, are at risk for DIC. However, that does not appear to be the issue in this patient's case, as evidenced by near-normal PT/PTT values and platelet count and only minimally elevated fibrin degradation product levels.

- The patient does have a mild, generalized coagulation factor deficiency as evidenced by slightly prolonged PT and PTT values. PT prolongations of less than 1.5 times the mid range of normal, or activated partial thromboplastin time (aPTT) prolongations of less than 2 times the upper limit of normal are unlikely to be a cause of significant postoperative bleeding.

Question 4: A

Explanation:

- The patient in this case has sustained a severe blood loss and has evidence of impending hemorrhagic shock (hypotension, tachycardia). In patients who experience significant bleeding, the first course of therapy is to replenish intravascular volume. This is generally accomplished using crystalloid (eg, normal saline) or colloid (eg, 5% albumin) volume-expanding solutions.
- Although variable from patient to patient, when one sustains a blood loss exceeding 25% of total blood volume, RBCs will oftentimes be required (to maintain oxygen-carrying capacity) in addition to volume expanders. As such, Whole Blood or RBCs are indicated. In this patient's case, Whole Blood could prove to be particularly useful as it provides both oxygen-carrying capacity and volume replenishment in the same package. However, Whole Blood is not readily available in most centers because of component preparation (RBCs, Platelets, FFP).
- Although the patient has a history of alcoholism and may suffer from associated hepatic dysfunction, there is no evidence that the patient has a coagulation factor deficiency. As such, FFP would not be indicated at this time. If, however, the patient continues to bleed and there is laboratory evidence of a coagulation factor deficiency (prolonged PT/PTT), then FFP would be indicated.

Question 5: D

Explanation:

- The patient has an extremely low platelet count (consistent with ITP) and a warm-reactive autoantibody. The patient, with coincident ITP and autoimmune hemolytic anemia, has Evans syndrome.
- TTP and acute leukemia would both be in this patient's differential diagnosis and would need to be ruled out. On clinical grounds alone, both of these diagnoses would be less likely given the fact that, aside from bleeding, the patient is asymptomatic. From a laboratory perspective, examination of a peripheral blood smear would be useful. The peripheral smear of a patient with Evans syndrome might demonstrate giant platelets (with ITP) and spherocytes (with autoimmune hemolytic anemia). However, schistocytes (with TTP) and blast cells (with acute leukemia) would be absent. If a diagnosis of acute leukemia was seriously entertained, a marrow examination would be mandatory. This would not be indicated, however, for any of the other diagnostic choices.
- The patient is anemic. To determine if this is at least in part caused by active hemolysis, appropriate additional testing would be required. This could include a reticulocyte count and lactate dehydrogenase, bilirubin (total, conjugated), and haptoglobin tests.

Question 6: A

Explanation:

- The patient's likely diagnosis is Evans syndrome, coincident ITP, and autoimmune hemolytic anemia. He is young and, other than his nosebleed, is asymptomatic. Transfusion is not indicated at this time.
- Platelet transfusion generally is not indicated in ITP, as the transfused platelets are almost instantaneously removed from the circulation by immune-mediated clearance. Platelet transfusion should be reserved to treat significant bleeding episodes though their utility, even in this setting, is questionable. Fortunately, patients with ITP

CLINICAL TRANSFUSION PRACTICE   245

do not often experience severe bleeding episodes, even with extremely low platelet counts.
- RBC transfusion is rarely indicated in asymptomatic patients with hemoglobin >7.0 g/dL who do not have a history of coronary or cerebral vascular insufficiency. The patient should be monitored with consideration given to transfusion if the hemoglobin is rapidly dropping or there are signs and symptoms of inadequate oxygen delivery that are not responsive to conservative therapy (O_2 therapy and limiting exertion).
- Therapeutic plasmapheresis is the treatment of choice for TTP. It would not be indicated for a patient with Evans syndrome.

Question 7: E

Explanation:

- DIC is a syndrome characterized by excessive protease activity in the blood, which results in soluble fibrin formation and accelerated fibrinolysis. DIC is an epiphenomenon, almost always caused by a serious underlying illness. Clinical conditions that may be associated with DIC include, but are not limited to, sepsis, trauma, organ destruction such as severe pancreatitis, malignancy, amniotic fluid embolism, vascular abnormalities, Kasabach-Merritt Syndrome, severe hepatic failure, and hemolytic transfusion reactions.
- The bleeding that may accompany DIC results from the depletion of coagulation factors, fibrinogen, and platelets that accompany this prothrombotic process. Fibrin degradation products are almost always detectable and result from fibrinolysis.
- The best screening tests for DIC are measurements of fibrin degradation products (elevated), PT (prolonged), fibrinogen level (decreased), and platelet count (decreased). Fibrin degradation products may also be elevated in trauma, following recent surgery, and with venous thromboembolism. Therefore careful attention to the patient's underlying condition is necessary when interpreting the results of these tests.
- Although each of the alternate choices is associated with thrombocytopenia (except HSP) and the possibility of bleeding, the additional laboratory abnormalities found in DIC are not routinely seen.

- Posttransfusion purpura is a severe platelet destructive process resulting from platelet antibody formation following transfusion. HSP is a systemic vasculitis characterized by nonthrombocytopenic purpuric lesions, transient arthralgias or arthritis, colicky abdominal pain, and nephritis. HSP most commonly occurs in children 3 to 7 years of age, often following an upper respiratory infection.

Question 8: E

Explanation:

- The patient in Question 7 has a diagnosis of DIC. He has an underlying clinical condition (pancreatitis) associated with DIC and a characteristic constellation of laboratory findings. He is actively bleeding and has severe anemia. Transfusion in this setting is justified.
- The primary therapy for DIC is to treat the underlying illness responsible for the coagulopathy. However, sometimes treating the causative disease itself is not enough to prevent serious bleeding or thrombosis. In such cases, treatment of the coagulopathy can be lifesaving.
- The indications for the treatment of DIC depend on the nature and treatability of the underlying disease and the severity of the coagulopathy. The mainstay of treatment is replacement therapy.
- The patient in this case has a severe coagulopathy requiring treatment with a combination of blood components. FFP is indicated to replenish depleted coagulation factors. Cryoprecipitated AHF may also be required depending on the rate of fibrinogen consumption and the patient's response (both clinical and as measured by fibrinogen level) to FFP transfusion. Platelet transfusion is indicated to counteract ongoing consumption. Replacement therapy is generally indicated for those patients who are actively bleeding, may be undergoing invasive procedures, or have a risk for bleeding. Replacement therapy should not be provided on the basis of laboratory values alone.
- Finally, red cell transfusions will almost certainly be needed to treat the patient's severe anemia.
- Pharmacologic inhibitors of coagulation and/or fibrinolysis represent an adjunct treatment option. These agents include heparin, antithrombin III concentrate, and recombinant tissue factor pathway

inhibitor, among others. However, the use of these agents remains controversial and/or still under investigation. Their use should probably be reserved for patients with clinical evidence of thrombosis.

Question 9: D

Explanation:

- The patient's history and laboratory findings are that of a warm autoimmune hemolytic anemia. The possibility exists that an underlying alloantibody could be present, a finding reported to occur in 13% to 40% of cases where an autoantibody is present.
- Rabbit erythrocyte stroma can be used to absorb cold autoantibodies, especially anti-I and anti-IH, as these antigens are present on rabbit red cells. Some alloantibodies, including anti-B, anti-D, anti-E, and anti-Vel, have been reported to be absorbed by rabbit erythrocyte stroma. A warm autoantibody would not be absorbed.
- Prewarming is used to prevent the binding of cold autoantibodies to red cells during collection, transport, and testing of samples. The patient's sample is collected and maintained at 37 C. During testing, the red cells, serum, and saline used to wash the red cells are warmed to 37 C. By doing this, cold-reacting autoantibodies cannot bind and fix complement and give positive test results. Some clinically significant cold-reactive alloantibodies such as some examples of anti-N and alloanti-P may not be detected with this technique; therefore, the prewarming technique should be used with caution.
- Absorption studies are used when it is necessary to separate two or more antibodies. Absorptions are most commonly used to remove autoantibodies from a sample so that it may be evaluated for the presence of alloantibodies.
- Autoabsorption uses the patient's enzyme-treated red cells to remove autoantibodies from the patient's serum, leaving alloantibodies behind. The resulting absorbate can then be used to identify alloantibodies and to crossmatch units. Enzyme-treated red cells are used because enzyme treatment enhances autoantibody binding. This method is applicable only to patients who have not been transfused within the preceding 3 months, because the presence of allogeneic red cells from recent transfusions can result in the absorption of alloantibodies.

- Alloabsorption involves the use of three reagent red cells of complementary phenotype to absorb the autoantibody while leaving the alloantibody behind. Alloabsorption is more complex than autoabsorption and is used when a patient has been recently transfused. Some laboratories find it desirable to manipulate the phenotype of the absorbing allogeneic cells by using enzymes to destroy MNS and Duffy system antigens and dithiothreitol to destroy Kell system antigens. The three cells are also selected to have complementary Kidd phenotypes.
    - In the first tube, patient's serum is absorbed with R_1R_1 (DCe/DCe) cells. This will remove the autoantibody as well as anti-D, anti-C, and anti-e but will leave anti-c, anti-E, and any other antibodies to antigens for which the absorbing cell is negative.
    - In the second tube, R_2R_2 (DcE/DcE) cells are used. This will remove anti-D, anti-c, and anti-E, leaving anti-C and anti-e as well as antibodies directed at any antigen for which the cell is negative.
    - In the third tube, rr (ce/ce) cells are used. This will remove anti-c and anti-e but will leave anti-D, anti-C, and anti-E as well as antibodies directed at any antigen for which the cell is negative.
    - The alloabsorbtion yields three absorbed sera, which are then tested in parallel against antibody screening cells and/or panel cells. The autoantibody-free absorbed sera will exhibit a differential pattern of reactivity that allows identification of alloantibody specificity.
    - The absorbed sera may also be used to perform crossmatches.
- Elution is a technique used to remove bound antibody from red cells. The eluate (antibody in solution) is tested against antibody screening cells and panel cells to identify the specificity of autoantibodies or alloantibodies. It is not used to crossmatch RBCs as alloantibodies may be present in the patient's serum that are not attached to red cells in the patient's circulation.

Question 10: A

Explanation:

- Most warm autoantibodies are broadly reactive and are directed at common epitopes within the Rh system.

- Warm autoantibody specificity may also be directed at antigens in the Kell, Kidd, MNSs, ABO, Vel, and LW blood group systems.
- As shown in Table 7-10, autoimmune hemolytic anemia can be any of the following:
  - Warm autoimmune hemolytic anemia (WAIHA).
  - Cold autoimmune hemolytic anemia (CAIHA) or cold agglutinin syndrome (CAS).
  - Paroxysmal cold hemoglobinuria (PCH).

Table 7-10.

Autoantibody	WAIHA Warm auto-antibodies	CAIHA or CAS Cold auto-antibodies	PCH Biphasic hemolysin
% of AIHA	$\cong$ 80%	$\cong$ 18%	$\cong$ 2%
Immunoglobulin	IgG	IgM	IgG
Optimum temperature of reactivity	37 C	4 C	4 C followed by 37 C
Immune destruction	Extravascular	Extravascular	Intravascular
Most common specificity	Antigens of the Rh system	Anti-I	Anti-P
DAT+ due to:	1. IgG: 30 to 40% 2. IgG + C3: 40 to 50% 3. C3: 10%	C3	C3 during attacks; DAT− in between attacks

AIHA = autoimmune hemolytic anemia; WAIHA = warm AIHA; CAIHA = cold AIHA; CAS = cold agglutinin syndrome; PCH = paroxysmal hemoglobinuria; DAT = direct antiglobulin test; IgG = immune globulin G; C3 and C3d = complement component.

Question 11: B

Explanation:

- Warm autoimmune hemolytic anemia may be idiopathic, but cases are also commonly seen in association with a variety of clinical conditions including leukemias/lymphomas, autoimmune disorders, and chronic inflammatory conditions. A large number of medications have also been implicated.
- Serologically, warm-reactive autoantibodies are broadly reactive with all reagent red cells tested (positive indirect antiglobulin test) and the patient's own red cells (positive DAT). These are typically IgG antibodies.
- With strongly reactive warm autoantibodies, the crossmatched RBC units are invariably incompatible. However, this does not mean that transfusion is contraindicated.
- There is little evidence that transfused red cells are more rapidly removed from the patient's circulation than their own red cells *unless* the patient has an underlying blood group alloantibody. The evaluation of the patient's sample for alloantibodies (underlying the autoantibodies) is a primary blood bank concern.
- IgG-sensitized red cells are removed from the circulation by extravascular mechanisms, primarily by the spleen. Partial phagocytosis of circulating red cells, by macrophages, results in spherocytic red cells.
- Splenectomy, intravenous immune globulin, steroids, and other immunosuppressive agents represent the most common therapies for warm autoimmune hemolytic anemia. Plasma exchange has not been proven to be effective.

Question 12: B

Explanation:

- The patient in this case presentation is severely symptomatically anemic and in urgent need of oxygen-carrying capacity. He is at high risk for ischemic tissue injury and will likely not benefit sufficiently

from either crystalloid or colloid infusion. The transfusion of 2 units of crossmatch-incompatible blood is warranted.
- It is unlikely that this patient's apparent brisk hemolysis will be exacerbated by the transfusion of incompatible units of blood for two primary reasons. First, there is no convincing evidence that transfused red cells are hemolyzed more quickly than the patient's own red cells or that transfusion "feeds the fire" unless the patient has underlying blood group alloantibodies. Second, it is highly unlikely that a male patient who has never been transfused would have alloantibodies that could put him at risk for delayed hemolysis (beyond that associated with the autoantibody).
- Warm-reactive autoantibodies typically react with all red cells tested, and all crossmatches are incompatible.
- There is no reason to believe that additional crossmatching would result in the identification of a compatible unit of blood. In reality, this would likely only serve to delay transfusion.
- Similarly, a new blood sample is unlikely to be informative in any way. Infusion of a crystalloid or colloid is not advised as primary therapy as the patient needs an increase in oxygen-carrying capacity.
- See also the explanation for Question 11.

Question 13: B

Explanation:

- Once an RBC unit is issued by the blood bank, it should be transfused as soon as possible. Although the desirable rate of infusion depends on a number of factors (eg, patient's blood volume, cardiac status, and hemodynamic condition), 4 hours is the maximum duration for an infusion. If additional time will be required (eg, as in a patient with severe congestive heart failure), the blood bank should split the unit.
- Red cells can be modified in a number of ways in order to meet the needs of transfusion recipients. It is unlikely that an otherwise healthy patient with colon cancer would benefit from irradiated, leukocyte-reduced, or washed red cells, as colon cancer would not be a general indication for their use.
- Blood warmers are reserved for two primary clinical situations:

- Patients who rapidly receive multiple units of refrigerated blood; this can cause or contribute to hypothermia with attendant consequences (eg, cardiac arrhythmias, coagulopathy).
- Patients with CAS for whom exposure to refrigerated blood could incite or exacerbate a hemolytic episode.

Question 14: D

Explanation:

- vWD, one of the most common inherited bleeding disorders, is caused by a deficiency or abnormality of von Willebrand factor (vWF). As a result, platelets do not adhere normally to damaged endothelial surfaces, and primary hemostasis is impaired.
- The prevalence of vWD is 1% to 2%, but this may be an underestimation because of difficulties in the laboratory diagnosis of the disease. The standard laboratory workup for vWD includes five tests: vWF activity (ristocetin cofactor activity), vWF antigen, Factor VIII activity, bleeding time, and vWF multimeric analysis. The PTT may be prolonged, as Factor VIII circulates with vWF and may be variably reduced, but the PT and platelet count are normal.
- The laboratory tests used to diagnose vWD should easily rule out Factor-VIII- or Factor-IX-deficient states. A Factor VII deficiency would be expected to prolong the PT, not the PTT.
- Glanzmann's thrombasthenia, a rare hemorrhagic disorder, is caused by a deficiency of platelet glycoprotein IIb/IIIa. This results in an inability of platelets to aggregate in a normal manner. The bleeding time is prolonged, but other tests used to diagnose vWD would not be abnormal. The diagnosis of Glanzmann's thrombasthenia is usually suspected after platelet aggregometry studies.
- The platelet-specific antigen system is described in Table 7-14. Patients with congenital absence of platelet glycoproteins can develop antibodies to these antigens.

Table 7-14.

HPA	Carrier	Receptor	Disease Association with Congenital Absence of Glycoproteins
HPA-1, -4, -6, -7, -8, -10, -11, -14, -16	GPIIIa	Fibrinogen, fibronectin, vitronectin	Glanzmann's thromb-asthenia
HPA-3, -9	GPIIb		
HPA-2, -12	GPIb	vWF*	Bernard-Soulier syndrome

*GPIb/IX/V is a receptor for vWF and congenital absence is associated with Bernard-Soulier syndrome.
HPA = human platelet antigen; GPIIIa = glycoprotein IIIa; vWF = von Willebrand factor.

Question 15: E

Explanation:

- The patient in Question 14 has vWD and will require therapy before wisdom tooth extraction. The type of therapy chosen to prevent or control bleeding in persons with vWD is dependent on the type and severity of vWD, the severity of the hemostatic challenge, and the nature of the bleeding or potential bleeding.
- Therapeutic approaches include increasing plasma vWF thru desmopressin-stimulated release of endogenous endothelial cell vWF stores, administering factor concentrates to replace vWF, and use of agents that promote hemostasis and wound healing but do not alter plasma vWF levels.
- DDAVP (1-deamino-8-D-arginine vasopressin, a synthetic vasopressin analog) is the treatment of choice for most patients with vWD. DDAVP stimulates the release of vWF from endogenous stores (primarily capillary endothelial cells) and avoids the need to transfuse factor concentrates such as Humate-P (CSL Behring, King of Prussia, PA)

and Alphanate SD/HT (Grifols USA, Los Angeles, CA) or Koate DVI (Talecris Biotherapeutics USA, Research Triangle Park, NC).
  - DDAVP is available in intranasal and intravenous forms. To ensure that a patient will benefit from its use, a trial infusion is performed before any operative procedure in which its use is contemplated. If a patient responds appropriately, with adequate increases in vWF activity and antigen levels, then DDAVP may be administered just before surgery.
  - Standard dosing for desmopressin is 0.3 µg/kg given intravenously in 30 to 50 mL of normal saline over 30 minutes. Peak increments in Factor VIII and vWF are seen 30 to 90 min after the infusion. Nasal administration of high-dose desmopressin acetate (Stimate, CSL Behring) is often effective for minor bleeding, but intravenous administration is the preferred route for prophylaxis of surgical bleeding.
- A Factor IX concentrate would provide no therapeutic benefit for a patient with vWD. FFP, on the other hand, does contain all plasma factors, including vWF. However, 2 units would not be a therapeutic dose.

Question 16: E

Explanation:

- In general, FFP is indicated as a source of coagulation factors to treat bleeding patients who have factor deficiencies, as evidenced by prolonged PT and/or PTT values.
- Even if it is determined that this patient is bleeding (or at risk for bleeding, as with an invasive procedure), there is no evidence of a coagulation factor deficiency.
- When an unusual order for a blood component is received, the best general strategy is a direct interaction with the ordering physician before taking any action. If it is determined that FFP is only being ordered as a source of volume replacement, then use of a crystalloid solution should be recommended.
- FFP is indicated to treat bleeding or to prepare for an invasive procedure or surgery in the following:
  - Patients with multiple coagulation factor deficiencies (indicated by PT >1.5 × midrange of normal, or aPTT >2 × upper limit of nor-

mal); examples include liver disease, DIC, and coagulopathy secondary to massive transfusion.
- Patients with an isolated factor deficiency for which specific therapy is unavailable (eg, Factors II, V, X, XI).
- Patients requiring emergency reversal of warfarin therapy, when medical necessity does not allow time for reversal by vitamin K. Prothrombin Complex Concentrates and recombinant Factor VIIa are more effective than FFP for reversal of warfarin and are recommended for those situations where complete and rapid reversal are warranted.
- Contraindications for transfusion of FFP:
  - Prophylactic use in massively transfused or cardiac surgery patients.
  - Volume expansion.
  - Nutritional support.
  - Bleeding with no evidence of factor deficiency.
  - Increased PT/PTT alone with or without liver disease.

Question 17: C

Explanation:

- The Rh-negative individual who is transfused with Rh-positive cellular blood components (red cells, platelets) is at risk for developing an anti-D immune response. Although there are many factors that contribute to the absolute risk with any exposure, the volume of Rh-positive red cells is probably the most important factor. Currently available apheresis platelets generally have only trace amounts of red cell contamination; however, even trace amounts may be immunogenic in immunologically intact patients.
- Although the risk of this patient developing an anti-D immune response is low (she is profoundly immunosuppressed and was exposed to a very low volume of Rh-positive red cells), she is at risk and should receive appropriate treatment.
- RhIG is human anti-D primarily used to prevent maternal sensitization to the D antigen. Another important application is the prevention of anti-D formation in Rh-negative females of child-bearing potential who are inadvertently exposed to Rh-positive red cells.

- Preparations of RhIG are available for either intramuscular (eg, RhoGAM, Ortho-Clinical Diagnostics, Raritan NJ) or intravenous administration (eg, WinRho, Baxter Healthcare, Deerfield, IL). One standard dose (single vial) of intramuscular RhIG will prevent sensitization to the D antigen with exposures of up to 15 mL of Rh-positive red cells. This product could be administered to the child in this case but would not be the best choice because of the intramuscular injection that would be required. Aside from being painful, an intramuscular injection in a thrombocytopenic patient could result in bleeding complications.
- The preferred route for RhIG administration in this case is the intravenous route, and the appropriate dose (for this indication) is 18 µg (90 IU)/mL of Rh-positive red cells transfused. If the Rh-positive platelets that the child received were devoid of any obvious red cell content (ie, <1 mL of red cells in the product), then coverage of a 1-mL Rh-positive red cell exposure would be adequate therapy (ie, provide ~100 IU of RhIG).

Question 18: A

Explanation:

- In the trauma setting, initial fluid resuscitation is accomplished with high-volume crystalloid (colloid, less commonly) solutions. As a general rule, hemodynamic normalization and clinical stabilization following a 1- to 2-L infusion usually indicates that a patient has not sustained a significant blood loss and that future blood loss will be minimal.
- The patient in this case failed to respond to crystalloid infusion and has clinical evidence of impending hemorrhagic shock. This indicates that the patient has likely suffered a massive hemorrhage or that blood loss is rapid and ongoing. This is a patient in critical need of extra oxygen-carrying capacity who should receive emergency transfusion.
- Although it is standard practice to perform complete serologic testing (ie, ABO grouping, antibody screening, crossmatching) before transfusion, this may not be possible in emergency situations because of time limitations. Full compatibility testing will take at

least 30 to 45 minutes, which may be too long for the patient in critical need of transfusion.
- Whole blood has the benefit of providing oxygen-carrying capacity and volume. As such, it is an ideal replacement fluid for massively bleeding patients. However, there are two potential drawbacks to its use: 1) whole blood is generally not available as whole blood donations are routinely fractionated into therapeutic blood components, and 2) whole blood, because it contains a significant volume of plasma, should be group-specific to avoid problems with plasma antibody incompatibilities.
- The best choice in this case is to obtain and transfuse group O red cells as quickly as possible. In many centers it is common practice to emergently transfuse male trauma victims with group O-positive red cells in order to preserve group O-negative units for females of childbearing potential. This has proven to be a safe and efficacious clinical practice.

Question 19: B

Explanation:

- The patient received a group O-negative, uncrossmatched red cell transfusion.
- The genotype of this component is most likely *ce/ce* or *r/r*.
- The genotype of the recipient is *CDe/CDe*.
- The antibody most likely to develop is anti-c.
- Other choices:
  - Anti-d does not exist.
  - It is unlikely that the recipient was exposed to the E antigen.
  - The recipient is positive for the e antigen. He will not develop anti-e.
  - The development of anti-Wr^a is unlikely because it is a low-frequency blood group antigen of relatively low immunogenicity.

Question 20: C

Explanation:

- Transfusions are indicated in patients with SCD for:
  - Reduction in morbidity and improvement of quality of life.
  - Prevention of complications, which include:
    - Primary stroke.
    - Neurologic injury.
    - Acute chest syndrome.
    - Chronic pain syndrome.
    - End-stage organ failure.
- Complications of transfusion in SCD include the following:
  - Iron overload: Automated RBC exchange may prevent or dramatically slow down iron accumulation. Any patient who is frequently transfused for anemia unrelated to bleeding is at risk of developing iron overload;
  - Alloimmunization: Patients with SCD have the highest rates of alloimmunizaton of any patient group.
  - Hemolytic transfusion reactions: These reactions are typically of the delayed extravascular type and are caused by IgG antibodies.
  - Autoantibody formation: Alloimmunization is associated with an increased incidence of RBC autoantibodies.
- As a result of developing multiple alloantibodies, patients with SCD use 20% of the units stocked by rare donor registries. Even in this group of patients, antibodies to high frequency antigens are uncommon.
- A lack of phenotypic compatibility is the major contributing factor for alloimmunization.
  - The majority of blood bank donors are of European ethnicity.
  - The majority of patients with SCD are of African ethnicity.
  - Interracial frequencies of RBC antigens are indicated in Table 7-20.
- Transfusion of blood phenotypically matched for common clinically significant antigens greatly reduces the incidence of alloimmunization, but for some institutions this may not be feasible because of the lack of availability of desired phenotypes. Common practice for nonalloimmunized patients is to perform a full patient phenotype before transfusion and then match for the C, E, and K antigens. Once

Table 7-20.

	Frequencies (%)	
Red Cell Phenotype	European-American (Majority of Blood Bank Donors)	African-American (Majority of SCD Patients)
D	85	92
C	70	33
E	30	20
K	9	2
Jk^b	72	39

SCD = sickle cell disease.

the patient exhibits alloimmunization, more extended phenotype matching is recommended (eg, Fy, Jk, and S antigens)
- Identification of phenotyped, matched units requires serologic screening of large numbers of units and is labor and time intensive. In the future, large scale genotype screening by microarray-based methodologies may provide a more efficient manner for identifying suitable donor units.

Question 21: C

Explanation:

See Question 22.

Question 22: E

Explanation for Questions 21 and 22:

- CMV is a leukocyte-associated virus. LR blood components are effective in preventing CMV transmission. Other established indications of LR are:
  - To prevent alloimmunization to HLA and leukocyte antigens in patients without alloimmunization.
  - To prevent febrile nonhemolytic transfusion reactions.
- Although numerous studies indicate that leukocyte reduction reduces transfusion-related immunomodulation (TRIM), avoidance of TRIM is not yet considered an established indication for leukocyte reduction. Nonestablished but potential benefits of universal leukocyte reduction include:
  - A decrease in the incidence of cancer recurrence, postoperative infections, postoperative morbidity, and length of hospital stay.
  - Prevention of vCJD or other prion disease transmission.
  - Prevention of human T-cell lymphotropic virus, types I and II; Epstein-Barr virus; human herpesvirus-8; or other unknown infectious agent transmission.
- Leukocyte-reduced cellular products may be of value for patients who have experienced TRALI reactions while the evaluation is still in process.
- Leukocyte reduction does not prevent reactivation of endogenous HIV and/or CMV.
- LR will not prevent TA-GVHD. At this time, irradiation is the only acceptable means of preventing TA-GVHD.

Question 23: D

Explanation:

- Mucosal bleeding may result from a quantitative or a qualitative platelet abnormality but is not characteristic of coagulation factor deficiencies, including Factor VIII (hemophilia A).

- vWF supports platelet adhesion to damaged endothelial surfaces, playing a major functional role in primary hemostasis. A quantitative or qualitative deficiency of vWF is associated with platelet-type mucosal bleeding.
- Coagulation factor deficiencies are more commonly associated with deep tissue bleeding (eg, joints, muscles) and may occur several hours after the inciting trauma.
- Abnormal hemostasis is commonly seen in chronic renal disease, although the pathogenesis remains obscure. Qualitative abnormalities of vWF, evidenced by decreased ristocetin cofactor activity, are seen with the possibility of associated mucosal bleeding. Cryoprecipitated AHF and DDAVP may prove effective in treating bleeding episodes accompanying uremia, though it is also important to correct the underlying disorder.

Question 24: D

Explanation:

- Cryo (Cryoprecipitated AHF) is the cold-insoluble portion of plasma that precipitates when FFP is thawed at 1-6 C. A unit of cryo has a volume of 10 to 15 mL and a fibrinogen content of at least 150 mg and as high as 400 mg. Cryo also contains a minimum of 80 units of Factor VIII, vWF, Factor XIII, and fibronectin. Cryo is the product of choice for fibrinogen replacement because therapeutic doses of fibrinogen may be provided in a much smaller volume than with plasma.
- Standard dosing for adults and children is usually a pool of at least 10 or 5 units, respectively. Dosing on the basis of 1 unit/7-10 kg body weight (10 units for the classic 70-kg man) is acceptable, but variability in the fibrinogen content of single units warrants caution when transfusing fewer than 3 units to pediatric patients—the increase in fibrinogen levels may not be as expected. Dosing may also be determined by calculating the number of milligrams of fibrinogen needed to raise the plasma fibrinogen to the desired level, then dividing by 250 mg (average fibrinogen content of a unit) to obtain the number of units to transfuse.

- Response to cryo transfusion may be variable as a result of both product and patient factors. Response should always be assessed by measuring fibrinogen levels after transfusion.
- Indications for the transfusion of cryo include the following:
  - Hypofibrinogenemia, congenital or acquired.
  - Dysfibrinogenemia.
  - vWD (unresponsive to DDAVP; concentrates that contain vWF factor are not available).
  - Uremic bleeding unresponsive to DDAVP.
  - Factor XIII deficiency.
  - Fibrin sealant (thrombin + Ca + cryo) for topical use.
  - Hemophilia A (only when AHF concentrates are not available).
- Contraindications for the transfusion of cryo include hemophilia A and vWD when factor concentrates are available.
- Hazards of cryo transfusion include:
  - Transfusion-transmitted infectious diseases.
  - Allergic reactions to plasma proteins.
- Fibrinogen levels in Plasma Frozen Within 24 Hours After Phlebotomy are the same as in FFP.

Question 25: B

Explanation:

See Question 26.

Question 26: C

Explanation for Questions 25 and 26:

- Indications for granulocyte transfusion in adult patients:
  - Transient (reversible) marrow depression and neutropenia <500/µL.
  - Bacterial or fungal infection unresponsive to antimicrobial therapy for more than 48 hours.
- Indications for granulocyte transfusion in neonatal and pediatric patients:

- Neutropenia <3000/µL.
- Bacterial or fungal septicemia not responsive to antimicrobial therapy.
• Controversial indications:
  - Prophylaxis during cancer chemotherapy or stem cell transplantation.
• Contraindicatons:
  - Viral or parasitic infections.

Question 27: A

Explanations:

- Because of their potent bactericidal activity, granulocytes would be expected to have greatest efficacy against bacterial and, possibly, fungal infections.
- Clear clinical data supporting the use of granulocyte transfusions are lacking. Published trials demonstrate modest or no improvement in outcomes, but many of these studies are limited by a small number of patients and low granulocyte yields in the products transfused. Donor stimulation using a combined protocol of corticosteroids and granulocyte colony-stimulating factor results in granulocyte collections with yields that may be 10-fold greater than previously available. Experience with higher-yield products is limited but encouraging.
- Granulocytes do not play a role in the clearance of viral and parasitic infections. Accordingly, granulocyte transfusions are not indicated in their treatment, even in those who are profoundly neutropenic.
- The pathophysiology of infectious prion proteins is only now beginning to be understood, but it seems unlikely that granulocytes would play any role in moderating infection.

Question 28: A

Explanation:

- Patients with PNH have lost glycosylphosphatidylinositol-linked proteins from the surface of their red cells. Among the proteins lost are

CD55 (decay accelerating factor, or DAF) and CD59 (membrane inhibitor of reactive lysis, or MIRL). These molecules inhibit lysis of red cells by complement. CD59 interacts with the membrane attack complex (MAC) and blocks the aggregation of C9. CD55 accelerates the rate of destruction of membrane-bound C3 convertase. Hemolysis in PNH results from the increased susceptibility of PNH red cells to complement.
- Patients with PNH may develop hemoglobinuria after transfusion. Although the exact mechanism of hemolysis is not known, it is presumed that some element of the transfused blood component activates complement. It was once held that patients with PNH required washed products in order to avoid complement activation and attendant hemolysis. It has been subsequently demonstrated that transfusion with type-specific products is as safe as using washed products. Selection of type-specific products avoids transfusion of soluable ABO antigens that can bind with recipient ABO antibodies and promote complement activation. Washing cellular blood products for patients with PNH is necessary only when type-specific products are unavailable.
- Other choices:
  - B and C: Washing removes the causative antibody from the component.
  - D: Irradiation will cause a more rapid rise in supernatant potassium and hemoglobin than normally occurs over the course of storage. When irradiated units are required for large-volume RBC neonatal transfusion, the units should be irradiated as close to the time of transfusion as possible. If the unit is stored for more than 24 hours after irradiation, washing to remove excess potassium is recommended. Similarly, washing is recommended for removing excess potassium whenever aged red cells are used for large volume neonatal transfusion. The amount of potassium delivered in routine small-volume transfusions does not pose a risk; washing is not needed in that setting.
  - E: Allergic reactions most commonly result from the infusion of foreign plasma proteins to recipients who have been sensitized to those proteins. Washing removes the causative antigen.

Question 29: C

Explanation:

- The clinical presentation of severe thrombocytopenia, bleeding, and neurologic symptoms is consistent with acute myelogenous leukemia (AML). Symptomatic thrombocytopenia is an indication for the transfusion of platelets.
- With the negative history of previous blood transfusions and pregnancy, platelet refractoriness caused by HLA antibodies is unlikely. HLA-matched or crossmatched platelets are not indicated. Randomly selected apheresis platelets or pooled whole-blood-derived platelets may be used interchangeably for transfusion of nonalloimmunized patients.
- This patient's presentation (clinial and laboratory) is *not* an indication for the transfusion of granulocytes, RBCs, or Cryoprecipitated AHF.
- Platelet transfusion is indicated for:
  - Prophylaxis in patients with counts of <10,000/µL (eg, settings of myelosuppression from chemotherapy or primary aplasia).
  - Treatment of patients with counts <50,000/µL who are actively bleeding or are preparing to undergo an invasive surgical procedure.
  - Trauma requiring massive transfusion (preemptively).
  - Treatment of patients with a documented history of platelet dysfunction.
- Transfusion of platelets is generally *not* indicated for:
  - Prophylactic use during cardiac surgery or massive transfusion.
  - Platelet dysfunction caused by extrinsic factors (eg, uremia, von Willebrand disease) in the absence of thrombocytopenia.
  - Treatment of TTP, hemolytic uremic syndrome, or heparin-induced thrombocytopenia.
  - ITP.

Question 30: E

Explanation:

- TRALI is a form of acute lung injury (ALI) that occurs upon administration of plasma-containing blood components. Any component that contains plasma, even the small amount present in additive RBC units, may precipitate a TRALI reaction.
- TRALI is the leading cause of transfusion-related deaths.
- Definition:
  - For purposes of categorization and study, TRALI is defined as ALI—hypoxemia with a partial pressure of oxygen in arterial blood/inspired oxygen concentration (PaO_2/FiO_2) ratio of ≤300 mm Hg or hemoglobin oxygen saturation as measured by pulse oximetry (SpO_2) ≤90% on room air and the following:
    - No preexisting ALI before transfusion.
    - Onset within 6 hours of transfusion.
    - No temporal relationship to an alternative risk factor for ALI.
  - Possible TRALI is defined as above but *with* an alternate risk factor for ALI.
  - Patients with other risk factors for ALI are also at increased risk of TRALI (see pathophysiology); therefore, the diagnosis of TRALI in clinical practice is often difficult.
- Incidence:
  - The incidence of TRALI is not clearly established but appears to be in the range of 1:1300 to 1:5000 transfusions.
- Clinical Presentation:
  - Clinical symptoms include fever, chills, dyspnea, cyanosis, hypotension, and pulmonary edema. Transient neutropenia or leukopenia may also occur.
    - Onset of symptoms is within 6 hours of transfusion; most cases are within 2 hours.
  - Lung injury is usually transient with approximately 80% of patients improving within 48 to 96 hours.
    - 20% of patients have a more protracted course or death.
- Pathophysiology:
  - Antibodies to leukocyte antigens and/or infusion of biologic response modifiers (BRMs) is thought to account for activation of neutrophils. Activated neutrophils then bind to pulmonary vascu-

lar endothelial cells and release granule contents and other biologic response modifiers, resulting in injury to endothelial cells. The injured alveolar capillaries leak protein-rich fluid into the alveolar airspaces, compromising oxygen diffusion.
- Antibodies may be directed at neutrophil antigens or HLA Class I or II antigens.
- Antibodies are usually of donor origin.
- Lysophosphatidylcholines are BRMs implicated in the pathophysiology of TRALI.
○ Two events are thought to be necessary for TRALI to occur:
- First, endothelial cells are activated and neutrophils primed by conditions that are associated with increased inflammation, such as surgery, sepsis, massive transfusion, and other physiologic stressors.
- Second, infusion of neutrophil-reactive antibodies or BRMs leads to activation and adherence of neutrophils in the pulmonary vasculature, with attendant injury.
- Differential Diagnosis:
  ○ Anaphylaxis:
    - Bronchospasm, severe hypotension, erythema, and urticuria should differentiate this from TRALI. Fever and pulmonary edema are not expected.
  ○ Transfusion-associated circulatory overload:
    - Respiratory distress with jugular venous distenstion, dependent edema, and increased blood pressure.
    - Brain natriuretic peptide may increase.
  ○ Sepsis:
    - Fever, decreased blood pressure, and vascular collapse.
    - Respiratory distress is possible but infrequent.
  ○ Unrelated to transfusion:
    - Myocardial infarct and pulmonary embolus.
- Therapy:
  ○ Respiratory support.
  ○ Steroids, although frequently administered, have not been shown to improve clinical outcome.
- Prevention:
  ○ Prevention focuses on 1) identifying donors who have or may have neutrophil or HLA antibodies (from previous pregnancy or transfusion) and excluding them from donating unmodified plasma-containing components, and on 2) reducing unnecessary transfusions.

REFERENCES

1. Nichols WL, Hultin MB, James AH, et al. von Willebrand disease (VWD): Evidence-based diagnosis and management guidelines. The National Heart, Lung, and Blood Institute (NHLBI) Expert Panel Report (USA). Haemophilia 2008;14:171-232.
2. Stanworth SJ, Massey E, Hyde C, et al. Granulocyte transfusions for treating infections in patients with neutropenia or neutrophil dysfunction. Cochrane Database Syst Rev 2005;3:CD005339.
3. Price TH. Granulocyte transfusion: Current status. Semin Hematol 2007; 44:15-23.
4. Brecher ME, Taswell HF. Paroxysmal nocturnal hemoglobinuria and the transfusion of washed red cells: A myth revisited. Transfusion 1985;29:681-5.
5. Mazzei C, Popovsky M, Kopko P. Noninfectious complications of blood transfusion. In: Roback JD, Combs MR, Grossman BJ, Hillyer CD, eds. Technical manual. 16th ed. Bethesda, MD: AABB, 2008:715-49.

8

Hematopoietic Progenitor Cells, Cord Blood, and Growth Factors

QUESTIONS

Question 1: Graft-vs-host disease (GVHD) following hematopoietic progenitor cell (HPC) transplant occurs as a result of:

A. ABO incompatibility between the donor and recipient.
B. Advanced patient age.
C. Differences between donor and recipient sex.
D. HLA incompatibility between the donor and recipient.
E. Inadequate recipient conditioning regimen.

Question 2: Which cell type primarily mediates GVHD?

A. B lymphocytes.
B. T lymphocytes.
C. Monocytes.
D. Granulocytes.
E. Progenitor cells.

Question 3: Allogeneic transplantation with major-ABO-mismatched HPCs can be expected to result in delayed recovery of which of the following?

A. Lymphocytes.
B. Granulocytes.
C. Platelets.
D. Red cells.
E. All of the above.

Question 4: When used for stem cell mobilization in allogeneic donors, which of the following will result in the highest increase in circulating CD34+ cells?

A. Granulocyte-macrophage colony-stimulating factor (GM-CSF).
B. Granulocyte colony-stimulating factor (G-CSF).
C. Cyclophosphamide.
D. Cyclophosphamide combined with G-CSF.
E. Erythropoietin combined with G-CSF.

Question 5: Adequacy of collection of HPCs from apheresis (HPC-A) is best assessed by enumerating the number of cells bearing which of the following antigens?

A. CD33.
B. CD4.
C. CD55.
D. CD34.
E. CD19.

Question 6: Which of the following is the most frequently reported side effect of G-CSF administration in HPC-A donors?

A. Fatigue.
B. Nausea.
C. Fever.
D. Bone pain.
E. Myalgia.

Question 7: Which of the following would make a prospective allogeneic HPC donor ineligible for donation?

A. Positive for antibodies to cytomegalovirus (CMV).
B. Positive for antibodies to hepatitis B virus (HBV) surface antigen (HBsAg).
C. Positive for antibodies to HBV core antigen (HBc).
D. Donor is a male who had sex with a male in 1990.
E. Donor lives in same household with someone who has asymptomatic hepatitis C virus (HCV) infection.

Question 8: Which of the following is a required HPC donor screening test?

A. Antibodies to Epstein-Barr virus (EBV).
B. Human T-cell lymphotropic virus (HTLV), types I and II nucleic acid testing (NAT).
C. Anti-HBsAg.
D. A serologic test for *Treponema pallidum*.
E. Human immunodeficiency virus (HIV), types 1 and 2 NAT.

Question 9: The minimum number of CD34+ cells that may be administered in an HPC-A transplantation without potentially compromising engraftment or speed of engraftment is closest to:

A. 2×10^5 CD34+ cells/kg.
B. 2×10^6 CD34+ cells/kg.
C. 2×10^7 CD34+ cells/kg.
D. 2×10^8 CD34+ cells/kg.
E. 2×10^9 CD34+ cells/kg.

Question 10: Which of the following is *true* regarding autologous HPC transplantation?

A. Higher incidence of CMV disease compared to allogeneic transplant recipients.
B. Autologous peripheral blood progenitor cells (PBPCs) stimulated by G-CSF engraft earlier than unstimulated, autologous, marrow-derived HPCs.
C. Not associated with veno-occlusive disease.
D. Prior pelvic irradiation is a contraindication for transplantation of HPCs from marrow (HPC-M).
E. Does not require irradiated cellular blood components when transfused.

Question 11: Which of the following regarding the CD34 antigen is *true*?

A. Represents a transmembrane glycoprotein restricted to hematopoietic progenitor cells.
B. Expressed on less than 1% of normal marrow cells.
C. Not normally found on cells in peripheral blood.
D. Is an adhesion molecule.
E. Found only on uncommitted HPCs in marrow.

Question 12: Which of the following statements regarding autologous HPC-A collection is *true*?

A. Collection is contraindicated in patients who have received multiple courses of chemotherapy.
B. Collection may stimulate platelet release with resultant increase in platelet counts.
C. Timing of collection is best predicted by the white cell (WBC) count.
D. The number of viable CD34+ cells in the combined products determines when to discontinue collection.

E. The best predictor of time to engraftment is total WBC cell content in the graft.

Question 13: A group B recipient receives a group A allogeneic HPC transplant. Which of the following would describe the best choices for transfusion support during the transplant?

A. Group O red cells and AB plasma/platelets.
B. Group O red cells and A plasma/platelets.
C. Group B red cells and A plasma/platelets.
D. Group B red cells and AB plasma/platelets.
E. Group A red cells and AB plasma/platelets.

Question 14: Which of the following is useful for evaluating the quality of an HPC graft at the time of collection or infusion?

A. Granulocyte count.
B. CD34+ cell enumeration.
C. Colony-forming assays.
D. Red cell count.
E. Plasma volume.

Question 15: Which of the following is associated with minor-ABO-mismatched (donor-plasma-incompatible) allogeneic HPC transplants?

A. Decreased risk of GVHD.
B. Hemolysis 7 to 14 days after transplantation.
C. Hemolysis 40 to 60 days after transplantation.
D. Delayed red cell recovery.
E. Delayed granulocyte engraftment.

Question 16: Which of the following is *true* regarding matched unrelated donor (MUD) HPC transplantation?

A. The most common indication is chronic myelogenous leukemia (CML).
B. The risk of GVHD is greater with HLA Class I disparity than with Class II.
C. Associated with a 70% to 80% incidence of chronic GVHD.
D. Associated with a graft-vs-leukemia (GVL) effect.
E. Progenitor cells from a matched unrelated donor can be obtained only by apheresis collection.

Question 17: Which of the following is *true* regarding transplantation with cryopreserved HPCs?

A. 15% dimethyl sulfoxide (DMSO) is used for cryopreservation.
B. Storage in liquid-phase nitrogen at −196 C will prevent cross-contamination of products.
C. HPCs are thawed at 37 C and must be transfused within 24 hours.
D. Cryopreserved HPCs expire 10 years from the date of freezing.
E. Nausea, vomiting, and bradycardia are associated with DMSO toxicity.

Question 18: Which of the following is *true* regarding a cord blood collection?

A. The mother's and father's medical history and consent must be obtained.
B. Viral testing must be performed on a maternal sample within 48 hours of the collection.
C. The collection volume is typically 50 mL.
D. Total CD34+ cell content is typically 2 to 4×10^6 cells.
E. A collection contains enough cells for reliable engraftment of recipients weighing up to 70 kg.

Question 19: Which of the following is *true* regarding allogeneic HPCs from cord blood (HPC-C) transplants vs other allogeneic HPC transplants?

A. Higher representation of minorities.
B. Higher risk of GVHD.
C. HPC-C may be stored for only 10 years.
D. Similar degree of donor risk.
E. More rapid platelet engraftment.

Question 20: In the setting of allogeneic HPC transplantation, HLA-identical (six-antigen-matched) sibling donors are identified for approximately what proportion of patients?

A. <1%.
B. 5%-10%.
C. 30%-40%.
D. 60%-70%.
E. >90%.

Question 21: Which of the following is *true* regarding donor lymphocyte infusions (DLIs, or Therapeutic Cells, Apheresis by ISBT-128 terminology)?

A. They are administered before transplantation to desensitize the recipient to donor antigens.
B. They are used to induce GVL in relapsed stem cell transplant patients.
C. They are not effective in related allogeneic transplants.
D. They are most often used to treat relapse in patients with non-Hodgkin lymphoma.
E. None of the above.

Question 22: Complications that may occur during HPC-A collection include all of the following *except*:

A. Syncopal reactions.
B. Hypomagnesemia.
C. Hypocalcemia.

D. Hyperkalemia.
E. Chills.

Question 23: A patient is to undergo autologous HPC-A collection. He is discovered to be positive for HCV by enzyme immunoassay. The infection is subsequently confirmed by radioimmunoblot assay. Which of the following statements concerning his donation is *true*?

A. He is not eligible for collection and an allogeneic donor should be identified.
B. His donation should be stored in a liquid-nitrogen freezer in liquid-phase nitrogen.
C. His donation should be stored in a liquid-nitrogen freezer in vapor-phase nitrogen.
D. His donation should be stored in a mechanical freezer at –70 C.
E. He is not eligible for transplantation and therefore a collection should not be performed.

Question 24: T-cell depletion of allogeneic HPC collections is performed for the purpose of decreasing the incidence of:

A. Infections.
B. GVHD.
C. GVL effect.
D. Relapse.
E. Graft failure.

Question 25: Reduced-intensity HPC transplantations are performed in preference to myeloablative transplantations when:

A. An HLA-matched donor cannot be identified.
B. The patient is young and wishes to reduce chemotherapy exposure in order to preserve fertility.
C. The patient is older and has comorbid conditions that limit the use of high-intensity regimens.

D. The transplant is for the purpose of adjunct therapy in a patient with complete remission.
E. The donor is HLA identical to the recipient, and therefore the risk of graft rejection is trivial.

ANSWERS

Question 1: D

Explanation:

- Major histocompatibility complex (MHC) incompatibility between donor and recipient is the most important risk factor for GVHD. (See also the explanation for Question 2.)
  - Mature donor-derived T lymphocytes recognize donor MHC antigens as foreign and mount an immune response.
- Sex differences between donor and recipient affect stem cell transplant outcomes:
  - F→M transplants are associated with:
    - Higher chronic GVHD and transplant-related mortality.
    - Reduced relapse rate for chronic myelogenous leukemia (CML), acute myelogenous leukemia (AML), and multiple myeloma.
    - Decreased overall survival in aplastic anemia, AML, and CML.
  - M→F transplants are associated with:
    - Increased graft rejection.
    - Decreased overall survival in aplastic anemia.
  - Observational and experimental evidence indicates that T cells specific for male minor histocompatibility antigens encoded by Y-chromosome genes contribute to GVHD, graft rejection, graft-vs-tumor complications, and survival in sex-mismatched transplantations.
- Other minor histocompatibility antigen differences also contribute to the risk of GVHD.
- Advanced patient age (>60 yrs) has been associated with higher transplant-related morbidity and mortality, including GVHD, although this appears largely attributable to existence of comorbid conditions.
- ABO incompatibility is not a risk factor for GVHD.

Question 2: B

Explanation:

- Marrow- and peripheral-blood-derived HPC products contain mature CD4+ and CD8+ T lymphocytes. Although these cells are necessary to reconstitute T-cell immunity and mediate antitumor effects, they are also the cause of GVHD, a broad attack against host tissues mediated by donor T lymphocytes.
- There are three requirements for the development of GVHD:
  - The graft must contain immunologically competent cells.
  - The recipient must be incapable of rejecting the transplanted cells.
  - The recipient must express tissue antigens that are not present in the donor.
- Interaction between donor and host cells results in activation and clonal expansion of donor T lymphocytes.
  - Following activation, there is a complex pattern of cytokine release, recruitment of secondary effector cells, and destruction of recipient cells and tissues.
- GVHD has acute and chronic forms.
  - Acute GVHD occurs within the first 100 days after transplantation and affects tissues of the host's immune system, including thymus, skin, gastrointestinal tract, and liver tissues.
    - Patients receiving nonmyeloablative transplants may develop acute GVHD beyond 100 days after transplantation.
  - Chronic GVHD occurs 100 days after transplantation, and, in addition to symptoms associated with acute GVHD, has diverse manifestations that can resemble autoimmune syndromes such as scleroderma-like skin disorders and biliary cirrhosis.
  - Acute GVHD occurs in 10% to 50% of patients receiving transplants from HLA-matched donors.
  - Chronic GVHD occurs in 20% to 50% of HLA-matched transplants.
    - Acute and chronic GVHD are both more common in incompletely matched transplants.
  - Acute GVHD is the most important risk factor for developing chronic GVHD.

Question 3: D

Explanation:

- Allogeneic transplantation with ABO-major-mismatched marrow results in delayed red cell recovery due to destruction of engrafted red cell progenitors by recipient isohemagglutinins.
  - Delayed donor erythropoiesis is most frequently reported in type O recipients of type A grafts.
- As titers of recipient isohemagglutinins decline, donor reticulocytes and red cells appear in the peripheral blood.
- Red cell recovery is generally delayed 40 to 60 days after transplantation and correlates with decreased antidonor isoagglutinin levels.
- Engraftment and recovery of the other cell lines is not affected by ABO compatibility.

Question 4: D

Explanation:

- Under steady state conditions, less than 0.05% of circulating white cells are CD34+.
  - Stem cell mobilization regimens are used to increase the levels of circulating CD34+ cells in preparation for HPC collection by apheresis.
  - Mobilization is not routinely used for marrow harvesting.
- G-CSF (filgrastim) and GM-CSF (sargramostim) are the hematopoietic growth factors most commonly used for stem cell mobilization. These factors increase the number of circulating HPCs greater than 50- to 200-fold.
  - G-CSF mobilizes more stem cells and has less toxicity than GM-CSF and for this reason has become the most commonly used single agent regimen for stem cell mobilization.
  - GM-CSF, when used, is typically used in combination regimens and on its own is considered a relatively poor mobilizer.

- G-CSF is administered subcutaneously once daily at doses ranging from 5 to 20 µg/kg/day (most commonly 10 µg/kg/day), beginning 4 days before collection and continuing with daily collections starting on day 5.
- Chemotherapy (eg, cyclophosphamide, etoposide) is used for mobilization in patients with malignant diseases undergoing autologous stem cell transplantation. As patients recover from therapy-induced leukopenia, circulating HPCs may increase 20- to 50-fold.
- The combination of chemotherapy and hematopoietic growth factors, specifically G-CSF, results in the greatest increase in CD34+ cells.
- Erythropoietin does have some ability to mobilize CD34+ cells and may be used in combination with G-CSF, but mobilization is not as effective as G-CSF combined with chemotherapy.
- Table 8-4 compares different mobilization regimens.

Table 8-4.

Regimen	Approximate Day When Peak HPC Concentrations Are Reached	Increase in HPCs above Steady State
Chemotherapy	Day 14 after completion of chemotherapy	20-50 times
Cytokines (G-CSF and GM-CSF)	Day 5 after initiation of cytokine therapy	50-200 times
Chemotherapy and cytokines	Day 5 after initiation of cytokine therapy	200-1000 times

G-CSF = granulocyte colony-stimulating factor; GM-CSF = granulocyte-macrophage CSF.

- Plerixafor (AMD3100), which became available for use in 2009, is a CXCR4 chemokine antagonist that disrupts its interaction with stromal-derived factor 1 (SDF-1, also called CXCL12), thereby releasing HPCs into the circulation. In multiple myeloma and non-Hodgkin lymphoma patients who have failed to mobilize with G-CSF alone or in combination with chemotherapy, CD34+ cell yields have been shown to increase five- to 100-fold with the combination of plerixafor and G-CSF. Plerixafor administration begins after 4 days of daily G-CSF, approximately 11 hours before apheresis, and continues for up to 4 consecutive days. The recommended dose is 0.24 mg/kg body weight subcutaneously, not to exceed 40 mg/day. Dosing should be decreased for renal failure.

Question 5: D

Explanation:

- CD34 is a glycoprotein found on the surface of early hematopoietic stem cells and other cell types (eg, endothelial cells). The CD34 content of HPC-A collections, enumerated by flow cytometry, has been shown to correlate with rapidity and durability of neutrophil and platelet engraftment.
- Other answers:
  - CD33 is a committed myeloid marker.
  - CD4 is a T-helper-cell marker.
  - CD55 is decay-accelerating factor, which regulates complement activation. It is decreased in paroxysmal nocturnal hemoglobinuria.
  - CD19 is a B-cell marker.

Question 6: D

Explanation:

- In order of frequency, symptoms commonly associated with G-CSF administration include bone pain, myalgia, headache, fatigue, insomnia, nausea, flu-like symptoms, sweats, and loss of appetite.
  - Bone aches and myalgia are usually mild and can usually be controlled with over-the-counter nonsteroidal anti-inflammatory drugs (NSAIDS) or acetaminophen.
  - Less common symptoms include fever, abdominal pain, local reactions, and allergic reactions.

- Normal donors may also demonstrate asymptomatic mild splenomegaly, mild elevations in alanine aminotransferase, lactate dehydrogenase, and alkaline phosphatase, as well as thrombocytopenia.
- Thrombocytopenia associated with G-CSF administration is usually mild and reversible. Apheresis, which also lowers the platelet count, contributes to the thrombocytopenia.
- More severe but rare side effects include splenic rupture, capillary leak syndrome, retinal hemorrhage, acute iritis, gouty arthritis, and thrombotic events.
- Symptoms resolve soon after stopping G-CSF.
- G-CSF should not be administered if the leukocyte count is more than 60,000/µL (6×10^9/L), as this could lead to leukostasis and increased blood viscosity.
- Onset of severe life-threatening sickle crisis and death (more than one case) have been reported in patients with sickle disorders who have received G-CSF. Acute elevations in granulocyte counts or increased granulocyte adhesiveness is thought to have played a role in the development of vaso-occlusive crisis. Administration of G-CSF should be avoided in patients with sickle cell disease or sickling disorders.
- Administration of G-CSF to donors with sickle cell trait has been reported to be safe.

Question 7: C

Explanation:

- Donor-eligibility determination is a conclusion that an allogeneic donor is either eligible or ineligible to donate based on the results of Food and Drug Administration (FDA)-specified donor screening and testing. The term "eligible" indicates that the donor has passed all FDA screening and testing requirements.
- Prospective allogeneic HPC donors are ineligible if they test positive for anti-HBc or for the presence of HBsAg.
- Ineligible donors may still be accepted for donation if the clinical circumstances justify making exceptions to donor eligibility criteria, eg, the only HLA match available for a recipient is a donor who is anti-HBc positive.

- Testing for antibodies to CMV is required; however, a positive result does not make the donor ineligible for donation. It may make the donor unsuitable for a recipient who is CMV negative.
- Men who have had sex with men in the preceding 5 years are ineligible for HPC donation. In contrast, male prospective blood donors are ineligible if they have engaged in male-male sex, even once, since 1977.
- See explanation for Question 3 in Chapter 15 for a complete listing of the differences between eligibility criteria for blood donors and tissue donors.

Question 8: D

Explanation:

- The following communicable disease tests are required for HPC donors:
  - Antibodies to HIV-1/2.
  - NAT test for HIV-1.
  - Antibodies to HCV.
  - NAT test for HCV.
  - HBsAg.
  - Antibodies to HBc.
  - Serologic test for *T. pallidum*.
  - Antibodies to HTLV-I/II.
  - Antibodies to CMV (IgM and IgG).
  - As of the time of writing, NAT for West Nile virus (WNV) was recommended by the FDA and implemented by donor collection centers but was still awaiting codification.
- Donors are ineligible if they are confirmed to be positive for HIV antibodies or nucleic acid, HCV antibodies or nucleic acid, antibodies to HBc, HBsAg, antibodies to HTLV, or WNV nucleic acid.
- Donors who test positive on a serologic test for syphilis may be determined to be eligible if they test negative on a specific treponemal confirmatory test (eg, fluorescent treponemal antibody with absorption test).
- When clinically justified, an ineligible donor may be determined to be acceptable for a specific intended recipient.

Question 9: B

Explanation:

- CD34 doses of less than 2×10^6 cells/kg may compromise the probability of engraftment and the speed of engraftment.
- Generally, target doses for HPC-A transplants are $\geq 5 \times 10^6$ CD34+ cells/kg. For poor mobilizers, collections may be stopped when yields reach 2×10^6 cells/kg.
- Transplants are performed with lower numbers of CD34+ cells (eg, 1×10^6 CD34+ cells/kg) when necessary, especially when marrow or cord blood are cell sources. Patients who receive lower doses typically experience a prolonged time to engraftment.

Question 10: B

Explanation:

- Autologous PBPCs stimulated by G-CSF are associated with granulocyte engraftment (median) on day 10 and platelet engraftment on day 14. Engraftment is several days to a week sooner than that seen with autologous marrow. If the donor receives G-CSF before marrow harvest, engraftment is equivalent.
- Autologous HPC transplantation is associated with a 1% to 2% risk of CMV disease, compared with 10% to 20% in the allogeneic setting.
- Veno-occlusive disease is a hepatic complication of high-dose chemotherapy characterized by weight gain, right upper quadrant pain, ascites, and hyperbilirubinemia. Histologically, fibrous obliteration of the central venules in the hepatic lobule is seen. This complication can occur in any patient receiving high-dose chemotherapy.
- Prior pelvic irradiation may lead to marrow necrosis and fibrosis, thereby reducing the chances of a successful marrow harvest, but it is not on its own a contraindication to marrow transplantation.
- Autologous transplant recipients are immune compromised as a result of the transplant-conditioning regimen (the chemotherapy and/or radiation given before transplantation). Allogeneic lymphocytes infused with nonirradiated blood components are capable of mediat-

ing transfusion-associated (TA)-GVHD in the autologous transplant recipient. For this reason, irradiated cellular components should be used for transfusion.

Question 11: D

Explanation:

- Approximately 115 kD in size, CD34 is a transmembrane sialo-mucin-like glycoprotein. CD34 is an adhesion molecule with a functional role in cell differentiation and mediating cell adhesion.
- 1% to 3% of normal marrow cells express the CD34 antigen. The large majority of these cells are committed progenitors.
- The CD34 antigen can be found in both hematopoietic cells and non-hematopoietic cells such as endothelial cells and stromal cells.
- CD34+ cells represent 0.01% to 0.1% of peripheral blood leukocytes in the normal state. Mobilization of an individual with G-CSF and chemotherapy can dramatically increase the proportion of CD34+ cells in the peripheral blood.
- Monoclonal antibodies to the CD34 antigen have been developed and allow enumeration of CD34+ cells in marrow, peripheral blood, or cord blood by flow cytometry.
- The CD34 antigen is expressed on both pluripotent hematopoietic cells and committed cells such as CD33+CD34+ myeloid cells. The pluripotent stem cell represents only a small portion of the CD34+ cell population in the marrow.

Question 12: D

Explanation:

- While some patients who have been heavily pretreated with chemotherapy or radiation mobilize poorly, this is not always the case. Repeat dosing with G-CSF or increasing the dose of G-CSF alone or in combination with GM-CSF has successfully mobilized patients who have failed prior attempts.

- Factors that *negatively* influence mobilization include:
  - Age. Age is not important if HPCs are mobilized by chemotherapy. However, when G-CSF is given alone, younger donors/patients mobilize better than older ones.
  - Presence of marrow involvement.
  - Prior radiation therapy.
  - Type and number of cycles of chemotherapy, particularly alkylating agents.
  - Patient diagnosis. Patients with AML have lower levels of peripheral CD34+ cells.
  - Premobilization platelet count.
  - Gender. Some studies have reported a higher probability of mobilization failures in females but others have failed to reproduce this finding.
- Timing for collection best correlates with the number of CD34+ cells in the peripheral blood. Collection should be timed to when the CD34+ count is 5/µL or higher. CD34+ cell measurements in peripheral blood of 10 cells/µL can be expected to yield at least 1×10^6 CD34+ cells/kg from a single collection.
- In the absence of a peripheral CD34 count, the collections should be timed to occur when the WBC count reaches 5000/µL or above.
- Platelet counts decrease during autologous HPC-A collection.
- The combined CD34+ cells/kg of the HPC-A products determines whether the collection is considered satisfactory or not. Target doses are usually $\geq 5 \times 10^6$ CD34+ cells/kg. Doses $\geq 2 \times 10^6$ CD34+ cells/kg are associated with rapid engraftment. Doses as low as 0.75×10^6 to 1.0×10^6 have resulted in engraftment but this is often delayed and prolonged.

Question 13: A

Explanation:

- An A donor to B recipient transplant represents both a major (donor RBCs are incompatible) and minor (donor plasma is incompatible) mismatch. Thus, red cells and plasma selected for transfusion must be compatible with both donor and recipient blood types. This strategy minimizes the chances of hemolysis occurring 7 to 14 days after

transplantation (due to passenger lymphocytes) and at 40 to 60 days after transplantation at the time of red cell engraftment.
- Other choices:
  - B: Plasma is not compatible with the recipient.
  - C: Red cells are not compatible with the donor and plasma is not compatible with the recipient.
  - D: Red cells are not compatible with the donor.
  - E: Red cells are not compatible with the recipient.

Question 14: B

Explanation:

- CD34+ cell dose is the best predictor of engraftment.
- AABB *Standards for Cellular Therapy Product Services* requirements for evaluation of HPC collections include a relevant cell count (eg, mononuclear cell count), antigen expression analysis appropriate for the product (eg, CD34 for HPC, CD3 for T-cell collections), cell viability, and product sterility.
- A positive culture does not necessarily require that the graft be discarded because these may be irreplaceable cells. Positive culture results need to be reviewed by a physician and evaluated on a case-by-case basis.
- Colony-forming assays take 2 weeks or more to perform and, thus, do not provide practical value in evaluating the quality of a graft. However, they may be useful for retrospective quality review.
- Red cell content is not used as a marker of graft quality. Red cells are not desirable in cryopreserved HPC products and are problematic in a fresh product if the donor cells are incompatible with the recipient. Red cell volumes in HPC-A products are typically less than 10 mL, so red cell reduction is rarely necessary. HPC-M and HPCs from cord blood (HPC-C) collections start with higher volumes of red cells. Red cells may not be effectively preserved by dimethyl sulfoxide (DMSO); therefore, these products are red-cell-volume-reduced before cryopreservation. Red cells are removed from HPC-M collections whenever the donor is ABO incompatible with the recipient or if tumor purging is to be performed.
- Plasma volume is not used as a marker of graft quality. Plasma is routinely removed from all products undergoing cryopreservation, and

from fresh products when the plasma is incompatible with recipient red cells, or when the product is undergoing further processing.

Question 15: B

Explanation:

- Minor-ABO-mismatched transplants may be associated with immediate hemolysis from passively transfused donor ABO antibodies, and with delayed hemolysis after 7 to 14 days caused by red cell antibodies produced by mature passenger lymphocytes in the graft. Hemolysis is associated with the development of a positive direct antiglobulin test (DAT), most commonly caused by ABO antibodies of the IgG class. Hemolysis is usually mild and transient but can be severe.
- Passenger lymphocyte hemolysis caused by donor antibodies to other red cell antigens may also occur.
- The onset of passenger lymphocyte syndrome (minor-ABO-incompatible hemolysis) frequently heralds the onset of GVHD. Both are a result of immune reconstitution.
- Red cell recovery is not delayed in minor-ABO-incompatible transplants.
- Delayed red cell recovery [pure red cell aplasia (PRCA)], not delayed engraftment, is typical of a major-ABO-mismatched transplant. Reconstitution of red cells is delayed because of recipient isoagglutinin-mediated destruction of emerging red cells; however, in-vitro colony assays reveal early erythroid progenitors in marrow samples from patients with delayed red cell recovery.
- Granulocyte and platelet engraftment or recovery is not affected by donor/recipient ABO compatibility.

Question 16: D

Explanation:

- GVHD has been associated with a decreased risk of disease relapse. This is thought to be mediated by the GVL effect. T cells of donor ori-

gin mount a cellular immune response not only to normal patient tissues (GVHD) but also to residual tumor cells (GVL). Research is underway to enhance the GVL effect while minimizing GVHD.
- Acute myelogenous leukemia (AML) is the most common indication for MUD transplantation.
- HLA Class II disparity is associated with a higher risk of GVHD compared with a HLA Class I mismatch. Molecular typing is routinely performed for DRB, DQ, and DP.
- Chronic GVHD occurs in 20% to 50% of patients undergoing MUD transplantation who survive more than 100 days. Chronic GVHD may involve the skin, gastrointestinal tract, or liver. Patients who develop chronic GVHD are predisposed to infectious complications.
- The National Marrow Donor Program has protocols for providing HPC-M or HPC-A MUD transplants. The advantages of HPC-A collection include less risk and inconvenience for the donor (general anesthesia is avoided, lower RBC loss, less pain and discomfort). Allogeneic HPC-A transplantation is associated with improved engraftment kinetics and an enhanced GVL effect but higher chronic GVHD than marrow.

Question 17: E

Explanation:

- Nausea, vomiting, bradycardia, and hypotension or hypertension are some of the toxic effects of DMSO. These symptoms may be avoided or decreased by slowing the rate of infusion or washing the product before infusion. With any manipulation of HPC products there is a concern that progenitor cells may be lost during processing.
- HPCs are most often cryopreserved in a 10% solution of DMSO. Some studies have demonstrated that cryopreservation in 5% DMSO may be just as effective.
- HPCs are thawed at 37 C, in a waterbath near the patient's bed or in the laboratory, and are transfused as soon as possible. Room temperature exposure to DMSO decreases HPC cell viability; therefore, infusion should occur within one hour of thawing. When delays after thawing are inevitable, the product should be washed to remove DMSO. Infusion should occur as quickly as possible after washing.

- Storage in the liquid phase of liquid nitrogen does not prevent cross-contamination of products.
- AABB *Standards for Cellular Therapy Product Services* and federal regulations do not specify a maximum expiration for HPC products. In-vitro viability has been demonstrated in HPC products stored in liquid nitrogen for up to 14 years, and successful engraftment has occurred with products up to 15 years old. The maximum amount of time that an HPC product may be stored and still maintain the ability to produce engraftment is not yet known.
- HPC-M may be stored for up to 3 days at either 2 to 8 C or 18 to 24 C. HPC-A viability is best preserved at temperatures approximating 4 C, but storage at 4 to 15 C for up to 72 hours is acceptable. HPCs should not be stored at 37 C.

Question 18: D

Explanation:

- Only the birth mother's consent is required for cord blood donation. AABB *Standards for Cellular Therapy Product Services* require that consent for procurement be obtained before active labor and that consent for banking be obtained within 48 hours after procurement. Consent may be obtained prenatally or during early labor. Consent may also be staged so that consent for procurement is obtained first, and consent for banking occurs after delivery.
- A medical history is required for the birth mother. The father's medical history is desirable but not required.
- Only maternal infectious disease screening and testing is required. The birth mother's sample for testing must be obtained within 7 days before or after delivery. A sample is not required from the neonate.
- Collection volumes are typically 80 to 100 mL (range = 40-140 mL).
- The median CD34+ cell content is approximately 3 to 4×10^6.
- Clinical studies show that reliable engraftment occurs in recipients weighing less than 45 kg. Successful engraftment has been reported in larger children and adults, but CD34+ dose is a major limitation on cord blood transplantation in adults. Adult transplantations are often performed using two HPC-C grafts in order to improve the chances of engraftment. The cords may be of the same blood type or different blood types.

Question 19: A

Explanation:

- Cord blood can be obtained at delivery from any eligible mother and, thus, provides the opportunity to include ethnic minorities underrepresented among National Marrow Donor Program (NMDP) donors. To increase minority representation, HPC-C collections can be targeted to birthing centers that serve underrepresented groups.
- Allogeneic HPC-C transplantation is associated with a lower risk of GVHD compared to HLA-mismatched marrow-derived sources. It is postulated that the immature nature of cord blood cells may make them more tolerant.
- Other advantages of HPC-C transplantation include the following:
  - Collection of product poses no risk to donor (or mother).
  - Lower incidence of viral contamination, including CMV and EBV.
  - No concern about donor attrition, in contrast to NMDP donor registries. Cord blood products are frozen and available when requested.
  - Because cord blood is already banked, it is more rapidly available (about 2 weeks) than adult HPCs obtained through the NMDP, which take about 2 to 3 months. This may be an advantage for patients with aggressive disease.
- Disadvantages of HPC-C compared to other HPCs:
  - CD34+ counts are frequently below 2×10^6.
  - The limited CD34+ dose may contribute to failed or delayed engraftment and may limit use in the adult population.
    - HPC-C transplants in the adult population are often performed using two or more cord collections to ensure engraftment. Although two or more cords are infused, only one cord engrafts.
  - It is not feasible to collect additional cells for donor lymphocyte infusions or for patients who experience graft failure.
  - The median time to platelet engraftment for unrelated HPC-C transplants is 56 days, which is prolonged compared to allogeneic marrow transplants.
- As with HPC-M and HPC-A, the maximum amount of time that an HPC-C collection may be stored and still provide successful engraftment is not yet established. At the time of writing, there is no regulated expiration time.

Question 20: C

Explanation:

- Only 30% to 40% of allogeneic HPC transplant candidates have an HLA-identical sibling donor.
- Matched unrelated donors may be identified by a search through the NMDP database. For patients of European ancestry, approximately 85% find a phenotypic HLA match. Patients from racial or ethnic minorities have a substantially lower chance of finding a match. Cord blood transplantation offers therapeutic options for these patients.

Question 21: B

Explanation:

- DLIs are used as adoptive immunotherapy to enhance the GVL effect after allogeneic transplantation. The cells mediating the effect are most likely CD4+ T cells. The GVL effect is maintained when the CD8+ T cells are removed from the DLI infusion.
  - The greatest experience with this form of therapy has been in the setting of CML. Response rates for patients treated with DLI for relapsed chronic phase CML are in the range of 76%. Response rates for advanced phase CML are significantly poorer at 28% or less.
  - DLI infusions are also used for relapsed AML where remission rates are in the range of 20% to 25%.
  - DLI has also been applied to relapsed myelodysplasia, lymphoma, and multiple myeloma. Response rates and remission duration with these diseases are less well defined.
- Donor lymphocyte infusions have proven efficacy in related allogeneic transplantation. Experience in unrelated transplantation is more limited, but results appear to be similar.
- Adoptive immunotherapy to prevent posttransplant EBV-associated lymphomas by infusion of virus-specific cytotoxic T lymphocytes (CTLs) has been successful in children receiving allogeneic marrow

transplants. The therapy has been similarly applied to CMV disease in the allogeneic transplant setting.
- DLIs are not given before transplantation. The risk of sensitizing a stem cell transplant recipient to donor major or minor histocompatibility antigens precludes exposing the recipient to the donor before transplantation.

Question 22: D

Explanation:

- Patients undergoing HPC-A procedures more frequently develop hypokalemia due to the combined effects of diuretic therapy, platinum-based chemotherapy, and citrate metabolism. (See also Question 26 in Chapter 13.)
- Syncopal reactions most frequently occur as a result of peripheral vasodilation from a vasovagal reaction. Treatment includes placing the patient in a Trendelenburg position and administering cold compresses and intravenous fluids.
- Citrate infusion may lower ionized calcium levels and magnesium levels to the point that the donor may become symptomatic. Symptoms include perioral numbness, tingling, nausea, vomiting, and chills. Symptoms may progress to facial spasm (Chvostek's sign), carpopedal spasm (Trousseau's sign), convulsion, or arrhythmias. Slowing the infusion of citrate and/or providing oral calcium supplements can usually treat early mild symptoms. Parenteral calcium and/or magnesium should be given when more severe symptoms occur.

Question 23: C

Explanation:

- Patients with infectious diseases are eligible for stem cell transplantation—autologous or allogeneic, whichever suits the patient best—even though the presence of the disease may complicate the patient's clinical course.

- Autologous donors with positive infectious disease results may not be excluded from donation if the attending physician chooses to proceed with transplantation.
- If a donor has positive test results for HBsAg, anti-HBc, HIV-1/2, HCV, or HTLV-I/II, the product must be labeled with a biohazard label (AABB *Standards for Cellular Therapy Product Services*).
- HPCs must be stored at less than –80 C. Products with positive test results and those for which test results are pending are best stored in vapor-phase nitrogen to minimize the risk of contaminating other products.

Question 24: B

Explanation:

- T lymphocytes within the graft (HPC-M or -A) mediate acute GVHD. In the setting of allogeneic transplantation, acute or chronic GVHD occurs in 30% to 60% of genotypically HLA-matched transplants. GVHD is responsible for significant morbidity and mortality. In an attempt to minimize this, T lymphocytes can be removed from the progenitor cell source. The benefit must be balanced with a number of negative consequences.
- Excessive T-cell depletion of HPC grafts (eg, via positive selection of CD34+ cells) may be associated with prolonged lymphocytopenia and a high rate of opportunistic infections.
- Graft failure and higher rates of disease relapse are both associated with T-cell depletion of grafts.
- The challenge of minimizing the severity of GVHD and maintaining the GVL effect is ongoing. Ongoing research is examining the role of subpopulations of T cells and/or cytokines in potentiating the GVL effect.

Question 25: C

Explanation:

- Many potential HPC transplant patients are excluded from transplantation because of advanced age or the presence of comorbid conditions, which may lead to higher transplant and nonrelapse mortality (NRM). Reduced-intensity regimens, including nonmyeloablative regimens, extend this treatment option to a larger group of patients. The most important benefit of nonmyeloablative transplants is the reduction of transplant morbidity and NRM.
- Patients with indolent disease, or who are transfusion dependent because of repeated courses of chemotherapy, are also candidates for reduced-intensity transplants.
- The conditioning regimen is intended to be sufficiently immunosuppressive to prevent graft rejection.
- The GVL effect is the mechanism of disease control.
- Postgrafting immunosuppression is used to enhance engraftment and control GVHD.
- The majority of patients achieve full donor chimerism within 6 months. Full donor chimerism is associated with better progression-free survival.
- Nonmyeloablative/reduced-intensity regimens are associated with a reduced incidence of acute GVHD, but the incidence of chronic GVHD remains the same.

REFERENCES

1. Szczepiorkowski ZM. Transfusion support for hematopoietic transplant recipients. In: Roback JD, Combs MR, Grossman BJ, Hillyer CD, eds. Technical manual. 16th ed. Bethesda, MD: AABB, 2008:679-95.
2. Davis-Sproul J, Haley RN. McMannis JD. Collecting and processing marrow products for transplantation. In: Roback JD, Combs MR, Grossman BJ, Hillyer CD, eds. Technical manual. 16th ed. Bethesda, MD: AABB, 2008:765-85.

3. Lane T, McMannis JD. Hematopoietic progenitor cells collected by aphereis. In: Roback JD, Combs MR, Grossman BJ, Hillyer CD, eds. Technical manual. 16th ed. Bethesda, MD: AABB, 2008:787-807.
4. McKenna DH, Kadidlo DM, McCullough J. Umbilical cord blood. In: Roback JD, Combs MR, Grossman BJ, Hillyer CD, eds. Technical manual. 16th ed. Bethesda, MD: AABB, 2008:809-31.
5. Billingham RE. The biology of graft versus host reaction. Harvey Lecture 1966;62:21-78.
6. Scott BL, Deeg HJ. Hematopoietic stem cell transplantation for acquired nonmalignant diseases and myelodysplastic syndrome. In: Hoffman R, Furie B, Benz E, et al, eds. Hematology: Basic principles and practice. 5th ed. Philadelphia: Elsevier Churchill Livingstone, 2009:1684-701.
7. Adler BK, Salzman DE, Carabasi MH, et al. Fatal sickle cell crisis after granulocyte colony-stimulating factor administration. Blood 2001;97:3313-14.
8. Antonenas V, Garvin F, Webb M, et al. Fresh PBSC harvests, but not BM, show temperature-related loss of CD34 viability during storage and transport. Cytotherapy 2006;8:158-65.
9. Donnenberg AD, Koch EK, Griffin DL, et al. Viability of cryopreserved BM progenitor cells stored for more than a decade. Cytotherapy 2002;4:157-63.
10. Porter D, Levine J. Graft-versus-host disease and graft-versus-leukemia after donor leukocyte infusion. Semin Hematol 2006;43:53-61.
11. Sadmaier B, Mackinnon S, Childs R, Reduced intensity conditioning for allogeneic hematopoietic cell transplantation: Current perspectives. Biol Blood Marrow Transplant 2007;13(Suppl 1):87-97.
12. Food and Drug Administration. Guidance for industry: Eligibility determination for donors of human cells, tissues, and cellular and tissue-based products (HCT/Ps). (August 2007) Rockville, MD: CBER Office of Communication, Training, and Manufacturers Assistance, 2007.
13. Bensinger W, DePersio JF, McCarty JM. Improving stem cell mobilization strategies: Future directions. Bone Marrow Transplant 2009;43:181-95.

9

Hemolytic Disease of the Fetus and Newborn, and Rh Immune Globulin

QUESTIONS

Question 1: Which of the following antigens is strongly expressed on newborn red cells?

A. A.
B. I.
C. Le^a.
D. Fy^b.
E. P$_1$.

Question 2: A pregnant woman's serum contains hemolytic anti-Le^a. Her husband's red cell type is Le(a+). What is the chance that her fetus will develop immune-mediated hemolysis and hemolytic disease of the fetus and newborn (HDFN)?

A. 100%.
B. 75%.
C. 50%.
D. 25%.
E. 0%.

Question 3: Mothers of infants with ABO HDFN are usually of which blood group?

A. A.
B. B.
C. AB.
D. O.
E. Equally likely among ABO groups.

Question 4: Forward and reverse ABO grouping results performed on a 2-day-old infant are shown in Table 9-4. The direct antiglobulin test (DAT) is positive and the eluate is positive for anti-A,B. The mother's and infant's ABO groups are:

Table 9-4.

Anti-A	Anti-B	Anti-A,B	A₁ Cells	B Cells
4+	—	4+	2+	2+

A. Infant, B; mother, A.
B. Infant, AB; mother, A.
C. Infant, O; mother, AB.
D. Infant, A; mother, O.
E. Infant, O; mother, B.

Question 5: Which of the following statements is *true*?

A. Rh incompatibility is the most common cause of HDFN.
B. Presence of the D antigen on the mother's red cells confers the risk of HDFN caused by anti-D.

C. Rh Immune Globulin (RhIG) administration is the first-line treatment for HDFN.
D. Absence of the D antigen on the mother's red cells confers the risk of HDFN caused by anti-d.
E. Antibodies to the D antigen are responsible for the most severe form of HDFN.

Question 6: A 26-year-old Rh-negative woman is seen 16 weeks into her second pregnancy. She has an anti-D titer of 16. You advise:

A. Intrauterine transfusion (IUT).
B. Amniocentesis or fetal middle cerebral artery flow study.
C. Follow titers every 2 weeks until >64.
D. Administer RhIG.
E. Repeat titer in 1 month.

Question 7: Which of the following statements concerning the rosette test is *true*?

A. Anti-D is incubated with a maternal sample. Rh-negative reagent red cells are added to the sample. A positive test can be used to calculate the dose of RhIG.
B. Anti-D is incubated with a maternal sample. Rh-positive reagent red cells are added to the sample. A positive test can be used to calculate the dose of RhIG.
C. Anti-D is incubated with a maternal sample. Rh-positive reagent red cells are added to the sample. A positive test cannot be used to calculate the dose of RhIG.
D. Anti-D is incubated with a maternal sample. Rh-negative reagent red cells are added to the sample. A positive test cannot be used to calculate the dose of RhIG.
E. Anti-D is incubated with Rh-positive reagent red cells. Sensitized cells are added to the maternal sample. A positive test can be used to calculate the dose of RhIG.

Question 8: A Kleihauer-Betke acid elution test can be used to determine the dose of RhIG in cases of fetomaternal hemorrhage (FMH). This test allows for the detection of:

A. D antigen.
B. Hemoglobin F.
C. I antigen.
D. Anti-D.
E. Adherent Wharton's jelly.

Question 9: A Kleihauer-Betke acid elution test identifies 40 fetal red cells in 2000 maternal red cells. The mother's blood volume is 5000 mL. How many doses of RhIG do you recommend?

A. 1.
B. 2.
C. 3.
D. 4.
E. 5.

Question 10: A 25-year-old woman is brought to the emergency room with severe bleeding following a motor vehicle accident. Transfusion with group O-negative blood is started and 10 units of crossmatch-compatible blood are ordered. Review of the blood bank history indicates that she delivered a group O-positive infant a year ago. She received RhIG at 28 weeks. The Kleihauer-Betke test was reported as 2.7% after delivery, and 5 doses of RhIG were administered intramuscularly within 60 hours. Type and screen testing now shows that she is group A, Rh negative with anti-D in her serum. No other blood group antibodies are identified.

The patient's anti-D is best attributed to:

A. Failure to administer enough RhIG.
B. The residual effect of RhIG administration.

C. Anti-G.
D. Untimely administration of RhIG.
E. Failure to administer RhIG by the intravenous route.

Question 11: In reference to Question 10, one out of 10 Rh-negative units are crossmatch incompatible. This is best attributed to:

A. Anti-K.
B. Anti-Jk^a.
C. Anti-Wr^a.
D. Anti-C.
E. Anti-Jk^b.

Question 12: A 28-year-old woman of European ethnicity is referred for high-risk obstetric care during her first pregnancy because of gestational diabetes. She is Rh negative and received antenatal RhIG at 28 weeks. The results of an antibody screen and identification, obtained at 30 weeks of gestation, are given in Table 9-12. Which of the following statements is *true*?

A. The patient should not receive RhIG at delivery.
B. The anti-D represents passive antibody from RhIG administration.
C. Two antibodies are present, anti-M and anti-D.
D. The immediate-spin reactivity represents a cold-reactive autoantibody.
E. The test should be repeated because check cells were not run with all cells.

Table 9-12.

Cell	D	C	c	E	e	f	V	Cw	K	k	Kpa	Kpb	Jsa	Jsb	Fya	Fyb	Jka	Jkb	Lea	Leb	P1	M	N	S	s	Lua	Lub	Xga	IS	AHG	CC
I	+	+	0	0	+	0	0	0	+	+	0	+	0	+	+	+	0	+	0	+	+	+	+	+	+	0	+	0	W+	1+	
II	+	0	+	+	0	0	0	0	0	+	0	+	0	+	0	+	+	0	+	0	+	+	+	0	+	0	+	+	W+	1+	
1	+	+	0	0	+	0	0	+	+	+	0	+	0	+	+	+	+	0	+	0	+	+	+	0	+	0	+	+	W+	1+	
2	+	+	0	0	+	0	0	0	0	+	0	+	0	+	+	+	+	0	+	0	+	+	0	0	+	0	+	0	W+	1+	
3	+	0	+	0	+	+	0	0	0	+	0	+	0	+	0	0	0	+	0	+	+	+	0	0	+	0	+	+	W+	1+	
4	+	+	0	+	0	0	0	0	+	+	0	+	0	+	+	0	+	+	0	0	+	0	+	0	0	0	+	0	W+	1+	
5	0	0	+	0	+	+	0	0	0	+	0	+	0	+	+	+	0	+	0	+	+	+	+	+	+	0	+	+	0	0	+
6	0	0	+	+	0	+	0	0	+	+	0	+	0	+	+	+	+	+	+	0	+	0	+	0	+	0	+	0	0	0	+
7	0	0	+	0	+	+	0	0	0	+	0	+	0	+	0	0	+	+	+	0	+	+	+	0	+	+	+	+	0	0	+
8	0	0	+	0	+	+	0	0	+	+	0	+	0	+	+	+	+	+	+	0	0	0	0	+	0	0	+	0	0	0	+
9	0	0	+	0	+	+	0	0	0	+	0	+	0	+	+	0	0	+	+	0	+	+	+	+	0	0	+	+	0	0	+
10	0	0	+	0	+	+	0	0	0	+	0	+	0	+	0	0	0	+	0	0	+	0	+	0	+	0	+	0	0	0	+
Patient's cells																															

HEMOLYTIC DISEASE   305

Question 13: A 22-year-old female at 28 weeks of gestation, who is group B negative, para 0, and gravida 0, has a negative antibody screen. She is seen in the emergency room for a urinary tract infection the day before she is scheduled to receive RhIG. A nurse administered a standard 300-µg antepartum dose of RhIG to avoid a visit to the hospital the next day. The obstetric service wants to rule out the presence of immune anti-D in the maternal serum for the proper management of the pregnancy. Which of the following tests allows exclusion of the possibility of alloimmunization?

A. Anti-D titer.
B. Anti-D allotype.
C. Antibody screen at the antiglobulin phase of testing only.
D. Strength of reaction of serum with D-positive cells at the antiglobulin phase of testing.
E. Antibody screen at immediate spin and at the antiglobulin phase of testing.

Question 14: Sequentially increasing anti-c titers are detected in a 28-year-old female who is AB positive, gravida 3, and para 2. Amniocentesis reveals a change in optical density reading at 450 nm (ΔOD_{450}) of 0.8 at 20 weeks of gestation on the Liley curve. The laboratory test results are shown in Table 9-14.

Table 9-14.

	Anti-D	Anti-C	Anti-E	Anti-c	Anti-e
Mother	+	+	−	−	+
Father	−	−	−	+	+

All the following statements are correct *except:*

A. The genotype of the fetus is *R1/r* or *r'/r*.
B. A compatible blood type for IUT is group O, r'/r'.
C. A compatible blood type for IUT is group O, r/r.
D. The probability of the fetus being Rh positive is greater than that of the fetus being Rh negative.
E. The choice of r'/r' units will considerably reduce the number of units available for IUT. The D status determination of the fetus may alleviate the situation.

Question 15: Assuming that each unit of platelet concentrate prepared from 1 unit of whole blood contains 0.5 mL of red cells, how many units of D-positive platelets would be neutralized by 1 standard vial of RhIG?

A. 10.
B. 30.
C. 45.
D. 60.
E. 90.

Question 16: A 72-year-old Rh-negative man is found to have anti-D in his serum. He is undergoing revision of a quadruple coronary artery bypass graft. He is transfused with 10 units of platelets; 6 units are Rh positive and 4 units are Rh negative. Your advice to the clinician is:

A. Therapeutic intervention is not required.
B. Perform exchange transfusion with Rh-negative red cells.
C. Monitor the platelet count closely because of the administration of incompatible platelets.
D. Administer RhIG.
E. Arrange for a therapeutic plasma exchange to remove the anti-D.

HEMOLYTIC DISEASE

Question 17: Anti-D and anti-C are identified in the serum of a 25-year-old woman, gravida 2, para 1, during routine antenatal screening. The history of transfusions is negative. The hospital records indicated that a 300-µg dose of RhIG was administered 1 year ago, at 28 weeks of gestation, and after the delivery of an Rh-positive infant. The erythrocyte rosette test was negative at the time of delivery. Antigen testing of the patient, her husband, and the infant is shown in Table 9-17. Your advice to the clinician is:

Table 9-17.

	Anti-D	Anti-C	Anti-E	Anti-c	Anti-e
Patient	−	−	−	+	+
Father	+	−	−	+	+
Infant	+	−	−	+	+

A. RhIG prophylaxis was insufficient, and the patient has developed anti-D. The anti-D titer should be determined.
B. The antibody identified is anti-G. RhIG prophylaxis is indicated at 28 weeks of gestation.
C. RhIG is detected in the serum.
D. Anti-C is a naturally occurring antibody.
E. Anti-C reagent is defective.

Question 18: If blood transfusion is required for the patient (mother) in Question 17, the phenotype of the compatible blood should be:

A. D+C+E+c+e+.
B. D−C+E+c+e+.
C. D−C−E−c+e+.
D. D+C+E−c+e+.
E. D+C+E−c−e+.

Question 19: A 28-year-old pregnant female presents to an obstetrician for her first prenatal visit. It is established that she is at the 10th week of gestation. Blood samples are drawn for routine laboratory testing. In addition, a sample is sent to the blood bank for type-and-screen analysis. The patient is group O positive and an anti-K is identified. Possible management strategies include:

A. Antigen typing of the presumed father.
B. Serial antibody titers.
C. Amniocentesis.
D. Periumbilical blood sampling (PUBS).
E. All of the above.

Question 20: The K antigen is:

A. A high-frequency antigen.
B. Strongly immunogenic.
C. Destroyed by enzymes.
D. Known to have a frequency of 50% in random populations.
E. Absent in patients with paroxysmal nocturnal hemoglobinuria (PNH).

Question 21: The patient with anti-K1 requires K-negative red cells for transfusion. What proportion of units would you expect to be K1 antigen-negative?

A. None.
B. 10% of all units.
C. 25% of all units.
D. 90% of all units.
E. 99% of all units.

HEMOLYTIC DISEASE   309

Question 22: Anti-k (anti-K2) is *not* a common cause of HDFN because:

A. The antibody is of little clinical significance.
B. The k antigen is *not* well developed at birth.
C. Anti-k is an IgM antibody.
D. The k antigen is of high frequency; hence, anti-k is a rare antibody.
E. The antibody always causes death in utero.

Question 23: Anti-k specificity is identified in the serum of a patient. The most probable genotype is:

A. KK.
B. Kk.
C. kk.
D. $Jk^a Jk^b$.
E. $Js^a Js^b$.

Question 24: Assuming ABO and Rh compatibility, who is the best potential source to provide compatible blood for an infant with severe HDFN caused by an antibody to a high-incidence antigen?

A. The mother.
B. The mother's siblings.
C. The American Rare Donor Program.
D. A random donor.
E. The infant's siblings.

Question 25: An AB-positive mother has an infant with anemia and a positive DAT. The mother's antibody screen is negative. You advise:

A. To screen the mother's serum for antibody against a high-incidence antigen.
B. To screen the mother's serum against the father's red cells.

C. To perform an antibody panel on the infant's serum.
D. To perform an eluate of the infant's red cells and test against a panel of low-incidence antigens.
E. To screen the mother's serum for antibody against a low-incidence antigen.

Question 26: A group A, D-positive woman, gravida 2, para 1, delivered a group O, D-negative infant, her second child. The first child had no features of HDFN. The maternal antibody screens at the first antenatal visit and at 28 weeks of gestation were negative. The cord blood of the newborn (second child) has a positive DAT, using anti-IgG, and the hemoglobin concentration is 6.0 g/dL. Reactions of the mother's serum with selected cells are shown in Table 9-26.

Table 9-26.

	Saline (IS at RT)	PEG, 37 C AHG	CC
Paternal red cells	2+	3+	NT
Red cells of the first infant	0	2+	NT
Red cells of the newborn	0	2+	NT
Maternal red cells	0	0	4+

IS = immediate spin; RT = room temperature; PEG = polyethylene glycol; AHG = antihuman globulin; CC = check cells; NT = not tested.

Which of the following is the most likely explanation for the findings?

A. ABO incompatibility.
B. Rh incompatibility other than anti-D (eg, anti-c and/or anti-E).
C. Anamnestic immune response secondary to re-exposure to paternal antigen in the first pregnancy.
D. Neonatal alloimmune thrombocytopenia (NAIT).
E. Incompatibility involving a low-incidence antigen.

Question 27: The line in Fig 9-27 represents the spectrophotometric analysis of a sample of amniotic fluid. Which of the following statements is *true*?

A. The slope of the line is in the reverse direction.
B. The horizontal axis represents the optical density.
C. The vertical axis represents the wavelength.
D. The sloping line represents the expected optical density in the absence of an elevated bilirubin.
E. ΔOD at 410 nm (ΔOD_{410}) represents a measure of bile pigment concentration.

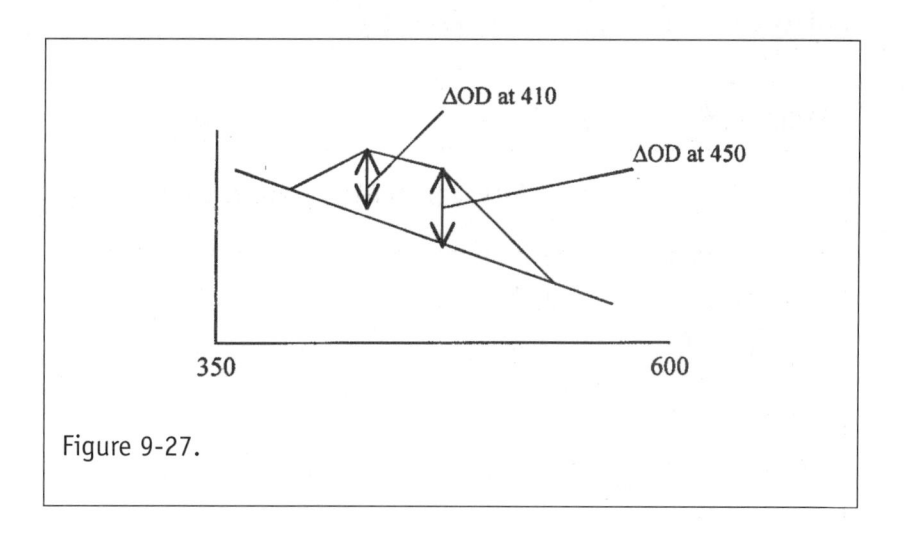

Figure 9-27.

Question 28: Figure 9-28A shows the plots of the absorbance values, at 450 nm, of amniotic fluid sampled at different periods of time from five different pregnancies in which alloantibodies were detected.

Fig 9-28A.

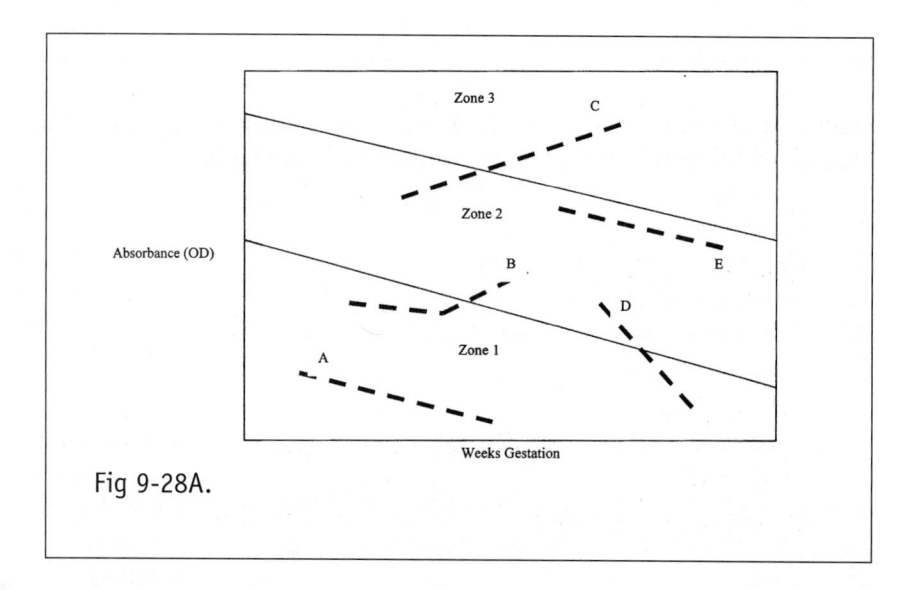

Which infant would be expected to be most severely affected by HDFN?

A. Infant from pregnancy A.
B. Infant from pregnancy B.
C. Infant from pregnancy C.
D. Infant from pregnancy D.
E. Infant from pregnancy E.

Question 29: In a child severely affected by HDFN, which of the following would not increase the risk of kernicterus?

A. Hypoalbuminemia.
B. Penicillin treatment.
C. Hypoxemia.
D. Prematurity.
E. Acidosis.

HEMOLYTIC DISEASE 313

Question 30: AABB *Standards for Blood Banks and Transfusion Services (Standards)* requires that red cells selected for IUT should be:

A. Irradiated.
B. Washed.
C. Leukocyte-reduced.
D. Transfused with a hematocrit ≤55%.
E. ≤3 days old.

Question 31: Which factor(s) contributing to HDFN are removed during exchange transfusion?

A. Antigen.
B. Antigen and antibody.
C. Antigen, antibody, and bilirubin.
D. Antibody.
E. Antigen and bilirubin.

Question 32: Which of the following statements is *true* about NAIT?

A. HLA-matched platelets should be used for transfusion.
B. The maternal platelet count is usually low.
C. The antibody has human platelet antigen (HPA)-1b specificity in most cases.
D. The antibody is IgM.
E. Genetic restriction is responsible for a lower incidence of the offending antibody than expected.

Question 33: Which of the following statements concerning NAIT is *true*?

A. The incidence of NAIT is approximately 1:10,000 births.
B. In contrast to ABO HDFN, the first infant or fetus is rarely affected.
C. HLA Class I antibodies are a common cause of NAIT.

D. Serial measurements of maternal platelet antibody titers are a useful predictor of the severity of fetal thrombocytopenia.
E. The most serious complication is fetal intracerebral hemorrhage (ICH).

Question 34: While performing utilization review of platelet transfusions, requests for patients with each of the following diagnoses are noted. Platelet transfusion is more often indicated for which of these diagnoses?

A. Gestational thrombocytopenia.
B. Immune thrombocytopenic purpura (ITP).
C. HELLP syndrome.
D. Patient with fetus at high risk for NAIT.
E. Thrombotic thrombocytopenic purpura (TTP).

ANSWERS

Question 1: D

Explanation:

- The antigens of the Rh, K, Fy, Jk, MNSs, Di, Do, and Sc systems, as well as Co^a, Au^a, and i are fully expressed on newborn red cells.
- The i antigen is strongly expressed on fetal and cord (newborn) red cells and has a linear biochemical structure. From birth to 2 years, i antigen expression gradually decreases while I antigen expression increases. The I antigen has a branched structure. The enzyme encoded by the *I gene* is responsible for this branching effect.
- A, B, P_1, Le^a, Le^b, Lu^a, Lu^b, Yt^a, Xg, Sd^a, I, and Vel are weakly expressed on newborn red cells.
- ABH antigens on the red cells of 6-week-old fetuses are weakly detectable. Full adult expression is reached by 2 to 4 years of age.

Question 2: E

Explanation:

- Lewis antibodies are not associated with HDFN for the following reasons:
  - Most examples of anti-Le^a and anti-Le^b are IgM and do not cross the placenta.
  - IgG anti-Le^a and anti-Le^b (capable of crossing the placenta) do not cause HDFN because fetal red cells have poor expression of Lewis antigens.
  - Lewis antigens are also expressed in plasma and on other tissues, providing additional targets for Lewis antibodies and reducing the risk of hemolysis.
- Similar to Lewis antigens, P and I are carbohydrate-based antigens. The immune responses to these antigens do not cause HDFN because the antigens are poorly expressed on fetal red cells. In addition, the antibodies are predominantly IgM.

- Anti-I, anti-Le^a, and anti-P$_1$ are often present in the serum of patients with no history of transfusion or pregnancy (ie, they are naturally occurring).
- The antibodies most commonly associated with severe HDFN are anti-D (RH1), anti-c (RH4), and anti-K (KEL1)
- Red cell antibodies that may occasionally cause HDFN include the following:
  - Other Rh system antibodies—usually mild.
  - Other Kell system antibodies—usually mild.
  - Anti-S (MNS3), -s (MNS4), -U (MNS5)—uncommon, but may be severe.
  - Anti-Fy^a (FY1), -Jk^a (JK1), -Jk^b (JK2)—uncommon, usually mild.
  - Anti-M (MNS1)—rare, but may be severe.
- Red cell antibodies *not* implicated in HDFN include anti-Le^b (LE2), anti-P (GLOB1), anti-Lu^a (LU1), anti-N (MNS2), anti-Xg^a (XG1), antibodies with high-titer, and low-avidity characteristics.

Question 3: D

Explanation:

- ABO HDFN is most common among group O mothers because group O individuals have ABO antibodies (anti-A, anti-B, and anti-A,B) that are approximately 50% IgG and 50% IgM. A, B, and AB individuals have predominately IgM ABO antibodies. Because only IgG antibodies can cross the placenta, neonates of group O mothers are at greatest risk for HDFN.
- Maternal-fetal ABO incompatibility is the most common cause of HDFN.
- ABO HDFN is usually mild because fetal cells have weak expression of ABH antigens, and because ABO antibodies are likely to be bound to ABO antigens expressed on the placenta and other fetal tissues. Full antigenic expression of ABH antigens is reached by the age of 2 to 4 years.
- The frequency of mild ABO HDFN is 1:150 births.
- The frequency of severe ABO HDFN is 1:3000 births.
- First pregnancies can be affected because antibodies to the ABH blood group antigens are naturally occurring and are present in the serum of normal, healthy individuals.

HEMOLYTIC DISEASE

- Maternal-fetal ABO incompatability occurs in approximately 20% of pregnancies and has been shown to provide protection against maternal alloimmunization to the D antigen. Incompatible fetal cells in the maternal circulation are hemolyzed by anti-A and anti-B specificities before an immune response (to D) is triggered.
- Group O fetuses and newborns are not affected by ABO HDFN. Because their red cells are compatible with the mother, protection against alloimmunization to paternal antigens is also not present.
- Large numbers of spherocytes are present on the peripheral blood smear of neonates with ABO HDFN.
- Treatment for ABO HDFN:
  - Treatment is usually not required.
  - Phototherapy is required in <5% cases.
  - Exchange transfusion is very rarely indicated.

Question 4: D

Explanation:

- The infant's ABO group is A (4+ reaction with anti-A and anti-A,B).
- Reverse grouping reactions indicate that anti-A and anti-B and/or anti-A,B are present in the infant's serum.
- Isoagglutinins are *not* present in serum of infants who are only 2 days old. The mother's IgG anti-A,B and/or anti-A and anti-B are present in the infant's serum. The mother's ABO group is O.
- Isoagglutinins appear after stimulation by cross-reacting antigens present in the environment (eg, on gut bacteria). Isoagglutinins are usually first detectable at 3 to 6 months of age and reach their maximal titer at 5 to 10 years of age.
- Newborns are usually typed by forward (cell) grouping reactions only. Reverse grouping reactions are not typically performed.

Question 5: E

Explanation:

- **D Antigen.** The presence or absence of the D antigen, an antigen of the Rh blood group system, defines the Rh positive or negative phenotype. In populations of European ethnicity, 85% of individuals are Rh positive. Only red cells express Rh antigens, including D.
- There is no d antigen.
- The *RH* locus is on chromosome 1 and contains *RHD* and *RHCE* genes, which are homologous and closely linked.
- The D+ phenotype is a result of the codominant inheritance of *RHD* genes.
- The genotype of D+ individuals is *RHD/RHD* or *RHD/–* (phenotype D/D or D/–).
- Rh-negative individuals of European ethnicity (D– phenotype) result from a deletion of the *RHD* gene.
- In African-American and other populations, the Rh-negative phenotype results from a single-point mutation, a partial deletion or a recombination event.
- The D antigen is a powerful immunogen; anti-D is commonly implicated in severe HDFN.
- **D Sensitization.** D– mothers, carrying D+ fetuses are at risk for HDFN caused by anti-D.
- Rh-negative women carrying ABO-compatible Rh-positive infants who do not receive RhIG will become sensitized at the following frequency:
  - 7% with first pregnancy.
  - 17% with subsequent pregnancies.
  - 15% to 22% total lifetime risk.
- Sensitization results from maternal-fetal hemorrhages, most important at the time of delivery. Once sensitized, subsequent pregnancies can be affected, usually with increasing severity.
- There is a 75% to 90% chance that an Rh-negative individual will form anti-D after receiving an Rh-positive blood transfusion.
- The immune response to the D antigen consists predominantly of IgG antibodies, usually IgG1 and/or IgG3; the majority of these antibodies do not fix complement.

- **RhIG.** RhIG administration prevents primary sensitization to the D antigen. The mechanism of action is not completely understood but is thought to include increased clearance of fetal red cells, competitive antigen blocking, and negative modulation of the primary immune response.
- RhIG administration does not reverse immunization, or prevent HDFN in an already immunized woman.
- Other antigens of the Rh system can cause Rh HDFN. This is usually less severe.
- Although some preparations may contain anti-C, anti-E, and other blood group alloantibodies, RhIG administration does not prevent formation of non-D antibodies.
- **HDFN.** Because of the use of RhIG, the most common cause of HDFN is no longer sensitization to the D antigen. Currently, ABO incompatibility is the most common cause of HDFN.
- HDFN results from the extravascular destruction of fetal/neonatal red cells by maternal red cell alloantibodies. Antibodies are directed against paternal antigens inherited by the infant and absent in the mother.
- Only IgG antibodies directed against antigens expressed on fetal/neonatal red cells can cause HDFN, as these are antibodies capable of crossing the placenta.
- Morbidity/mortality of HDFN results from the following:
  - High-output congestive heart failure, in utero or during the neonatal period, caused by anemia.
  - Neonatal kernicterus caused by elevated bilirubin levels.

Question 6: B

Explanation:

- Amniocentesis may be performed to assess bilirubin concentrations (ΔOD_{450}), by spectrophotometric analysis. This correlates with the severity of hemolytic disease of the fetus. Alternatively, Doppler ultrasonography of fetal middle cerebral artery peak systolic velocity may be used as a noninvasive method to assess fetal anemia.
- The assessment of the significance of an antibody titer is dependent on the antibody specificity and whether or not the patient has had a previously affected fetus.

- For patients who have not had affected fetuses, or who are in their first pregnancy, the titers are important for determining the type of fetal evaluation that will be performed. Once sensitization is detected, titers are repeated on a monthly basis until about 24 weeks, then every two weeks thereafter.
- The data correlating antibody titers and clinical findings are largely derived from experience with anti-D. Recommendations based on anti-D are largely applicable to other specificities associated with HDFN, with the possible exception of anti-K (see Question 19).
- In women who have had affected fetuses, antibody titers are no longer adequately predictive of HDFN. The paternal antigen type may be used to determine whether fetal typing is necessary. If the fetal genotype is positive, fetal assessment for evidence of HDFN should begin no later than at 18 weeks gestation.
- The critical titer is defined as the lowest titer that is associated with a significant risk of fetal hydrops. Each facility should define its own critical titer, but generally anti-D titers are considered critical when they reach 16 or 32. An anti-D titer of 32 is always considered critical. Waiting for titers of 64 or greater before initiating further management will endanger the fetus.
- Once a critical titer has been reached, further risk assessment may include the paternal antigen type, the fetal antigen type, Doppler ultrasonography to determine middle cerebral artery peak velocities, and spectral analysis of amniotic fluid. Increased middle cerebral artery peak velocity is predictive of fetal anemia.
- Decisions regarding intrauterine transfusion are based on ΔOD_{450} values in relation to the gestational age of the fetus, as described by the Liley graph.
- **Contraindications to the administration of RhIG:**
  - RhIG is not indicated for patients who are actively immunized to the D antigen.
  - RhIG is not indicated for Rh-negative women carrying or delivering Rh-negative infants.
  - RhIG is not indicated for Rh-positive women with weak D phenotype due to decreased expression of a normal D antigen (ie, quantitative decrease in D antigen sites); they do not make anti-D.
- **Partial D:**
  - Rh-positive individuals with a partial D phenotype lack one or more epitopes of D the antigen. D^{VI} is perhaps the most significant partial D; these individuals can make anti-D, yet test as weak D positive when testing is performed with antisera in common use.

HEMOLYTIC DISEASE

Increasingly, transfusion services are choosing not to perform weak D testing on patient samples. This approach avoids the risk that a D^{VI} variant individual will be transfused with D-positive cells and become alloimmunized. Although there is still some controversy about whether partial D women require Rh prophylaxis, not testing for weak D eliminates the dilemma.
- RhIG is not indicated for patients who are Rh positive except for the treatment of immune thrombocytic purpura (ITP).
- RhIG may be used to prevent alloimmunization in Rh-negative individuals exposed to Rh-positive cellular blood products. This intervention is most commonly reserved for females of child-bearing potential, and is uncommonly used for males or postmenopausal females.
- Possible hazards of RhIG administration:
  - RhIG contains IgA and has caused hypersensitivity reactions in IgA-deficient individuals with IgA antibodies.
  - In the past, rare lots of RhIG were implicated in viral infectious disease transmission.

Question 7: C

Explanation:

- **Indication:** The erythrocyte rosette test is a screening test indicated in Rh-negative women giving birth to Rh-positive infants.
- **Principle and Procedure:** The number of Rh-positive fetal red cells may be too small to detect in a mother's sample by the direct addition of anti-D. In the rosette test, a chemically modified anti-D is incubated with the mother's sample. The cells are then washed and Rh-positive indicator cells are added. If fetal cells are present, they will have been coated by anti-D. Indicator cells (D-positive) and D-positive fetal cells are bridged by the anti-D, forming microscopic rosettes, which are counted.
- **Interpretation of positive and negative rosette tests:**
  - A positive result is a qualitative measure indicating that at least 10 mL of Rh-positive fetal red cells may have entered the maternal circulation. This result cannot be used to determine the necessary dose of RhIG. This requires a quantitative evaluation such as the Kleihauer-Betke test.

- If the test is negative, then <<10 mL of fetal red cells are present and a standard dose of 300 µg of RhIG is sufficient to prevent sensitization to the D antigen.
- One vial (300 µg) of RhIG offers protection against 30 mL of D-positive whole blood or 15 mL of D-positive red cells. A microdose of RhIG (50µg) offers protection against 2.5 mL of D-positive red cells. The protective effect probably results from interference with antigen recognition in the induction phase of primary immunization.
- Doses of less than 300 µg may be used for pregnancy terminations up to and including 12 weeks gestation.
- A standard dose of 300-µg RhIG is indicated for the following:
  - Antepartum dose at 28 to 32 weeks of gestation.
  - Amniocentesis at any time during the pregnancy.
- A minimum of 1 300-µg vial and testing to assess the need for additional vials is indicated for the following:
  - Postpartum administration.
  - All other obstetric procedures.

Question 8: B

Explanation:

- The Kleihauer-Betke test is based on the ability of fetal hemoglobin (hemoglobin F) to withstand the denaturing effect of an acid solution. The test is used to determine the volume of FMH and calculate the appropriate dose of RhIG.
- The Kleihauer-Betke acid elution test identifies fetal hemoglobin, *not* blood group surface antigens, including D.
- Maternal hereditary persistence of fetal hemoglobin (HPFH) may cause a falsely elevated Kleihauer-Betke test caused by the presence of maternal red cells with hemoglobin F (Hb F).
- The I antigen is identified by testing red cells with anti-I.
- Wharton's jelly is a thick gelatinous substance that coats the umbilical cord. Wharton's jelly, if present in the cord blood sample, can cause the following:
  - Rouleaux.
  - ABO discrepancies.
  - False-positive DATs.

HEMOLYTIC DISEASE   323

Question 9: D

Explanation:

- The Kleihauer-Betke test is performed if the rosette test is positive.
- **Principle:** The Kleihauer-Betke acid elution test is used for quantification of FMH in order to provide adequate RhIG immunoprophylaxis (to Rh-negative mothers who deliver Rh-positive infants).
- **Procedure:** Upon exposure of a maternal blood smear to an acid buffer, fetal hemoglobin resists elution and appears bright pink and refractile. Adult maternal hemoglobin is eluted and the red cells appear as "ghost cells" with intact red cell membranes. The percent of fetal (pink) cells are determined by counting the number of pink cells present out of 2000 total cells examined.
- **Calculation:** 2000 cells are counted and the number of cells with fetal hemoglobin are noted.
    - Percentage of fetal red cells:
      (Number of fetal cells ÷ 2000) × 100
      (40 ÷ 2000) × 100 = 2%
    - Example of calculation of vials of RhIG required for 2% fetal red cells in a mother with 5000-mL blood volume:
      2/100 × 5000* mL [or 2 × 50* (% fetal cells × maternal blood volume/100)] = 100 mL fetal blood
      100 mL fetal blood ÷ 30 mL fetal blood/vial of RhIG = 3.33 vials
      *When the maternal blood volume is not known, 5000 mL is commonly used as an estimate of average maternal blood volume. Use of the mother's actual blood volume is recommended as it provides a more accurate determination of the number of doses of RhIG needed.
- Because of the error inherent in the Kleihauer-Betke test and the risk of underestimating an FMH, the number of doses is adjusted to provide a safety margin. Once the number of doses is determined, then rounding rules must be applied:
    - If the digit to the right of the decimal is less than 5, round down and add 1 dose (eg, 3.33 = 3 + 1 = 4 doses).
    - If the digit to the right of the decimal point is equal to or greater than 5, round up and add 1 dose (eg, 3.75 = 4 + 1 = 5 doses).

Question 10: A

Explanation:

- The patient received sufficient RhIG protection at 28 weeks.
- The Kleihauer-Betke test determines the volume of FMH and is used to calculate the dose of RhIG. One dose of RhIG protects against the immunizing effects of 30 mL of Rh-positive whole blood.
- RhIG dose calculation:
  - FMH in milliliters = (% fetal cells × 50) = 2.7 × 50 = 135 mL.
  - Number of RhIG doses = FMH/30 mL = 2.7 × 50/30 = 4.5.
  - Number of doses of RhIG required: 4.5, rounded up to 5 + 1 = 6 doses.
- The patient received 5 doses. Inadequate postpartum dosing likely caused the RhIG failure in this case, resulting in immune anti-D formation.
  - Using 5000 mL as an estimate of the mother's blood volume may also underestimate the amount of RhIG necessary. Whenever possible the mother's actual blood volume should be used in the calculation.
- In pregnant women receiving RhIG at 28 weeks of gestation and within 72 hours of delivery, the RhIG failure rate is 0.1%.
- Causes of RhIG failure include:
  - Inadequate dosing.
  - Failure to give the RhIG dose to the mother (eg, dose given to father or infant).
  - Failure to give the RhIG dose at 28 weeks.
  - Failure to give the RhIG dose within 72 hours of delivery, procedure, or transfusion.
- In the case of postpartum administration, administration up to 13 days after delivery has been found to be effective in preventing alloimmunization. Therefore, in situations where RHIG was not provided within 72 hours because of error or other unplanned circumstances, the RHIG should still be administered as soon as possible for up to 28 days after delivery.
- RhIG is available in two forms:
  - **IM (intramuscular):** Up to 6 doses of RhIG can be given by the IM route at one time. For larger quantities, the injections are spaced over a period of 72 hours for patient comfort. IM preparations (eg,

Rhogam, Ortho-Clinical Diagnostics, Raritan, NJ) must not be given intravenously as they contain aggregates of immunoglobulin that may activate complement.
- **IV (intravenous):** IV preparations [eg, WinRho (Baxter Healthcare, Deerfield, IL), Rhophylac (CSL Behring, King of Prussia, PA)] are filtered to disrupt immunoglobulin aggregates. A standard IV dose is 1500 IU, which is the equivalent to the 300-μg IM dose. (Note: Intravascular RhIG preparations are available in vials containing 600 or 1500 IU.)

Question 11: C

Explanation:

- The Wr^a antibody is commonly found in patients with hyperactive immune systems, who are exposed to Wr^a+ red cells. The antibody is commonly seen in the sera of:
  - Recently delivered women who have formed anti-D.
  - Patients with autoimmune hemolytic anemia (AIHA).
  - Patients alloimmunized to other blood group antigens.
- Anti-Wr^a and Anti-Wr^b are naturally occurring antibodies and react best by the indirect antiglobulin test (IAT).
- Anti-Wr^a is present in 1 of 100 serum samples but rarely causes HDFN or hemolytic transfusion reactions.
- Wr^a (WR1) is a low-prevalence antigen with a frequency of 0.001% (1:100,000).
- The antithetical Wr^b (WR2) antigen is a high-prevalence antigen with a frequency of 99.999%.
- Wr^a (WR1) and Wr^b (WR2) have a codominant pattern of inheritance and require an interaction with glycophorin A for expression.
- Anti-C, -Jk^b, -Jk^a, and -K are antibodies to common antigens, which are identified by the antibody panel. Antibodies to low-prevalence antigens, such as Anti-Wr^a, are usually not identified by the antibody screen because the antigens are not typically present on the screening cells.
- A reaction between anti-Wr^a (in serum) and the Wr^a (WR1) antigen on the red cells of the donor unit may have resulted in the incompatibility seen with one crossmatched unit.

Question 12: A

Explanation:

- The antibody screen and panel demonstrate an antibody with anti-D specificity reacting at both immediate spin and the antihuman globulin (AHG) phases of testing. The presence of reactivity at immediate spin suggests that an IgM antibody is present. RhIG preparations, either IV or IM, contain IgG anti-D and not IgM. The presence of IgM anti-D is indicative of alloimmunization to the D antigen. The patient likely represents an RhIG failure that is reported to occur in 0.1% of patients receiving RhIG at 28 weeks and within 72 hours of delivery.
- Because the patient is alloimmunized against D, administration of RhIG at delivery is not indicated.
- Features that suggest active alloimmunization, and not passive anti-D from RhIG, include a titer greater than 4 and persistence of the antibody 3 months or more after administration. Weak reactivity ($\leq$1+) is also suggestive of passive immunization; however, this criterion should be interpreted with caution as polyethylene glycol, gel, and solid-phase adherence testing may all give 2+ or greater reactivity with passive antibodies. Strength of reactivity alone is not sufficient to differentiate between passive and active immunization. Unless the origin of the D antibody can be clearly established, it is best to err in the direction of administering the RhIG.
- There is no evidence for anti-M (see panel cell 8).
- The negative autocontrol, using patient's cells and serum, excludes a cold-reactive autoantibody. Check cells are used to verify that AHG was added to negative tubes. They are not added to positive tubes.

Question 13: B

Explanation:

- A frequently arising question is whether anti-D present in a serum sample represents passive anti-D (caused by RhIG) or active alloimmunization to the D antigen (as in this case).

HEMOLYTIC DISEASE

- The administration of RhIG results in a positive antibody screen. Repeating the screen will identify anti-D and will not differentiate between passively and actively acquired antibody.
- To definitively determine if an antibody represents passive antibody or an alloantibody, the allotype of the anti-D must be compared to the allotype of antibodies known to be produced by the patient (eg, antibodies generated as a result of childhood immunizations). If the allotype of these antibodies are different, then the anti-D is passive as RhIG is derived from the plasma of multiple sensitized individuals. If they are the same, then it is an immune alloantibody. All alloantibodies of a particular person are identical (with respect to allotype).
- Allotypic variants are generally the result of amino acid changes in the antibody constant regions. IgG antibodies have Gm and Km allotypes. IgM antibodies have Km allotypes.
- Allotype antibody testing is carried out at research institutions and is not routinely available.
- Other helpful but not conclusive characteristics of passive anti-D vs alloimmunizaton include the following:
  - Weakly reactive (≤1+; see also the explanation for Question 12).
  - Low titer (4 or less).
  - IgG anti-D only. The presence of an IgM antibody (reactivity at immediate spin) indicates a primary immune response and alloimmunization to the D antigen. The absence of an IgM component does not rule out alloantibody.
  - Short duration of detection. RhIG is usually no longer detectable by 3 months, with virtually all cases being negative by 6 months. Rare cases of persistence from 8 months to 1 year have been reported.
  - A positive history of RhIG administration.
- The presence of a high titer or strongly reactive antibody suggests alloimmunization.
- Obstetric indications for RhIG administration in Rh-negative women *not* alloimmunized to D include the following:
  - Antepartum status (28 weeks).
  - Postpartum status (if infant is Rh positive).
  - Termination of pregnancy (abortion).
  - Ectopic pregnancy.
  - Amniocentesis.
  - Percutaneous umbilical blood sampling.
  - Chorionic villous sampling.

- Obstetric complications (eg, abdominal trauma, abruptio placenta, placenta previa, manual removal of placenta, threatened abortion, antepartum vaginal bleeding, in-utero fetal demise, external cephalic version, and trophoblastic disease or neoplasia).
- Nonobstetric indications for RhIG administration include the following:
  - Transfusion of Rh-positive red-cell-containing blood components (red cells, platelets, granulocytes) to an Rh-negative individual not alloimmunized to the D antigen.
  - Treatment of ITP (in Rh-positive individuals).

Question 14: C

Explanation:

- A compatible blood type for intrauterine transfusion (IUT) is group O negative, c antigen negative (r'/r', Ce/Ce).
- The anti-c specificity in the fetal circulation may hemolyze ce/ce (r/r) RBCs.
- The genotype of the mother is *DCe/Ce (R1/r')* or *DCe/DCe (R1/R1)*.
- The frequency of the *R1/R1* genotype is 17.2%; the frequency of the *R1/r'* genotype is 0.77% (general population).
- The genotype of the father is *ce/ce (r/r)*.
- The genotype of the fetus is *R1/r* or *r'/r*.
- The probability that the mother is homozygous for D (R1/R1) is 22 times more likely than her being heterozygous for D (R1/r'). Hence, the probability that the fetus is Rh positive is greater than the fetus being Rh negative.
- The *r'/r'* genotype is rare, with a frequency of 0.01%, so D status determination of the fetus may be useful in selecting blood for IUT. If the fetus is Rh positive, group-specific R1/R1 or group O R1/R1 units can be used.
- The D status of the fetus can be determined by the following:
  - Polymerase chain reaction (PCR) to amplify the DNA of fetal cells derived from amniotic fluid or maternal blood samples.
  - PCR of biopsy-derived chorionic villous tissue.
  - Serologic reactions (D-antigen testing) of fetal blood obtained by cordocentesis.

Question 15: B

Explanation:

- One standard vial of RhIG contains 300 µg of predominantly IgG anti-D. This dosage offers sufficient protection to prevent sensitization to the D antigen in a D-negative recipient who receives a blood component containing up to 15 mL of D-positive red cells or 30 mL of whole blood.
- The D antigen is an integral membrane protein of D-positive red cells and is not present on platelets.
- A platelet concentrate unit typically contains ≤0.5 mL of red cells.
- Thirty units of pooled platelet concentrates could contain as much as 15 mL of red cells, which will be neutralized by 1 standard vial of RhIG.
- Leukocyte-reduced apheresis platelets generally have red cell contents of <0.01 mL. The risk of D sensitization after transfusion of Rh-positive leukocyte-reduced apheresis platelets may be negligible, especially when transfusing patients who are immune compromised because of underlying disease or therapy. Even so, it is prudent to provide RhIG prophylaxis for at least women of child-bearing potential.
- Intravenous preparations of Rh Immune Globulin are prepared for thrombocytopenic patients in order to avoid the risk of injection site intramuscular bleeding.

Question 16: A

Explanation:

- Hemolysis will occur only in an Rh-negative recipient with anti-D who receives blood components containing a significant amount of Rh-positive red cells. Antibodies to the D antigen are associated with extravascular hemolysis. The small amount of red cells present in platelet components (including Rh-positive platelets) will not result in any clinical consequences.

- Platelets do not posses Rh antigens, so the presence or absence of anti-D would not affect the survival of the transfused platelets. Only red cells possess Rh antigens.
- RhIG prophylaxis should be offered to all Rh-negative, premenopausal, female recipients who are not alloimmunized against D and who receive blood components containing Rh-positive red cells. Administration of RhIG to non-alloimmunized males or postmenopausal females is optional. Administration to alloimmunized individuals is contraindicated.
- Therapeutic plasma exchange is indicated for the reduction of unwanted antibody from the circulation of a patient. It has been used to remove anti-D from the circulation of pregnant women carrying Rh-positive fetuses. However, this therapy has rarely been effective and is not recommended for the treatment of HDFN by the American Society for Apheresis or AABB.
- The D antigen is the most immunogenic of all red cell antigens. More than 80% of Rh-negative recipients who receive a transfusion of a single unit of Rh-positive red cells would be expected to develop anti-D.

Question 17: B

Explanation:

- Immune anti-C is not present in the serum, as the patient has had no exposure to the C antigen.
- Anti-G (anti-CD) is an immune antibody and has apparent anti-D and anti-C specificity. The antibody recognizes an epitope associated with both the D and C antigens. Most individuals with the apparent combination of anti-D and anti-C also have anti-G in their serum. Anti-G is usually suspected in a woman whose serum contains anti-D and anti-C despite having received appropriate RhIG prophylaxis.
- The anti-G specificity is identified by sequential elution-absorption technique, as follows:
  - Absorb the serum with D+G+C− cells (absorption #1).
  - If a separate anti-C is present, the absorbate will contain anti-C. An antibody panel performed using absorbate #1 will demonstrate anti-C in the absence of anti-D reactivity.

HEMOLYTIC DISEASE 331

- If anti-G is present, the eluate of the absorbing cells will exhibit reactivity to D and reactivity to C. Because the absorbing cells were C negative and therefore unable to bind anti-C, the anti-C reactivity detected in the eluate is attributable to anti-G.
- Absorb the eluate with D−G+C+ cells (absorption #2).
- If a separate anti-D is present, the absorbate will contain anti-D. An antibody panel formed using absorbate #2 will demonstrate anti-D in the absence of anti-C reactivity.
- The eluate from absorption #2 may contain anti-G, ie, anti-D and anti-C reactivity eluted from a cell that is D negative; therefore, D reactivity is attributable to G.
- Anti-G specificity is confirmed using $r^G r$ (D−C−G+) cells and D^{IIIb} (D+C−G−) cells.
- The D^{IIIb} (D+C−G−) phenotype is very rare and expresses a partial D antigen.
- The accurate identification of anti-G is important in women of child-bearing age with apparent anti-D and anti-C. If these antibodies actually represent anti-G, RhIG prophylaxis would be indicated.
- The half-life of RhIG, in the absence of significant FMH, is 21 days. RhIG is usually detectable up to 3 months after administration and in some cases up to 6 months after administration.
- The Rh antigen profile of the trio is as follows:
  - Patient (mother): ce/ce (r/r).
  - Father: cDe/ce (Ro/r) or cDe/cDe (Ro/Ro).
  - Child: cDe/ce (Ro/r) or ce/ce (r/r).

Question 18: C

Explanation:

- The genes expressing the D and/or C antigens also express the G antigen, with few exceptions.
- Rare individuals with D+G− and D−C−G+ phenotypes have been described.
- Individuals with ce/ce (r/r), cE/cE (r"/r"), and ce/cE (r/r") can make anti-G.
- Individuals with anti-G should be transfused with r/r, r"/r", or r/r" red cells. Choice C is r/r.

Question 19: E

Explanation:

- Kell antigens are well-expressed on fetal cells. Anti-K and other Kell system antibodies are immune IgG antibodies capable of crossing the placenta and causing HDFN and hemolytic transfusion reactions (HTRs).
- Antibody titers are a minimally invasive way of predicting the risk of clinical HDFN. The antibody that has been best studied to date is anti-D, with a titer of 16 to 32 considered to be a "critical titer" with respect to fetal hemolysis.
- Although it has been well studied in the context of anti-D, data is scarce that would support a critical titer of 16 to 32 with other antibodies (with respect to this titer serving as the trigger to do more invasive testing). However, in the absence of data, it has been common practice to extrapolate the anti-D data to other blood group antibodies.
- Antibody titers are even less reliable when anti-K is involved. These antibodies have a tendency to behave in an unpredictable manner (ie, titer may not have much correlation with hemolysis in the antigen-positive fetus). At least one reason for this is that anti-K, in addition to causing anemia through a classic hemolytic process, may also cause fetal anemia through the inhibition of normal erythropoiesis. Anti-K antibodies suppress or inhibit erythroid progenitor cells. A lower critical value titer of 8 has been suggested for antibodies to the K and k antigens
- Paternal antigen testing can be very helpful in predicting the likelihood of anti-K HDFN. If the father's red cells type K antigen-negative (likely, as ~90% of all individuals type negative for this antigen), then the fetus would not be at risk for hemolysis.
- If the father's red cells type homozygous for K antigen expression (ie, k antigen-negative; unlikely, as only ~0.2% of all individuals are homozygous for the K antigen), then the fetus is at definite risk for HDFN.
- If the father's red cells type as Kk antigen positive (~8.8% of all individuals are heterozygous), then the fetus has a 50% chance of inheriting the K antigen with the associated risk of hemolysis.

HEMOLYTIC DISEASE

- The phenotypic frequency of Kell blood group antigens and risk of anti-K HDFN are shown in Table 9-19.

Table 9-19.

Paternal Phenotype	Frequency of the Phenotype — Whites	Frequency of the Phenotype — Blacks	Fetal Phenotype	Risk of Anti-K HDN
K–k+ (kk)	91%	98%	K–k+ (kk)	0%
K+k– (KK)	0.2%	Rare	K+k+ (Kk)	100%
K+k+ (Kk)	8.8%	2%	50% chance fetus will be K+k+	50%
			50% chance fetus will be k+k+	0%

- The frequency of the K (K1) antigen is 9% in people of European ethnicity and 2% in people of African ethnicity. The K antigen is a member of the Kell blood group system. The immune response to this protein determinant is typically IgG, so the antibody can readily cross the placenta. If the developing fetus is also K antigen-positive, then hemolytic disease of the newborn is a significant risk. However, it is important to note that this does not become an overriding concern until later in pregnancy (ie, >20 weeks). Overall, the risk that a K-negative woman will develop anti-K and be at risk of HDFN is lower than the risk of a D-negative woman developing anti-D and having anti-D-related-HDFN.
- Amniocentesis and PUBS (cordocentesis) are more direct methods for assessing fetal well-being (with respect to the degree of hemolysis and anemia). Amniocentesis is performed 1) to assess fetal status and need for cordocentesis in fetuses of homozygous fathers and 2) to determine the fetal genotype when the father is heterozygous or paternity may be questionable.
- Cordocentesis is performed when there is Doppler evidence of fetal anemia (increased middle cerebral artery flow), or amniotic fluid

bilirubin concentration (ΔOD_{450}) is increased. The red cell mean corpuscular volume (MCV) offers rapid confirmation that fetal blood has been sampled during cordocentesis. The average adult (maternal) MCV is ~91 fL, whereas that of the fetus is ~114 fL. However, the distinction between maternal and fetal MCV becomes obscured after the first intrauterine transfusion and later in gestation. The procedure-related rate of fetal loss associated with cordocentesis is 1% to 2%.

Question 20: B

Explanation:

- The K antigen is the second most immunogenic blood group antigen. Approximately 10% of K-negative individuals exposed to 1 unit of K-positive blood will form an anti-K antibody. In comparison, transfusion of a D-positive unit to a D-negative individual carries an 80% risk of sensitization. The relative immunogenicity of protein blood group antigens is: D >> K >> c >> E >> e >> Fy^a >> C >> Jk^a >> S >> Jk^b >> s.
- Proteolytic enzyme treatment does not destroy Kell system antigens. Reagents such as 2-mercaptoethanol (2-ME), dithiothreitol (DTT), and 2-aminoethylisothiouronium bromide (2-AET) can denature them.
- The Kell protein is a single-pass glycoprotein that is complexed with the Kx protein, a multipass transmembrane protein. Kell has considerable homology to other neutral endopeptidases.
- The Cromer system antigens are located on the complement regulatory protein decay accelerating factor (DAF), which is absent in PNH. Other antigens lost in PNH include John Milton-Hagen (JMH), Cartwright system antigens, and Dombrock system antigens.

Question 21: D

Explanation:

- Antigens K (K1, KEL1) and k (Cellano, K2, KEL2) are encoded by the antithetical codominant autosomal alleles *K* and *k*, respectively.

HEMOLYTIC DISEASE 335

- These genes are present at the *Kk* sublocus of the *KEL* complex locus on chromosome 7q33-q35.
- Kell system phenotypes and frequencies are shown in Table 9-21.

Table 9-21.

Antibody Produced After Sensitization	Phenotype	Antigens on Red Cells	Phenotype Frequency (%) Whites	Blacks
Anti k	KK, (*KK*)	K	0.2	Rare
—	Kk, (*Kk*)	K, k	8.8	2
Anti K	kk, (*kk*)	k	91	98

Question 22: D

Explanation:

- The high-frequency antigens are highly prevalent in all human populations. Therefore, antigen-negative individuals, in whom immune antibody can be produced, are rare. As such, antibodies to high-frequency antigens are rare causes of HDFN.
- The low-frequency antigens are very rare. Immune sensitization to low-frequency antigens is rare because of the rarity of exposure. Hence, low-frequency antigens are rare causes of HDFN.
- Anti-k is an immune, IgG, and potentially clinically significant antibody implicated in HDFN and HTRs. HDFN varies in severity and does not always cause death in utero.
- The Kell antigens are well expressed on the fetal red cells.
- k (K2) is a high-frequency antigen. Its prevalence is 99.8% in people of European ethnicity and >99% in people of African ethnicity.
- When anti-k is discovered (or other antibodies to high-frequency antigens), there may be difficulty in obtaining antigen-negative blood for transfusion. The American Rare Donor Program may be helpful in obtaining high-frequency antigen-negative units of blood.

- The mother and her siblings can be screened for antigen-negative, crossmatch-compatible blood.

Question 23: A

Explanation:

See explanations for Questions 21 and 22.

Question 24: A

Explanation:

- In HDFN caused by an antibody to a high-incidence antigen, the mother is homozygous for a low-incidence antigen and the infant/fetus is positive for the antithetical high-incidence antigen.
- The mother's or her siblings' irradiated, washed, antigen-negative, compatible red cells are a good source of fresh blood for the transfusion of the infant. The mother's red cells must be washed to remove the offending antibody present in the mother's plasma.
- Compatible donors can also be sought through a rare donor file.
- Random donors are not a good source of units as they are likely to be positive for the high-incidence antigen.
- If the father is heterozygous for the high- and low-incidence antigens in question, the infant's siblings can be screened for compatible red cells.

Question 25: B

Explanation:

- The etiology of HDFN:
  - A red cell antigen present on infant/fetal red cells (inherited from the father) and absent on the mother's red cells can elicit the immune response resulting in HDFN.

HEMOLYTIC DISEASE

- ○ The red cells of the infant/fetus enter the mother's circulation, either during gestation or the birth process.
- ○ The mother's immune system responds by producing IgG antibodies against the specific antigen on the infant/fetal red cells. The immune IgG antibodies cross the placenta and cause HDFN by opsonizing fetal red cells, resulting in extravascular hemolysis via splenic removal.
- The clinical situation in this question is consistent with HDFN caused by an antibody directed at a low-incidence antigen present on the father's and the infant's red cells and absent on the mother's red cells.
- The frequency of low-incidence antigens is typically ≤1:1000.
- The mother's antibody screen is negative because the screening cells lack the low-incidence antigen in question. The antibody screen detects most antibodies against high-incidence antigens and common blood group antigens.
- The immune antibody in the mother's serum will react with the antigen-positive red cells of the father and the infant/fetus.
- The infant has anemia and a positive DAT because of opsonization of red cells with the mother's IgG antibodies. If free antibody is present in the infant's serum, it will also react against screening cells in the same manner that the mother's antibody screen reacted. Testing against a panel of low-incidence antigens is not necessary because knowing the exact specificity of the antibody is not essential.
- The eluate prepared from the infant's red cells would react identically to the mother's plasma, ie, the antibody screen performed with the eluate would also be negative.
- Identification of the exact specificity of the mother's antibody is not essential.
- Transfusion of the infant, if clinically indicated, is easily accomplished using the mother's serum to identify crossmatch-compatible random-donor units of blood.
- Unlike the case of an antibody directed against a high-incidence antigen, it is not necessary to use the mother as a source of red cells, as most donors will not possess the low-incidence antigen.
- Because of the negative antibody screen, it is difficult to identify women with antibodies to low-incidence antigens during their pregnancies, unless there is a history of a previously affected pregnancy.

Question 26: E

Explanation:

- The positive DAT indicates coating of newborn red cells with maternal IgG antibody. It could be the result of ABO incompatibility, or incompatibility involving high-incidence or low-incidence antigens.
- The mean cord hemaglobin concentration of healthy newborn infants is 16.9 ±1.6 g/dL. A hemoglobin concentration of 6.0 g/dL indicates anemia.
- The negative maternal antibody screen for clinically significant antibodies rules out HDFN involving common antigens, including D, c, and/or E.
- The mother is group A with anti-B in the serum. The newborn is group O, and lacks A and B antigens on his/her red cells. ABO incompatibility is not responsible for HDFN.
- The HDFN is caused by an antibody directed against a low-incidence antigen.
- The father and children are positive for the low-incidence antigen. The mother was exposed to paternal antigen in the first pregnancy and mounted an anamnestic response during the second pregnancy, leading to HDFN.
- The IgM ABO antibodies are saline reactive. The mother and the biologic father are ABO incompatible, indicated by a 2+ reaction at room temperature.
- The mother is ABO compatible with the two children.
- The immune, IgG specificity in the mother's serum, directed at a low-incidence antigen on red cells of the father and the newborn, is responsible for the positive agglutination seen in the IAT with antihuman globulin.
- Neonates with NAIT have a low platelet count and are usually not anemic unless they have sustained severe hemorrhagic complications.

HEMOLYTIC DISEASE 339

Question 27: D

Explanation:

- Amniotic fluid spectrophotometric analysis is performed by first measuring the light absorbance of the fluid at wavelengths from 350 nm to 700 nm. The values at 365 and 550 are plotted on semilog graph paper, with optical density on the logarithmic vertical axis and wavelength on the horizontal axis. The straight line formed by connecting the two points represents the absorbance expected from unpigmented amniotic fluid. The correct direction of the slope is shown in Fig 9-27. The expected 450-nm absorbance derived from the line is compared to the actual measured absorbance. The difference is the ΔOD_{450}.
- Bile pigments, derived from hemolyzed fetal red cells, have peak absorbance at 450 nm.
- Bile pigments, oxyhemoglobin, and meconium all contribute to the optical density reading at 450 nm.
- Hemoglobin absorbs light at 410 and 450. To correct for the contribution of hemoglobin absorption, the ΔOD_{410} is calculated, multiplied by 0.05, and subtracted from the ΔOD_{450} to yield the corrected ΔOD_{450}. Multiplying by 0.05 accounts for the fact that hemoglobin absorption at 450 is only 5% of that at 410.

Question 28: C

Explanation:

- The figure pictured is the Liley graph. Amniotic fluid is sampled in women with evidence of possible HDFN (alloantibody present and titers greater than or equal to a value of concern—eg, 16 or 32); the change in optical density measured at 450 nm is a measure of the increase in amniotic fluid bilirubin. The Liley graph plots ΔOD_{450} on the vertical axis and weeks gestation on the horizontal axis.
- The slope of the line is downward. As pregnancy length increases, the absorbency at 450 nm decreases because of dilution by fetal urine. This results in the downward slope of the two solid lines. These lines

divide the graph into three zones that represent the anticipated severity of the hemolysis in the child. Zone 1 is unaffected to mildly affected, zone 2 is moderately affected, and zone 3 is severely affected.
- In addition to the zone in which a measurement falls, the trend of the lines over time also determines prognosis.
- The Liley graph was originally employed for the management of HDFN in the third trimester. The Queenan modification of the Liley graph (Queenan, 1993; see Fig 9-28B) applies ΔOD_{450} monitoring to the second trimester.

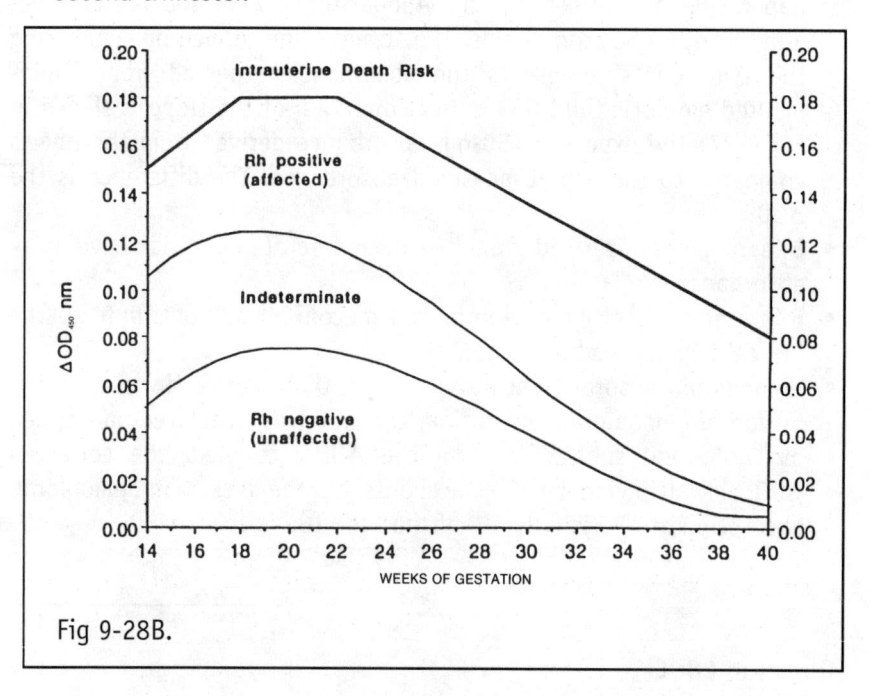

Fig 9-28B.

- Lines B and C demonstrate increasing absorbance, which means that the bilirubin levels are increasing, a sign of increasing hemolysis. Line C falls within the severely affected zone, indicating a worse prognosis.
- Line D demonstrates decreasing absorbance, a favorable trend suggesting decreasing hemolysis.
- Lines A and E parallel the solid lines separating the zones. This results from the dilution of the amniotic fluid by fetal urine.

Question 29: B

Explanation:

- Kernicterus refers to the deposition of bilirubin in neural tissues associated with neurologic injury. The regions of the brain that are most commonly affected are the basal ganglia, hippocampus, geniculate bodies, and cranial nerve nuclei, especially the oculomotor, vestibular, and cochlear nuclei. The cerebellum can also be affected. The long term consequences are cerebral palsy, mental retardation, hearing loss, and upward gaze paresis.
- The risk of kernicterus is increased when hyperbilirubinemia occurs in a setting where compromise of the blood-brain barrier permits higher than normal permeability to bilirubin. This can occur with prematurity, hypoxemia, or acidosis.
- Albumin binds bilirubin and is important for reducing the levels of free bilirubin in the circulation. The risk of kernicterus is higher in the setting of hypoalbuminemia, or when bilirubin is displaced from albumin by drugs such as sulfa antibiotics.
- The levels of bilirubin at which exchange transfusion may be required is dependent on the gestational maturity of the infant, the rate of bilirubin increase, whether hyperbilirubinemia is caused by hemolysis, and whether there are other associated risk factors.
- In general, term infants with isolated hyperbilirubinemia do not require exchange transfusion until the total serum bilirubin levels approach 25 mg/dL. Near-term infants (35 weeks) and sick infants may need exchange transfusion at levels approximating 20 mg/dL. Critical levels are lower for markedly preterm infants.

Question 30: A

Explanation:

- Cellular components used for intrauterine transfusion must be irradiated, according to *Standards*. Fetuses are not fully immune competent because of immaturity of their immune systems. Irradiation of

cellular blood components effectively prevents graft-vs-host disease (GVHD).
- Other characteristics that should be considered when selecting blood for intrauterine transfusion include the following:
  - Antigen negative (with respect to the mother's blood group antibody).
  - Hemoglobin S negative.
  - ABO and Rh compatible.
  - Fresh as possible to avoid elevated potassium levels and optimize posttransfusion red cell survival.
  - Hematocrit = 75% to 85%.
  - Washed (if antibody is present in the donor).
  - Cytomegalovirus (CMV)-negative or leukocyte reduced if the mother is nonreactive for CMV antibodies.

Question 31: C

Explanation:

- Exchange transfusion replaces fetal antigen-positive red cells sensitized with maternal antibody with adult antigen-negative cells; it removes maternal antibody in the infant's circulation and removes bilirubin from the intravascular compartment.
- Bilirubin concentrations may continue to rise after exchange transfusion because of the following:
  - Extravascular bilirubin migration into the intravascular compartment (following a concentration gradient).
  - Continuous destruction of remaining sensitized fetal red cells.
- A repeat exchange transfusion may be required if hyperbilirubinemia is clinically significant.

Question 32: E

Explanation:

- Human platelet-specific antigens HPA-1 through -16 are present on platelets but not on red and white cells.

- The most common causes of NAIT in people of European ethnicity (Whites) are antibodies to HPA-1a (Pl[A1]) (80%), HPA-5b (Br[a]) (10%), HPA1b (4%), and HPA-3a (Bak[a]) (2%), other antibodies are responsible for the remainder. Among people of Asian ethnicity (Asians), antibodies to HPA-4a (Yuk/Pen[a]) are the most common cause. This is because the HPA-1b/1b genotype is common in Whites and virtually absent in Asians. HLA incompatibility is a rare cause of NAIT.
- The pathology of NAIT is analogous to HDFN. The mother develops antibodies toward platelet-specific antigens present on fetal platelets. These antibodies cross the placenta and bind to the platelets, resulting in platelet destruction. In addition, some antibodies, such as those to HPA-1a, HPA-1b, and HPA-2a, interfere with platelet function.
- In NAIT, the mother's platelet count should be relatively normal.
- HPA-1a and HPA-1b are antithetical antigens. HPA-1a is a public or high-frequency antigen with a 98% phenotypic frequency in Whites. Its antithetical antigen, HPA-1b, is less common, with a 28% phenotypic frequency in Whites.
- Phenotypic frequencies of HPA-1 system antigens in Whites are shown in Table 9-32.

Table 9-32.

Alloantigen System	Allelic Forms	Phenotypic Frequency
HPA-1	HPA-1a	72% HPA-1a/1a
		26% HPA-1a/1b
	HPA-1b	2% HPA-1b/1b

- The HPA-1b/1b polymorphism is present in 2% of the population. Approximately 5% of HPA-1a antigen-negative mothers carrying an HPA-1a antigen-positive fetus become immunized. One reason for this low rate of sensitization is the genetic restriction of the formation of HPA-1a antibodies to individuals with DRW52a (DRB3 0101) HLA type. An amino acid substitution of leucine for proline at position 33 on the GPIIIa chain is responsible for the production of alloantibodies. The preferential presentation of this polypeptide with certain HLA molecules is postulated as the mechanism for the genetic restriction seen in NAIT.

- NAIT occurs in 1:1500 to 1:2000 pregnancies. In contrast to HDFN, first pregnancies are affected in NAIT.
- The treatment of choice during pregnancy is maternally administered intravenous immune globulin (IVIG) therapy, 1 g/kg/week with or without steroids. Of note, high doses of IVIG may interfere with the immunoassays used to detect infectious diseases. If the mother will be giving a platelet product for intrauterine transfusion, infectious disease testing should be performed before starting IVIG treatments.
- IVIG therapy in current and subsequent pregnancies successfully raises the fetal platelet count in most cases.
- IVIG nonresponders or severely affected fetuses are treated with intrauterine antigen-negative platelet transfusions. Maternal platelets (concentrated, washed, irradiated, and leukocyte-reduced) may be the most readily obtainable antigen-negative platelets. When available, routine volunteer antigen-negative platelets are preferred in order to avoid the need for washing.
- HPA-1a antibodies are also responsible for posttransfusion purpura.

Question 33: E

Explanation:

- NAIT varies in severity from mild thrombocytopenia with no clinical signs to overt bleeding. The most serious complication is fetal ICH, which has been reported to occur in 10% to 30% of cases. ICH is typically intraparenchymal and tends to occur when platelet counts fall below 20,000/μL. Bleeding of this type can occur as early as 20 weeks of gestation.
- The fetal platelet count is the most important predictor of the clinical severity of NAIT. In high-risk pregnancies (for NAIT) a fetal blood sample to determine the platelet count is obtained by cordocentesis. If thrombocytopenia is detected, compatible, irradiated, leukocyte-reduced, and CMV-safe platelets are transfused during the same procedure.
- Maternal antibody titers do not predict the severity of NAIT, though subclass analysis of the antibodies may be useful. Women with predominantly IgG3 anti-HPA-1a have more severely affected infants than those with predominantly IgG1 antibodies.

- The first infant or fetus is affected in 25% of NAIT cases. Subsequent pregnancies are affected 75% to 90% of the time.
- Platelets express HLA Class I antigens. Multiparous women may have high-titer HLA antibodies. HLA antibodies are implicated in rare cases of NAIT, but these cases tend to be clinically mild.

Question 34: C

Explanation:

- Approximately 4% to 12% of patients with eclampsia (severe toxemia of pregnancy) develop HELLP syndrome. Significant clinical findings include the following:
    - **H**emolysis.
    - **E**levated **L**iver enzymes.
    - **L**ow **p**latelet count.
- Platelet transfusion may be required for patients with HELLP syndrome at delivery (usually by urgent caesarean section) and postpartum.
- Most patients recover within a few days of delivery. A subset of patients requires plasma exchange.
- Gestational thrombocytopenia is seen in the third trimester in some women and is the most common cause of thrombocytopenia in pregnancy. It is characterized by a platelet count around 100,000/µL without evidence of hemorrhage. Infants of women with gestational thrombocytopenia are not thrombocytopenic. Maternal platelet transfusion is usually not required and not indicated. It should be noted that the maternal platelet count tends to fall throughout pregnancy.
- The presence of very low platelet counts (< 50,000/µL) suggests a diagnosis of maternal ITP. The autoantibodies present in ITP can cause thrombocytopenia in infants (around 12%) but are not associated with the high risk of ICH seen in NAIT. The incidence of ICH is 1% in ITP. Treatment of ITP consists of IVIG, corticosteroids, and postpartum splenectomy. Maternal platelet transfusion is very rarely indicated or helpful.
- Other common causes of thrombocytopenia in pregnancy include systemic lupus erythematosus, preeclampsia, and viruses, especially human immunodeficiency virus.

- Maternal platelet transfusion is not indicated in patients with a fetus at high risk for NAIT.
- Platelet transfusions have been considered contraindicated in TTP because of the concern that increasing the platelet count may lead to the formation of more platelet microthrombi. Although evidence is lacking to support or refute this concern, limiting platelet transfusions to those situations where bleeding is severe or life threatening is recommended.
- Other conditions where the transfusion of platelets is generally not indicated include the following:
  - Prophylactic use during cardiac surgery or massive transfusion.
  - Platelet dysfunction caused by extrinsic factors (eg, hypergammaglobulinemia, uremia).
  - Treatment of hemolytic uremic syndrome and heparin-induced thrombocytopenia.
  - Posttransfusion purpura, ITP, and compensated disseminated intravascular coagulation.

REFERENCES

1. Queenan JT, Tomai TP, Ural SH, King JC. Deviation in amniotic fluid optical density at a wavelength of 450 nm in Rh-immunized pregnancies from 14 to 40 weeks' gestation: A proposal for clinical management. Am J Obstet Gynecol 1993;168:1370-6.
2. Kennedy M. Perinatal issues in transfusion practice. In: Roback JD, Combs MR, Grossman BJ, Hillyer CD, eds. Technical manual. 16th ed. Bethesda, MD: AABB, 2008:625-37.
3. McFarland J. Platelet and granulocyte antigens and antibodies. In: Roback JD, Combs MR, Grossman BJ, Hillyer CD, eds. Technical manual. 16th ed. Bethesda, MD: AABB, 2008:525-45.
4. Poole J, Daniels G. Blood group antibodies and their significance in transfusion medicine. Transfus Med Rev 2007;21:58-71.
5. Urbaniak SJ, Greiss MA. RhD haemolytic disease of the fetus and the newborn. Blood Rev 2000;14:44-61.
6. Moise K. Management of Rhesus alloimmunization in pregnancy. Obstet Gynecol 2008;112:164-76.
7. Bowman JM, Pollock JM, Manning FA, et al. Maternal Kell blood group alloimmunization. Obstet Gynecol 1992;79:239-44.

8. Moise KJ. Red blood cell alloimmunization in pregnancy. Semin Hematol 2005;42:169-78.
9. Webster R. Reproductive function and pregnancy. In: McPherson RA, Pincus MR, Henry JB, eds. Henry's clinical diagnosis and management by laboratory methods. 21st ed. Philadelphia: WB Saunders Company, 2006. [Available at http://www.mdconsult.com (accessed September 8, 2008).]
10. Oepkes D, Seaword G, Vendenbussche F, et al. Doppler ultrasonography versus amniocentesis to predict fetal anemia. N Engl J Med 2006;555: 156-64.

10

Noninfectious Complications of Transfusion

QUESTIONS

Question 1: When a fatality occurs in association with blood collection or transfusion, the Director of the Office of Compliance and Biologics Quality of the Food and Drug Administration (FDA) must be notified by:

A. Telephone or e-mail only, as soon as possible.
B. Written report only, within 7 days.
C. Written report only, within 30 days.
D. Telephone or e-mail as soon as possible and written report within 7 days.
E. Telephone or e-mail as soon as possible and written report within 30 days.

Question 2: Most preventable fatal transfusion reactions are caused by:

A. Errors in the performance of donor disease testing.
B. Errors in patient or specimen identification.
C. Errors in the interpretation of serologic reactions.
D. Hemolytic antibodies of the Kidd blood group system.
E. Hemolytic antibodies of the Rh blood group system.

Question 3: The most common cause of transfusion-associated mortality reported to the FDA is:

A. Posttransfusion purpura (PTP).
B. Transfusion-associated graft-vs-host disease (TA-GVHD).
C. Hemolytic transfusion reactions associated with ABO incompatibility.
D. Transfusion-related acute lung injury (TRALI).
E. Transfusion-associated infections.

Question 4: Of the following, the least common cause of transfusion-associated mortality reported to the FDA is:

A. PTP.
B. TA-GVHD.
C. Hemolytic transfusion reactions associated with ABO incompatibility.
D. TRALI.
E. Transfusion-associated infections.

Question 5: Antibodies directed against which of the following blood group systems are most commonly implicated in intravascular hemolytic transfusion reactions?

A. Kidd.
B. ABO.
C. Kell.
D. Rh.
E. Duffy.

Question 6: The most common initial sign/symptom of an intravascular hemolytic transfusion reaction is:

A. Pain at the infusion site.
B. Fever.
C. Hypotension.
D. A feeling of impending doom.
E. Hemoglobinuria.

Question 7: Which of the following serologic evaluations is most important in the assessment of a possible acute hemolytic transfusion reaction?

A. Antibody screen.
B. Antibody identification panel.
C. Crossmatch.
D. Direct antiglobulin test (DAT).
E. Rh type.

Question 8: A 65-year-old woman is in the operating room for a complicated spinal surgical procedure. Multiple Red Blood Cell (RBC) units are expected to be required. The patient is blood group O positive. During the transfusion of the third unit of blood, the anesthesiologist notes that the patient is producing red urine. All vital signs are stable. The transfusion is stopped and a transfusion reaction investigation ensues. Which of the following is the least likely explanation for this patient's reaction?

A. Intravascular hemolytic transfusion reaction.
B. Mechanical damage to red cells secondary to use of a cell saver device.
C. Bladder irritation from catheterization causing hematuria.
D. Bacterial contamination of the third unit.
E. Osmotic damage to red cells caused by infusion of a nonisotonic solution.

Question 9: While receiving a platelet transfusion, a 25-year-old neutropenic man with acute leukemia develops a fever and rigors. The most likely diagnosis is:

A. Intravascular hemolytic transfusion reaction.
B. Anaphylactic transfusion reaction.
C. Bacterial contamination of the unit.
D. Allergic transfusion reaction.
E. Manifestation of the patient's underlying clinical condition.

Question 10: The most common cause of fever in the context of transfusion is:

A. TRALI.
B. PTP.
C. Febrile nonhemolytic transfusion reaction (FNHTR).
D. Intravascular hemolytic transfusion reaction.
E. Patient's underlying clinical condition.

Question 11: A 50-year-old man with a 5-year history of myelodysplastic syndrome is scheduled to undergo a hip replacement for severe osteoarthritis. He has not required transfusion previously. At the end of the operative procedure, the patient is noted to have a platelet count of 40,000/μL. His surgeon orders a platelet transfusion. The transfusion service provides a pool of 5 platelet concentrates that are transfused in the recovery room. Near the end of the transfusion, the patient experiences a temperature elevation, from a baseline of 98.5 F to 101 F, accompanied by chills. All other vital signs are stable except for an elevation in blood pressure from 126/82 mmHg to 158/88 mmHg. The patient is treated with an antipyretic and his fever promptly resolves. What type of transfusion reaction has this patient likely experienced?

A. Intravascular hemolytic transfusion reaction.
B. Delayed hemolytic transfusion reaction (DHTR).

C. Bacterial contamination.
D. FNHTR.
E. TRALI.

Question 12: A 50-year-old man with pancreatic cancer is undergoing chemotherapy and has a requirement for frequent red cell and platelet transfusions. During the transfusion of 6 units of pooled platelet concentrates, the patient suddenly develops a high fever accompanied by rigors, shock, facial flushing, abdominal cramping, nausea, and vomiting. This constellation of symptoms is most suggestive of:

A. An intravascular hemolytic transfusion reaction.
B. An FNHTR.
C. TRALI.
D. A bacterially contaminated unit.
E. A manifestation of the patient's underlying clinical condition.

Question 13: A 3-year-old girl with a metastatic tumor is admitted to the hospital for surgical evaluation of her disease. She received multi-agent chemotherapy and is now anemic, with a hematocrit of 20%. She receives a 150-mL aliquot of red cells after admission without incident. Within 30 minutes of a second red cell transfusion (also 150 mL) 24 hours later, the patient begins to cough and has increasing difficulty breathing. She also develops a fever with a temperature elevation of 2 C. All other vital signs are stable including heart rate and blood pressure. Eventually, the child requires intubation secondary to increasing respiratory effort and poor oxygenation. The most likely diagnosis is:

A. TRALI.
B. An anaphylactic transfusion reaction.
C. A hemolytic transfusion reaction.
D. Volume overload.
E. A manifestation of the patient's underlying clinical condition.

Question 14: TRALI is defined by which of the following features?

A. Preexisting acute lung injury before transfusion.
B. Onset of symptoms within 6 hours of transfusion.
C. Evidence of left atrial hypertension.
D. Presence of HLA antibodies in the transfused blood component.
E. A higher mortality rate in comparison with other types of acute lung injury.

Question 15: A 2-year-old child has a complex congenital heart defect in need of surgical repair. The procedure will require extracorporeal bypass and multiple units of blood will be needed. Near the end of the surgical procedure, a unit is transfused. Shortly thereafter, the anesthesiologist notes the development of red urine. A blood sample obtained for intraoperative laboratory testing also reveals red serum. All vital signs are stable. The transfusion is stopped and a transfusion reaction workup is initiated. The transfusion reaction investigation is negative (ie, clerical check is fine, pre- and posttransfusion DAT testing is nonreactive, and repeat ABO typing demonstrates no discrepancy) except for the visual inspection (ie, red serum). This child likely experienced what type of reaction?

A. Intravascular hemolytic transfusion reaction.
B. DHTR.
C. No hemolysis; red serum and red urine are unrelated to transfusion.
D. Mechanical hemolysis attributable to the bypass circuit.
E. Hematuria and hemoglobinuria related to bladder catheterization.

Question 16: Antibodies directed against which of the following blood group systems are most commonly implicated in DHTRs?

A. Kidd.
B. ABO.
C. Kell.

D. Rh.
E. Duffy.

Question 17: The transfusion service received an order for 1 RBC unit for an anemic patient with a history of four pregnancies. The patient received 6 units of crossmatch-compatible blood 16 days ago and had a negative antibody screen at that time. The current pretransfusion blood sample contains anti-Jk^a and anti-E. The patient has a 2+ reactive DAT with polyspecific antihuman globulin (AHG) reagent. Testing with anti-IgG is positive, whereas testing with anti-C3d is negative. The patient's red cell phenotype, using the original pretransfusion sample, is E negative and Jk^a negative. Red cells from the current sample demonstrate mixed-field reactivity for the E and Jk^a antigens. Nine out of 10 units are crossmatch-incompatible. The best interpretation of these findings is that:

A. An intravenous injection of penicillin given the previous day has caused the positive DAT.
B. The patient has warm autoimmune hemolytic anemia (WAIHA).
C. The patient has experienced a DHTR caused by anti-Jk^a and/or anti-E.
D. The DAT reactivity must be confirmed with an indirect antiglobulin test (IAT) in order to make sense of the serologic findings.
E. Since compatible blood is not available, the transfusion order should be cancelled.

Question 18: Which of the following statements about allergic transfusion reactions is *true*?

A. They occur in about 10% of all transfusion recipients.
B. They most commonly present with cutaneous manifestations.
C. True anaphylaxis is a common consequence.
D. Fever is a common finding.
E. They can be treated and prevented with Tylenol (McNeil-PPC, Fort Washington, PA).

Question 19: A 14-year-old boy with a diagnosis of acute leukemia is hospitalized to begin consolidation chemotherapy. He received multiple transfusions in the past (red cells and platelets) without incident. After infusion of 50 mL of a plateletpheresis product, the patient begins to cough and wheeze. His breathing is labored and his oxygen saturation falls to 80%. His blood pressure also falls from 114/68 mmHg to 84/42 mmHg, but he remains afebrile. The patient is treated with Benadryl, subcutaneous epinephrine, and an albuterol updraft and stabilizes rapidly. The signs and symptoms that he experienced are most likely the result of:

A. An acute hemolytic transfusion reaction.
B. TRALI.
C. Volume overload.
D. Anaphylaxis.
E. A manifestation of the primary disease process.

Question 20: Which of the following statements about IgA deficiency is *true*?

A. Most patients do not have anti-IgA.
B. Patients are at risk for acute hemolytic reactions.
C. It occurs at a frequency of approximately 1 in 70,000 to 1 in 80,000 people of European ethnicity.
D. Previous transfusion or pregnancy is required to develop IgA antibodies.
E. Washed platelets are the product of choice for IgA-deficient patients.

Question 21: TA-GVHD is characterized by which of the following?

A. The development of dermatitis, hepatitis, and enteritis.
B. Prevention through the provision of washed cellular blood components.

C. Prevention through leukocyte-reduction of cellular blood components.
D. A fatality rate similar to that seen with the GVHD accompanying marrow transplantation.
E. Destruction of recipient tissue by activated lymphocytes of recipient origin.

Question 22: Which of the following is a generally accepted indication for the irradiation of cellular blood components?

A. Patients with sepsis.
B. Patients with AIDS.
C. Patients with solid-organ malignancy undergoing chemotherapy.
D. Patients with IgA deficiency.
E. Recipients of directed donations from biologic relatives.

Question 23: For which of the following patient categories is gamma irradiation of cellular blood components *not* generally performed?

A. Recipients or candidates for marrow or progenitor cell transplants.
B. AIDS patients.
C. Patients with severely compromised cell-mediated immunity.
D. Recipients of intrauterine transfusion (IUT).
E. Blood components of donors selected for HLA compatibility.

Question 24: A 60-year-old woman with a history of five pregnancies receives a 2-unit red cell transfusion during a surgical procedure. She has no previous history of transfusion. Seven days later, the patient is noted to have extensive bruising of the extremities and bleeding gums. She has no other symptoms. Her platelet count is 5000/µL. The most likely diagnosis is:

A. Drug-induced thrombocytopenia.
B. PTP.
C. Immune thrombocytopenic purpura (ITP).

D. Thrombotic thrombocytopenic purpura (TTP).
E. Disseminated intravascular coagulation (DIC).

Question 25: Which of the following statements related to iron and red cell transfusion is *true*?

A. Each RBC unit contains approximately 2 g of iron.
B. There is no physiologic means to excrete excess iron.
C. Patients who acutely require massive volumes of red cells are at greatest risk for iron overload.
D. Chronically transfused patients are at no excess risk for iron overload.
E. Iron chelation therapy is an ineffective treatment for those with iron overload.

Question 26: The immunomodulatory effects of transfusion:

A. Are attributed to the infusion of leukocytes.
B. Are attributed to the infusion of immunoglobulins.
C. Are minimized with the use of irradiated cellular blood components.
D. Are amplified with the use of leukocyte-reduced cellular blood components.
E. Have profound negative clinical consequences for transfusion recipients.

Question 27: Which of the following represents a potential complication of massive transfusion?

A. Hypermagnesemia.
B. A hypercoagulable state.
C. Hyperthermia.
D. Hypotension.
E. Citrate toxicity.

NONINFECTIOUS COMPLICATIONS OF TRANSFUSION   359

Question 28: Which of the following statements regarding hypotensive transfusion reactions is *true*?

A. They are associated with the use of positively charged bedside leukocyte-reduction filters.
B. They have been seen in patients taking angiotensin-converting enzyme (ACE) inhibitors.
C. They are mediated by the infusion of cytokines.
D. They are most often seen in conjunction with Fresh Frozen Plasma (FFP) transfusions.
E. They are more often seen when prestorage leukocyte-reduced units are transfused.

Question 29: A 70-year-old man with a history of coronary artery disease is admitted to the hospital for a total hip arthroplasty. During the procedure, his vital signs are within normal limits, though he experiences significant bleeding. In the recovery room, he is found to have a hematocrit of 26%, so a 2-unit red cell transfusion is ordered. Halfway through the administration of the second unit of blood, the patient begins to cough and complains of tightness in his chest and a severe headache. He is afebrile, but his other vital signs are altered, as follows:

- Blood pressure—pretransfusion = 120/75 and posttransfusion = 165/85.
- Heart rate—pretransfusion = 78 and posttransfusion = 120.
- Respiratory rate—pretransfusion = 20 and posttransfusion = 32.
- The transfusion is discontinued, the patient is provided supplemental oxygen and, after 30 minutes, feels much better. Which of the following adverse reactions to transfusion has the patient most likely experienced?

A. TRALI.
B. Anaphylaxis.
C. Transfusion-associated circulatory overload (TACO).
D. Acute hemolytic reaction.
E. Bacterial contamination of the donor unit.

Question 30: Which of the following statements is *true* regarding acute pain transfusion reactions (APTRs)?

A. They most often occur in patients with sickle cell disease.
B. They are associated with the use of ACE inhibitors.
C. They most commonly last for several hours after the discontinuation of transfusion.
D. They are characterized by severe pain in the trunk and proximal extremities.
E. They are prevented by premedicating patients with acetaminophen.

ANSWERS

Question 1: D

Explanation:

- Fatalities related to blood collection or transfusion must be reported promptly to the Director, Center for Biologics Evaluation and Research, Office of Compliance and Biologics Quality of the FDA. The following contact methods may be used:
  - Email: fatalities2@fda.hhs.gov
  - Telephone: 301.827.6220
  - Delivery of report:
    FDA/Center for Biologics Evaluation and Research
    Office of Compliance and Biologics Quality
    Division of Inspections and Surveillance (HFM-650)
    1401 Rockville Pike, Suite 200 North
    Rockville, MD 20852-1448
- A report should be made by telephone or e-mail as soon as possible.
- A written report should be submitted within 7 days of the fatality.
- The initial report need not contain all of the pertinent information in final form, as additional studies (eg, cultures) and analysis may be pending. However, once finalized, this information must be sent to the FDA as soon as possible.
- Reporting is performed in accordance with the Code of Federal Regulations [21 CFR 606.170(b)].

Question 2: B

Explanation:

- Most preventable fatal transfusion reactions are caused by the transfusion of ABO-incompatible units of blood.
- Approximately 15 to 20 such reactions occur annually in the United States, as reported to the FDA.
- The underlying reason for all ABO-incompatible transfusions is human error: patients receive the wrong units of blood.

- These errors can result from problems in the correct interpretation of serologic reactions, but the majority relate to errors in either patient or specimen identification (ie, mistaken identity). Only 10% of these errors occur within the blood bank. The remaining 90% occur at the time of specimen collection or patient transfusion.
- The best hope for the prevention of ABO-incompatible transfusions lies in preventing or detecting errors in every phase of the transfusion process: from phlebotomy to all steps in laboratory testing, and to the issue of units and their ultimate transfusion.

Question 3: D

Explanation:

See explanation for Question 4.

Question 4: A

Explanation for Questions 3 and 4:

- Table 10-4A describes the incidence and mortality associated with noninfectious complications of transfusion.
- Table 10-4B describes the cases of transfusion-associated mortality reported to the FDA during fiscal years 2005 and 2006.

Table 10-4A.

Complication	Incidence	Mortality (%)
Hemolysis associated with ABO incompatibility	1:33,000	5
TA-GVHD	1:400,000	>90
TRALI	1:5,000	5
PTP	1:200,000	0 to 13
Microbial infection: RBCs / Platelets	1:250,000 / 1:75,000	70 / 5

Table 10-4B.

	FY2005		FY2006		Total (FY05+FY06)	
Complication	Number	Percentage (%)	Number	Percentage (%)	Number	Percentage (%)
TRALI	29	47	35	56	64	51
HTR (non-ABO)	16	26	9	14	25	20
Microbial infection	8	13	7	11	15	12
HTR (ABO)	6	10	3	5	9	7
TACO	1	2	8	13	9	7
Other*	2	3	1	2	3	2
Totals	62	100	63	100	125	100

*FY2005 includes one case of transfusion-associated graft-vs-host disease and one therapeutic plasma exchange error (use of a treatment column contraindicated because of the patient's medical history).
*FY2006 includes one case of anaphylaxis (patient had high-titer anti-IgA).
FY = fiscal year; TRALI = transfusion-related acute lung injury; HTR = hemolytic transfusion reaction; TACO = transfusion-associated circulatory overload.

- TRALI reactions are the most common cause of transfusion-related mortality reported to the FDA. The reporting of TRALI-related fatalities has increased over the last 5 to 10 years, which is likely the result of an increased recognition of this clinical entity.
- Hemolytic transfusion reactions, caused by the transfusion of ABO-incompatible red cells, continue to be a common type of fatal transfusion reaction reported to the FDA. Perhaps surprisingly, hemolytic transfusion reactions caused by non-ABO antibodies are also an important cause of reported fatal transfusion reactions.
- Bacterial contamination is an important cause of transfusion-associated mortality that is far more commonly associated with platelet products because they are stored at room temperature. It is very uncommon for red cell units to be contaminated, but transfusion of contaminated red cells is likely to have devastating effects for recipients.
- PTP is the least common cause of transfusion-associated mortality reported to the FDA. This is because PTP reactions are rare and have a low mortality. In contrast, TA-GVHD is also rare, but it is far more likely to be associated with a recipient death and, thus, more likely to be reported to the FDA.
- It is important to remember that, although fatal transfusion reactions are rare, transfusion reactions account for a greater morbidity that is *not* necessarily reported to the FDA. At present, there is only a requirement that fatal reactions be reported.
- The true incidence of any transfusion reaction is difficult to estimate because of probable underreporting and failure to make an accurate diagnosis.

Question 5: B

Explanation:

- Preformed, high-titer anti-A and/or anti-B are the most common antibodies implicated in acute intravascular hemolytic transfusion reactions.
- Anti-A and anti-B are naturally occurring antibodies that develop within a few months of birth. They are predominantly IgM antibodies, but they are reactive at 37 C.

- Anti-A and anti-B fix complement, having the ability to drive the complement cascade to completion and cause intravascular hemolysis.
- Antibodies directed against the Kidd, Kell, Rh, and Duffy blood group determinants are predominantly IgG. They have the ability to sensitize red cells but do not fix complement well, with the exception of Kidd antibodies. These IgG antibodies are more frequently implicated in delayed transfusion reactions with associated extravascular hemolysis.

Question 6: B

Explanation:

- All of the possible answers are signs/symptoms that may accompany intravascular hemolytic transfusion reactions, but fever is by far the most common initial presentation (75% of cases). Other signs and symptoms include rigors, chest pain, back pain, and nausea/vomiting.
- Symptoms of an intravascular hemolytic reaction may vary significantly in severity: some patients will experience minimal or no obvious clinical manifestations (even with the transfusion of multiple units of incompatible blood), while others may have severe reactions after only 10 to 15 mL of incompatible blood is transfused.
- The estimated mortality from acute hemolytic transfusion reactions is about 5%, although there is considerably more morbidity involved [eg, shock, renal failure, disseminated intravascular coagulation (DIC)].
- It has been estimated that for every 33,000 units of blood transfused, at least 1 unit is ABO incompatible with a recipient, placing the recipient at risk for an acute hemolytic transfusion reaction and associated clinical consequences.

Question 7: D

Explanation:

- There is significant morbidity and mortality accompanying intravascular hemolytic transfusion reactions. Because of this, quick clinical intervention and laboratory evaluation are essential.
- The DAT is the most important serologic test to perform in the early evaluation of an acute hemolytic transfusion reaction. A newly reactive DAT or a DAT that has increased in strength of reactivity in comparison with the pretransfusion sample strongly supports immune-mediated hemolysis.
- Other common serologic tests, including the antibody screen, the antibody identification panel, and Rh typing, are not likely to yield important information in the evaluation of an acute hemolytic transfusion reaction, as the vast majority of these reactions are caused by ABO antibodies.
- Repeat crossmatch testing is unlikely to be useful unless the root cause of the patient's reaction was a pretransfusion sample that actually belonged to another patient. In that case, crossmatching with a posttransfusion sample would be expected to confirm the incompatibility.
- The vast majority of intravascular hemolytic transfusion reactions are caused by clerical errors (ie, the intended recipient receives the wrong donor unit). As such, a clerical check is an early critical step in the evaluation of these adverse reactions.
- Visual inspection of serum (for evidence of hemoglobinemia) and a centrifuged urine specimen (for evidence of hemoglobinuria) are rapid tests that are commonly used to determine if intravascular hemolysis has occurred.

Question 8: D

Explanation:

- Any patient who develops red urine during transfusion must be considered to be experiencing an intravascular hemolytic transfusion

reaction until proven otherwise. Transfusion should be stopped immediately and a transfusion reaction workup should ensue.
- The critical components of a transfusion reaction workup include a clerical check (essentially, ensuring that the patient received the correct unit), a visual inspection of the serum (for hemoglobinemia), and appropriate serologic studies that include a DAT.
- Red urine should be analyzed after centrifugation to determine the cause for the discoloration. *Hematuria* refers to free red cells in the urine (urine is clear after centrifugation with a pellet of red cells at the bottom of the test tube) while *hemoglobinuria* refers to free hemoglobin in the urine (urine remains red after centrifugation).
- Hematuria is a *common* clinical finding and could result from bladder irritation secondary to an indwelling catheter. Hemoglobinuria is an *uncommon* clinical finding indicative of intravascular hemolysis.
- Intravascular hemolytic transfusion reactions often result in hemoglobinuria. This same finding can be seen with mechanical red cell damage (eg, secondary to a malfunctioning cell saver device) or osmotic damage (as with transfusion accompanied by a nonisotonic saline solution).
- Bacterial contamination in a red cell unit can result in hemolysis. This could, ultimately, result in hemoglobinuria, but the fact that there were no vital sign changes accompanying the development of red urine argues against this possibility. Transfusion of a bacterially contaminated RBC unit would be expected to be accompanied by serious clinical consequences, including high fever, shock, and even death.

Question 9: E

Explanation:

- Fever is the most common presenting sign of an intravascular hemolytic transfusion reaction. However, this is not the best explanation for the patient's reaction because he was receiving a platelet, not a red cell, transfusion. The infusion of ABO-incompatible plasma (with platelet transfusions) is associated occasionally with intravascular hemolysis, caused by high-titer anti-A and/or anti-B, but this is quite rare.

- Anaphylactic transfusion reactions are characterized by flushing of the skin, hypotension, substernal pain, and dyspnea but *not* fever. Some anaphylactic reactions occur in patients who are IgA deficient and have IgA-specific antibodies, but most reactions are associated with unknown allergens.
- Bacterial contamination, another severe and potentially life-threatening complication of transfusion, is classically characterized by the development of high fever, flushing of the skin, abdominal cramping, and shock. Platelet products, because they are stored at room temperature, are the most likely components to be bacterially contaminated.
- Allergic transfusion reactions are characterized by a pruritic skin rash. Occasionally, they are more severe and take on features of anaphylaxis (eg, laryngeal edema, dyspnea, and hypotension); however, a fever is not seen.
- A leukemic patient who is neutropenic could readily manifest a fever in conjunction with transfusion that is actually related to the underlying disease process (eg, a bacterial or fungal infection) and not related directly to the transfused blood component.

Question 10: E

Explanation:

- A patient's underlying clinical condition, including coincidental infection, is the most common cause of fever seen in the context of transfusion.
- FNHTRs are the second most common cause of fever. They may be seen in up to 3% of all transfusion recipients.
- Bacterial contamination, TRALI, PTP, and intravascular hemolytic transfusion reactions are significantly less common causes of fever. In cases of PTP and TRALI, fever may be caused by the presence of HLA antibodies which react with white cells and result in the release of pyrogenic cytokines. These cytokines may also be elaborated in the course of acute hemolytic transfusion reactions.

Question 11: D

Explanation:

- FNHTRs, along with urticarial transfusion reactions, are among the most common adverse reactions to transfusion. FNHTRs may occur in 1% of red cell transfusions and up to 30% of platelet transfusions.
- FNHTRs result from cytokines, such as tumor necrosis factor alpha (TNF-α), interleukin-1 (IL-1), and interleukin-6 (IL-6).
- There are two pathogenic mechanisms important to explaining the etiology of FNHTRs: 1) the recipient has leukoagglutinating antibodies (most commonly HLA antibodies) that react with donor-derived white cells leading to lysis of these cells and cytokine release and 2) the infusion of pre-formed pyrogenic cytokines that accumulate during blood storage as a result of the breakdown of white cells. The latter mechanism explains why FNHTRs can occur in men without any evidence of alloimmunization. Either mechanism could be at play in this clinical case.
- FNHTRs typically occur either during transfusion or up to 6 hours after the completion of transfusion. Chills may accompany them and rigors and mild hypertension are also common findings.
- FNHTRs can be treated and possibly prevented by the administration of antipyretic agents (eg, acetaminophen). Rigors may require the administration of meperidine.
- Leukocyte-reduced cellular blood components are useful in preventing FNHTRs in the chronically transfused and those who are predisposed to these adverse reactions.
- FNHTRs are diagnoses of exclusion. In addition to FNHTRs, intravascular hemolytic transfusion reactions, bacterial contamination, and the patient's underlying clinical condition must also be included in the differential diagnosis of those who develop fevers in association with transfusion. PTP and TRALI represent less common transfusion reactions that may be associated with fever.

Question 12: D

Explanation:

- Bacterial contamination of stored blood poses a serious risk to the transfusion recipient. Fatalities are reported each year to the FDA, although this almost certainly represents the most severe manifestation of a more common clinical problem.
- It is estimated that 1 in 5000 apheresis platelets are bacterially contaminated, as evidenced by positive microbiologic cultures, although clinically significant reactions are likely less common. There is also evidence that suggests that platelet concentrates are more likely to be bacterially contaminated than apheresis platelet products.
- Platelets are the most likely blood component to be contaminated for two related reasons: 1) they are stored at room temperature and 2) skin flora that may enter the blood bag at the time of donor phlebotomy or unit processing have an opportunity to proliferate before recipient transfusion.
- In the past, the most common organism isolated from contaminated RBC units was *Yersinia enterocolitica*, which was largely related to its growth characteristics (eg, ability to proliferate at 4 C and obligate requirement for iron). Currently, *Staphylococcus* species and enteric pathogens are the most common bacterial isolates associated with transfusion-related fatalities reported to the FDA.
- An AABB standard [5.1.5.1 in *Standards for Blood Banks and Transfusion Services, 26th edition (Standards)*] states that "The blood bank or transfusion service shall have methods to limit and to detect or inactivate bacteria in all platelet components." This is oftentimes accomplished by the bacterial culture of platelets at the donor center.
- Other transfusion reactions listed would be highly unlikely for the following reasons:
  - Intravascular hemolytic reactions are almost always associated with red cell transfusions, though they may be seen with ABO-incompatible platelet transfusions when donors have high-titer isohemagglutinins.
  - FNHTRs are not as severe clinically as the presentation in this case (ie, shock). A fever related to the patient's underlying clinical condition would also not likely be as severe.

- TRALI may present with fever, but no pulmonary signs or symptoms are present in this case.

Question 13: A

Explanation:

- TRALI is a form of noncardiogenic pulmonary edema accompanying transfusion. It is marked by respiratory distress during transfusion or within 6 hours after the completion of transfusion. Fever, rigors, and hypotension can also be seen. The pulmonary capillary wedge pressure in TRALI patients is usually normal.
- There are two pathogenic mechanisms that have been put forth to explain TRALI reactions:
  - HLA Class I and/or Class II antibodies and granulocyte antibodies in donor plasma reacting with recipient leukocytes.
  - A "two-hit" model whereby the patient's serious clinical condition serves to prime granulocytes (first hit) followed by the infusion of a biologically active lipids or antibodies in the transfused blood product that activates recipient leukocytes.
- Regardless of the mechanism, the result is a damaged pulmonary endothelium, a capillary leak syndrome, and consequent pulmonary edema.
- An anaphylactic transfusion reaction could present in a similar way, but fever would not typically be seen and the patient would likely be hypotensive.
- An intravascular hemolytic transfusion reaction merits consideration, but distinct pulmonary symptoms would be unusual.
- Volume overload, and resultant pulmonary edema, is an important diagnostic consideration. Other aspects of the patient's clinical presentation (eg, fever) make this less likely, but additional investigation is indicated. The pulmonary capillary wedge pressure in volume overload is usually elevated.
- Additional information regarding TRALI:
  - The chest radiograph reveals a normal cardiac size with bilateral pulmonary infiltrates caused by pulmonary edema. Left atrial and pulmonary wedge pressures are within normal limits or low. The diagnosis is supported by a test for granulocyte and HLA-specific

- antibodies in the donor, though a negative result does not rule out this diagnosis. TRALI is a clinical diagnosis of exclusion.
  - Treatment consists of immediate cessation of transfusion and the provision of respiratory support, including supplemetal oxygen and, in some cases, intubation. Vasopressors may be required. The value of corticosteroids is unclear. Cases involving donor antibodies require no future special transfusion requirements for the patient.
  - Prognosis: Most patients (~95%) recover and return to baseline within 48 to 96 hours.

Question 14: B

Explanation:

- TRALI is a clinical diagnosis with a defined set of features that include the following:
  - New acute lung injury.
  - No preexisting acute lung injury before transfusion.
  - Onset of symptoms within 6 hours of transfusion.
- Other clinical features of TRALI include:
  - Hypoxemia with a partial pressure of oxygen in arterial blood/inspired oxygen concentration (PaO_2/FiO_2) ratio of ≤300 mm Hg or hemoglobin oxygen saturation as measured by pulse oximetry (SpO_2) ≤90% on room air.
  - Bilateral infiltrates on frontal chest radiograph.
  - No evidence of left atrial hypertension.
- There is no specific diagnostic test for TRALI; it is a diagnosis of exclusion. However, the demonstration of lymphocytotoxic, HLA (Class I or II) or ganulocyte-specific antibodies in donor or recipient serum strongly suggests the diagnosis.
- Unlike other types of acute lung injury with mortality rates of 40% to 50%, the mortality attributed to TRALI is much lower, approximately 5%, provided that prompt and vigorous respiratory support is provided.
- Also see the explanation for Question 13.

Question 15: D

Explanation:

- It is highly unlikely that this child has experienced either an acute intravascular or a DHTR, as the transfusion reaction workup is negative. Most importantly, the DAT testing is nonreactive, making an immune-mediated hemolytic process distinctly unlikely.
- Hematuria (free red cells in the urine) could accompany bladder irritation caused by catheterization. It is much more likely, however, that the patient has hemoglobinuria, given the fact that her serum is also red (ie, hemoglobinemia).
- Mechanical trauma to the red cell can result in a nonimmune-mediated hemolytic process. This results from direct damage to the cell. Malfunctioning prosthetic heart valves, cell saver devices, and extracorporeal bypass circuits can cause mechanical red cell injury.
- Other causes of nonimmune hemolysis include:
  - Dilution of red cells with hypotonic solutions causing osmotic red cell injury.
  - Faulty blood warmers or the use of inappropriate blood warming devices (eg, towel warmers or microwave ovens not approved by the FDA for this purpose) causing thermal injury.

Question 16: A

Explanation:

- ABO antibodies are most commonly implicated in intravascular hemolytic transfusion reactions (also see the explanation for Question 5).
- Kidd, Kell, Rh, and Duffy antibodies are predominantly IgG and are most commonly associated with DHTRs.
- DHTRs result as follows:
  - Previous exposure to a red cell antigen through transfusion or pregnancy results in the development of an antibody.
  - This antibody may be of too low a titer to be detected or the titer may fall rapidly. Upon rechallenge with the antigen, an anamnes-

tic (secondary) immune response occurs with a rise in antibody titer leading to red cell destruction.
- The secondary immune response to an antigen results in IgG deposition on antigen-positive transfused red cells. Removal by the reticuloendothelial cells of the spleen results in extravascular hemolysis. Clinically, however, this is delayed in onset (with respect to the transfusion) as it takes days to mount a high-titer secondary immune response. Hemolysis generally peaks 1 to 2 weeks after transfusion.
- Kidd system antibodies are most commonly implicated in DHTRs for the following reasons:
  - They tend to quickly become undetectable after primary sensitization.
  - The secondary immune response is frequently quite potent.
  - Kidd antibodies are efficient complement activators.
- Kidd antibodies are responsible for over 75% of DHTRs.
- Primary means to prevent DHTRs: 1) evaluation of a recipient's transfusion history, even if the pretransfusion antibody screen is negative and 2) provision of antigen-negative RBC units if there is a history of clinically significant antibodies in the serum of the recipient.
- Anyone who has ever been transfused or pregnant is at risk for a DHTR.
- A delayed serologic transfusion reaction occurs when antibody and antigen are present together in the transfusion recipient but there is no clinical or laboratory evidence of hemolysis.

Question 17: C

Explanation:

- Approximately 3% of patients receiving large doses of intravenous penicillin develop a positive DAT. However, these patients will not have positive antibody screens unless the reagent red cells used in the screen are incubated with the drug. In this situation, the expected DAT findings are a positive reaction with anti-IgG and a negative reaction with anti-C3d. An eluate of the patient's cells would be negative.
- This patient has almost certainly experienced a DHTR. The classic features of DHTRs are as follows:
  - A history of pregnancy or transfusion in the recipient.

- A negative antibody screen and a compatible crossmatch with pre-transfusion serum.
- A positive antibody screen and incompatible crossmatch with pos-treaction serum.
- Clinical and/or laboratory evidence of hemolysis, including decreasing hemoglobin, increasing indirect bilirubin, and a positive DAT.
• A positive DAT indicates that red cells are coated with excess IgG and/or complement in vivo.
• A positive IAT (antibody screen or antibody identification panel) indicates a reaction between *free* serum antibodies and antigen-positive reagent red cells in vitro. With test tube-based agglutination, a negative IAT must be confirmed by a positive reaction with check cells (indicates that the AHG reagent has been added).
• A positive IAT is *not* required to confirm a positive DAT.
• The patient requires E-negative and Jk^a-negative red cells for transfusion.
• The phenotypic frequency of E-negative units in people of European ethnicity is 70%; it is 79% in people of African ethnicity.
• The phenotypic frequency of Jk^a-negative units is 23%.
• The proportion of units that are both E-negative and Jk^a-negative is calculated as follows: $0.7 \times 0.23 = 0.161$ (or 16%).
• A positive autocontrol and agglutination of all reagent red cells is observed in WAIHA. The autocontrol can also be positive in DHTRs, as the alloantibody reacts with the transfused red cells still present in the patient's circulation.
• Also see the explanation for Question 15.

Question 18: B

Explanation:

• Allergic transfusion reactions occur in about 1% of all transfusion recipients and range in severity from localized cutaneous manifestations (urticaria, hives, itching) to anaphylaxis (dyspnea, laryngeal edema, vasomotor instability). The cutaneous manifestations of these reactions are common, while true anaphylaxis is rare.

- Allergic reactions may occur when antibodies in sensitized recipients react with foreign plasma proteins in the transfused blood component. These reactions are histamine-mediated.
- Most allergic reactions are mild and self-limited and do not increase in severity with the additional infusion of blood.
- Mild allergic reactions are the only type of transfusion reaction where it is permissible to stop the transfusion, treat the patient, and restart the transfusion once the reaction has cleared.
- Antihistamines (eg, Benadryl) represent the most important treatment and preventive strategy for allergic transfusion reactions.
- The most commonly identified cause of anaphylactic reactions is the presence of IgA antibodies in IgA-deficient individuals. However, in most cases the implicated antigen and corresponding antibody are not identified.
- Although fever is a common sign accompanying many other adverse reactions to transfusion (eg, hemolytic transfusion reactions, FNHTRs, and TRALI), it is *not* seen commonly in allergic reactions.

Question 19: D

Explanation:

- Dyspnea, laryngeal edema, and hypotension (vasomotor instability) are classically seen in anaphylactic transfusion reactions, the most severe manifestation of allergic reactions.
- This would be a distinctly unusual clinical presentation for an acute hemolytic transfusion reaction, but volume overload and TRALI should always be considered in the differential diagnosis of a pulmonary syndrome accompanying transfusion.
- Volume or circulatory overload, also known as TACO (transfusion-associated circulatory overload), develops when too large a volume of blood is transfused too quickly (unlikely in this case as the patient had received only a small volume of blood). Signs and symptoms of volume overload include headache, plethora, dyspnea, tachycardia, and systolic hypertension.
- TRALI is a severe reaction to transfusion presenting clinically as non-cardiogenic pulmonary edema. In contrast to patients with anaphylaxis, those suffering from TRALI reactions typically develop fever and require mechanical ventilation. They would not be expected to

recover quickly with the multi-agent drug therapy that this patient received.
- Rare cases of anaphylaxis result from allergic reactions to infused IgA in severely IgA-deficient patients with anti-IgA. Special IgA-deficient plasma products are available, from known IgA-deficient blood donors, but should be reserved for the IgA-deficient patient with anti-IgA who has experienced an anaphylactic transfusion reaction.

Question 20: A

Explanation:

- IgA deficiency is the most common congenital immune deficiency, affecting approximately 1 in 700 to 1 in 800 individuals.
- From the perspective of a clinical immunology practice, a patient with a serum IgA level below 5 mg/dL is "IgA deficient." However, these patients do not recognize IgA as a foreign molecule and, therefore, do not make anti-IgA.
- From the perspective of a transfusion medicine practice, only patients with IgA levels below 0.05 mg/dL are "IgA deficient." These patients are at risk for developing class-specific IgA antibodies when exposed to IgA via pregnancy or transfusion.
- Up to 30% of severely IgA-deficient individuals have IgA class-specific (IgG or IgM) antibodies in their circulation.
- IgA-deficient transfusion recipients with anti-IgA are at risk for anaphylactic transfusion reactions.
- Anaphylactic reactions can occur suddenly and after transfusion of only a few milliliters of blood.
- The treatment of anaphylactic transfusion reactions includes discontinuation of transfusion, intravenous fluid infusion, and epinephrine administration. The patient's airway needs to be protected (eg, intubation). Patients may also require vasopressor support.
- The transfusion of blood components from IgA-deficient donors can prevent anaphylactic reactions in recipients who have experienced such reactions caused by IgA antibodies. These components can be obtained from larger blood centers. The transfusion of washed or deglycerolized RBCs are also used to prevent anaphylactic reactions.
- Although methods are available to wash platelets, they are cumbersome and washing may activate the platelets, making them less

effective from the standpoint of hemostasis. Platelets from IgA-deficient donors, obtained by apheresis, are the product of choice for IgA-deficient donors at risk for anaphylaxis.
- Individuals with acquired IgA deficiency (eg, multiple myeloma) are not at risk for these reactions.
- Also see the explanations for Questions 17 and 18.

Question 21: A

Explanation:

- TA-GVHD is a rare but almost uniformly lethal complication of transfusion.
- The pathogenesis is related to the infusion of immunocompetent lymphocytes (donor origin) into a recipient incapable of destroying these foreign cells. The donor lymphocytes recognize recipient tissues as foreign, become activated, and attack the recipient tissues.
- Activated immunocompetent donor lymphocytes "home" to recipient skin, liver, and gastrointestinal tract mucosa. In addition, there is marrow aplasia, the primary cause of mortality seen with TA-GVHD. This distinguishes this entity from the GVHD associated with marrow transplantation.
- TA-GVHD is prevented by irradiation of cellular blood components. Neither leukocyte reduction nor washing is considered to be an adequate preventive measure.
- AABB *Standards* (Standard 5.7.4.2), requires that a minimum dose of 25 Gy (2500 cGy) be delivered to the midplane of the irradiation canister or field. In addition, the minimum dose at any point in the canister or field must be 15 Gy (1500 cGy).
- The maximum storage time for irradiated RBC components is 28 days. Irradiated platelet components maintain their original expiration.

Question 22: E

Explanation:

- Patients with severe cellular immunosuppression are at greatest risk for transfusion-associated GVHD. This includes patients with marrow ablation (as with hematopoietic progenitor cell transplantation or myeloablative chemotherapy) and patients with abnormal T-cell function (eg, children with congenital T-cell immunodeficiency syndromes).
- TA-GVHD has *not* been identified in AIDS patients despite their profound state of immunosuppression. Thus, AIDS is not a clinical indication for irradiation. In like manner, TA-GVHD is not associated with septic patients, per se, or patients with humoral immunodeficiency states (eg, IgA deficiency).
- Immunocompetent patients can also be at risk for TA-GVHD. The risk is generally ascribed to the degree of HLA haplotype sharing between recipient and donor. Antigens of the HLA system are so polymorphic that, under the usual circumstances of transfusion, there is no sharing of HLA determinants. Thus, the recipient recognizes donor lymphocytes as foreign with consequent destruction. However, when the recipient is heterozygous for an HLA haplotype for which the donor is homozygous, donor lymphocytes may not be recognized as foreign (and are not destroyed). On the other hand, recipient tissues can be recognized as foreign with the potential for donor lymphocyte activation and subsequent recipient tissue injury (ie, GVHD). This situation is more likely to occur in populations with less genetic diversity (eg, Japan) or when a blood donor is a genetically related relative of an intended recipient (eg, context of directed blood donation).
- Patients receiving high-dose, nonmyeloablative chemotherapy for solid-organ malignancies would not generally be considered to be at increased risk for TA-GVHD.
- Also see explanations for Questions 20 and 23.

Question 23: B

Explanation:

- IUT recipients must receive irradiated cellular blood components. TA-GVHD has been reported in infants who received IUT followed by postnatal exchange transfusion. The hypothesis is that T lymphocytes present in the blood components received during IUT induce tolerance, impairing the rejection of lymphocytes in the subsequent exchange transfusion.
- Clinical indications for irradiated cellular blood components include the following:
  - Patients with severe deficiencies in cell-mediated immunity.
  - Immunocompetent patients who are recipients of direct-donor transfusion from genetically related relatives.
  - Blood components of donors selected for HLA compatibility.
  - Recipients of or candidates for marrow or progenitor cell transplants.
  - Patients with hematopoietic malignancies receiving myeloablative chemotherapy.
  - Premature infants or low-birthweight infants
- Clinical conditions not requiring irradiated cellular blood components include the following:
  - Conditions associated with only humoral immunodeficiency, such as agammaglobulinemia, or nonlymphoid cellular abnormalities such as chronic granulomatous disease.
  - AIDS; there are no reports of TA-GVHD in AIDS patients.
  - Full-term infants.
- Components not requiring irradiation are:
  - Fresh frozen plasma (FFP).
  - Cryoprecipitated AHF.

Question 24: B

Explanation:

- Each of the possible answers can be associated with severe thrombocytopenia and bleeding, but the patient's gender, pregnancy history, and severe thrombocytopenia 1 week after transfusion are features most consistent with PTP.
- PTP arises as a consequence of an anamnestic immune response to a platelet antigen. This accounts for the 1-week delay in platelet destruction.
- In most cases (>90%), the alloimmune response is directed against the platelet glycoprotein PL^{A1} (HPA-1a). However, this does not explain why the patient's own antigen-negative platelets are also destroyed.
- There are 3 theories that have been promulgated to explain the mechanism of autologous platelet destruction in PTP:
  - Immune complexes formed by the interaction of soluble platelet-specific antigen in donor plasma and antiplatelet antibody in the patient, which then bind to autologous platelets, causing their destruction.
  - Soluble platelet antigen in donor plasma absorbs to the recipient's platelets, rendering them "antigen-positive" and subject to destruction by the patient's platelet alloantibody.
  - Antibody with an autospecificity develops from an allogeneic immune response upon reexposure to an incompatible platelet alloantigen.
- Although ~2% of the population lacks the PL^{A1} antigen and would be at theoretical risk for PTP, this is a rare adverse consequence of transfusion. One reason for this relates to the genetic restriction of PL^{A1} antibodies to individuals with the HLA-B8 and HLA-DRw52 antigens.
- The treatment of choice for PTP is intravenous immune globulin therapy, 1 g/kg/day for 2 days. Plasmapheresis is now used as a secondary treatment modality. Over 90% of affected patients will respond to therapy, usually within 3 to 4 days of initiation.

Question 25: B

Explanation:

- Iron overload (secondary hemosiderosis) is most commonly seen in chronically transfused patients, especially those with hemoglobinopathies.
- Chronically transfused patients have progressive accumulations of iron, as there is no physiologic mechanism for the excretion of excess iron. Patients with massive acute blood needs are not at risk for iron overload as most of this blood is not retained in the body.
- Each milliliter of red cells contains 1 mg of iron. Therefore, a unit of blood with 250 mL of red cells contains approximately 250 mg of iron.
- When reticuloendothelial sites are saturated, excess iron deposits in solid organs (particularly the heart, liver, and endocrine glands) and eventually interferes with function. Hepatic failure and cardiac toxicity are the most common causes of the morbidity and mortality associated with iron overload.
- The iron overload accompanying chronic transfusion can be treated effectively with desferoxamine, an iron-chelating agent that can be given intravenously or by subcutaneous infusion.
- Until recently, there was no safe and efficacious oral iron chelator that would reliably put a patient into a negative iron balance. However, there is now an FDA-approved oral iron chelator called deferasirox. Although it is an effective chelator, serious side effects, including hepatotoxicity and nephrotoxicity, make it an unsuitable medication for some patients.

Question 26: A

Explanation:

- Immunomodulation refers to an alteration in a blood recipient's immune system as a result of transfusion.

- The immunomodulatory effect of transfusion was first recognized with the observation of improved renal allograft survival in transfused patients in the 1970s.
- Experimental studies in animals have demonstrated clearly that the immunomodulatory effect of transfusion can be ascribed to transfused leukocytes. Thus, the use of leukocyte-reduced cellular blood components would be expected to be associated with a minimization of this effect.
- Irradiation affects the proliferative capacity of transfused lymphocytes but is not associated with an immunosuppressive effect in the transfusion recipient.
- Although animal models of tumor progression and infection clearly demonstrate the negative effect of transfusion-associated immunomodulation, the clinical consequences in humans are less clear and remain the subject of current research efforts.

Question 27: E

Explanation:

- Citrate is universally used as an anticoagulant for blood components because of its calcium-chelating properties. The rapid infusion of citrated blood components can result in a significant decrease in ionized calcium levels. This can be associated with depressed cardiac function, hypotension, and cardiac arrhythmias. Citrate is rapidly metabolized by the liver to bicarbonate and is excreted by the kidneys. Thus, in addition to hypocalcemia, citrate toxicity can be associated with acid-base imbalances (eg, alkalosis). Close monitoring of ionized calcium levels should be part of the care of the massively transfused patient.
- Hypomagnesemia is a complication of extreme citrate toxicity. With severe hypomagnesemia, myocardial depression and ventricular arrhythmia can occur.
- Hemostatic abnormalities frequently occur in the massively transfused patient and may contribute to excess bleeding. These patients are at risk for a dilutional coagulopathy, and DIC is frequently seen (though it is not a direct consequence of massive transfusion). A hypercoagulable state has not been associated with massive transfusion.

- The rapid infusion of cold blood can complicate the care of patients who may already be hypothermic (eg, patients with severe traumatic injuries and surgical patients with open thoracic or abdominal cavities). Hypothermia has multiple potential adverse effects including depressed myocardial function, impaired oxygen delivery to peripheral tissues, impaired function of coagulation cascade enzymes and platelet dysfunction. High-flow blood warmers are commonly used in the setting of massive transfusion.
- Hypotension is more likely to be a manifestation of uncontrolled blood loss (hemorrhage) than a direct consequence of massive transfusion.
- The rapid infusion of large volumes of red cells may result in metabolic abnormalities including potassium and acid-base imbalances.
  - A transient hyperkalemia is sometimes seen but is not usually clinically significant unless the recipient has impaired potassium excretion (eg, neonates and adults with compromised renal function). Hypokalemia may also accompany massive transfusion. Close monitoring of potassium levels is warranted in these cases.
  - During storage, red cell components accumulate acid to the extent that, at the end of the storage period, pH levels may fall to approximately 6.5. The rapid infusion of red cells can be associated with a transient acidosis. However, significant acidosis in the context of massive transfusion is more commonly attributable to the consequences of uncontrolled hemorrhage (ie, severe hypovolemia and poor tissue perfusion). More typically, massive transfusion is associated with a metabolic alkalosis, which results from the accumulation of bicarbonate, the metabolic byproduct of citrate.

Question 28: B

Explanation:

- Primary hypotensive transfusion reactions are characterized by the following:
  - A drop in systolic or diastolic blood pressure (or both) by 30 mm Hg or more, compared with a pretransfusion blood pressure.
  - Hypotension occurring within minutes of starting a transfusion.
  - Hypotension that resolves quickly once the transfusion is stopped.

- Hypotensive transfusion reactions must be distinguished from septic reactions, TRALI, allergic reactions, hemolytic reactions, hypovolemia, and other medical causes of hypotension.
- Hypotensive reactions are most commonly associated with platelet and red cell transfusions.
- They appear to be mediated by bradykinin and des-Arg^9-bradykinin, vasoactive kinins that are generated by activation of the contact system. Contact system activation occurs when plasma comes into contact with a negatively charged surface or the surface of activated endothelial cells.
- Bradykinin has in-vivo effects characterized by hypotension, flushing, and abdominal pain without fever or chills.
- Most hypotensive reactions have occurred in patients receiving cellular blood components that have undergone filtration through negatively charged, bedside leukocyte-reduction filters. These may be responsible for the generation of kallikrein, which cleaves high-molecular-weight kininogen to release bradykinin.
- Hypotensive transfusion reactions much less commonly occur when prestorage leukocyte-reduced units are transfused.
- ACE inhibitor use is strongly associated with hypotensive transfusion reactions. ACE inhibitors block the action of angiotensin-converting enzyme, the principle degradation enzyme that transforms bradykinin into an inactive metabolite. ACE inhibitors can increase the half-life and bioavailability of bradykinin.

Question 29: C

Explanation:

- The patient in this vignette has signs and symptoms of a pulmonary syndrome accompanying transfusion. Though any of the possible answers are plausible, the best diagnostic fit for his reaction is TACO.
- Patients with a diminished cardiac reserve and/or significant anemia who receive blood too quickly are at risk for acute pulmonary edema secondary to congestive heart failure (ie, TACO).
- Older adults and infants are especially susceptible to fluid overload, but no recipient is immune and even small transfusion volumes have been associated with TACO, especially in infants.

- The differential diagnosis of acute respiratory distress accompanying transfusion includes TACO, TRALI, and anaphylaxis.
- TRALI is less likely to be the diagnosis in this patient's case as he experienced hypertension (rather than hypotension), was afebrile, and responded favorably to a discontinuation of the fluid infusion.
- Anaphylaxis is less likely to be the diagnosis in this patient's case as he experienced hypertension (rather than hypotension), had evidence of pulmonary edema (not seen in anaphylactic reactions), and had no cutaneous manifestations as part of his reaction.
- Acute hemolytic reactions and the infusion of a bacterially contaminated red cell unit would typically present very differently (eg, fever, hypotension, lack of pulmonary signs and symptoms).
- Although the risk of TACO is generally felt to be low, growing evidence suggests otherwise. In fact, in certain patient populations (eg, intensive care patients not requiring respiratory support at the time of transfusion), TACO may be very common.
- TACO reactions are managed as follows:
  - Stop the transfusion.
  - Provide supplemental oxygen.
  - Reduce the intravascular volume with intravenous diuretics.
  - Place the patient in a sitting position.
- TACO reactions are best prevented by transfusing susceptible patients slowly (1 mL/kg of body weight/hour) using the most concentrated form of the blood component possible. Alternatively, units can be split so that a given volume of blood can be infused over a greater period of time.
- Brain natriuretic peptide level assessment may prove to be a valuable laboratory tool in diagnosing TACO reactions and distinguishing them from TRALI.

Question 30: D

Explanation:

- APTRs are a recently described adverse consequence of transfusion characterized by the abrupt onset of severe pain in the trunk and proximal extremities shortly after the initiation of transfusion.
- APTRs typically occur within 30 minutes of starting a transfusion and last for approximately 30 minutes after the transfusion is stopped.

- No single diagnosis seems to predispose patients to APTRs, as they have been reported in association with a wide variety of illnesses including leukemia, solid malignancies, sickle cell disease, and cirrhosis.
- Various medications have been associated with APTRs, including antihistamines, acetaminophen, beta-blockers, and albuterol; however, ACE inhibitors have not been associated with these reactions.
- The cause of APTRs is unknown, but there seems to be an association with the use of prestorage leukocyte-reduction filters. This suggests that either some modification of the component by filtration or a substance released from the filter is causative.
- Because the cause of APTRs is unknown, no specific preventive measures are available, including premedication with acetaminophen.

REFERENCES

1. Mazzei C, Popovsky M, Kopko P. Noninfectious complications of blood transfusion. In: Roback JD, Combs MR, Grossman BJ, Hillyer CD, eds. Technical manual. 16th ed. Bethesda, MD: AABB, 2008:715-50.
2. Popovsky MA, ed. Transfusion reactions. 3rd ed. Bethesda, MD: AABB, 2007.
3. Price TH, ed. Standards for blood banks and transfusion services. 26th ed. Bethesda, MD: AABB, 2009.

In: Blackall D, Figueroa P, Winters J
Transfusion Medicine Self-Assessment and Review, 2nd Edition
Bethesda, MD: AABB Press, 2009

11

Infectious Complications of Transfusion and Positive Disease Markers in Blood Donors

QUESTIONS

Question 1: Which of the following is the correct estimated risk of transfusion-transmitted viral disease following the implementation of nucleic acid testing (NAT)?

A. Hepatitis B virus (HBV): 1:2,000,000.
B. Hepatitis C virus (HCV): 1:250,000.
C. Human immunodeficiency virus, types 1 and 2 (HIV-1/2): 1:2,000,000.
D. Human T-cell lymphotropic virus, types I and II (HTLV-I/II): 1:1,000.
E. West Nile virus (WNV): 1:1,000,000.

Question 2: NAT has reduced the "window period" for HCV by:

A. 5 days.
B. 10 days.
C. 20 days.

D. 50 days.
E. 80 days.

Question 3: Which infectious agent is transmitted by white cells within blood products?

A. HBV.
B. *Treponema pallidum.*
C. Cytomegalovirus (CMV).
D. *Plasmodium malariae.*
E. HCV.

Question 4: Which of the following organisms is a transfusion recipient most likely to be exposed to?

A. HIV.
B. *Yersinia enterocolitica.*
C. HBV.
D. Coagulase-negative *Staphylococci.*
E. HCV.

Question 5: Which of the following donors is eligible to continue donating?

A. Donor has a positive HIV-1/2 enzyme immunoassay (EIA) and a negative HIV NAT with an indeterminate Western blot.
B. Donor has a positive HIV-1/2 EIA and a negative HIV NAT with a negative HIV immunofluorescence assay (IFA).
C. Donor has a positive HIV-1/2 EIA and a negative HIV NAT with a negative HIV IFA. Testing 6 months later demonstrates a positive HIV-1/2 EIA, a negative Western blot, a negative HIV-1 EIA, and an HIV-1/2 EIA using whole viral lysates.
D. Donor has a positive HIV-1/2 EIA and a negative HIV NAT with a negative Western blot. Testing 6 months later demonstrates a negative HIV-1/2 EIA, a negative Western blot, negative HIV-1 and a

negative HIV-1/2 EIA using whole viral lysates, and a negative HIV NAT.
E. Donor has a negative HIV-1/2 EIA and a positive HIV NAT.

Question 6: Which of the following HIV Western blot patterns should be interpreted as positive?

A. p24 and gp41 bands are present.
B. p31, p17, and p55 bands are present.
C. p24, p31, p17, and p55 bands are present.
D. gp120/160, p31, and p55 bands are present.
E. gp41 band is present.

Question 7: Which of the following is *true* concerning HIV-1 p24 antigen testing?

A. It detects donors not identified by NAT.
B. A donor with a repeat-reactive HIV-1 p24 antigen test that neutralizes is eligible for requalification (reentry).
C. Since its implementation in 1996, HIV-1 p24 antigen testing has detected approximately 200 HIV-infected donors who are HIV negative by EIA.
D. Compared to the HIV EIA, HIV-1 p24 antigen testing resulted in reduction of the HIV window period by 6 days.
E. Once present, HIV-1 p24 antigen is detectable at high levels throughout the course of HIV infection.

Question 8: NAT has reduced the window period for HIV, compared to HIV-1/2 EIA, by:

A. 1 day.
B. 11-15 days.
C. 20 days.
D. 30 days.
E. 40 days.

Question 9: Which of the following is least likely to transmit HTLV-I/II?

A. Fresh Frozen Plasma (FFP) transfusion.
B. Breast feeding.
C. Intravenous drug abuse.
D. Sexual intercourse.
E. Red cell transfusion.

Question 10: Which of the following statements concerning HTLV-I/II infection is *true*?

A. After 30 to 50 years, 30% to 50% of individuals infected with HTLV-I at birth develop adult T-cell leukemia/lymphoma (ATL).
B. Between 2% and 5% of individuals infected with HTLV-I develop tropical spastic paraparesis (TSP)/HTLV-I associate myelopathy (HAM), usually in the fourth decade.
C. The infectivity of blood components decreases with storage.
D. ATL has never been seen in recipients infected by transfusion.
E. TSP/HAM may occur after a longer latent period in individuals infected by transfusion.

Question 11: Which of the following donors is eligible to donate?

A. Donor has tested repeatedly reactive for HTLV-I/II on a single previous donation.
B. Donor has tested repeatedly reactive for antibodies to hepatitis B core antigen (HBc) on two previous donations.
C. Donor has a repeatedly reactive rapid plasma regain test (RPR) and a positive fluorescent treponemal antibody test (FTA) and has not undergone treatment.
D. Donor has tested repeatedly reactive for hepatitis B surface antigen (HBsAg), which was neutralizable.
E. Donor has tested repeatedly reactive with an HCV EIA, with an indeterminate recombinant immunoblot assay (RIBA).

INFECTIOUS COMPLICATIONS

Question 12: Which of the following is a DNA hepatitis virus?

A. Hepatitis A virus (HAV).
B. HBV.
C. HCV.
D. Hepatitis D virus (HDV).
E. Hepatitis E virus (HEV).

Question 13: A 28-year-old male patient has mild scleral icterus, fatigue, and loss of appetite. Mild tender hepatomegaly is detected. The patient lives with his brother, who was diagnosed with hepatitis 3 weeks ago. Given the natural history and frequency of various hepatitis viruses, which test would most likely be positive in this patient?

A. HBsAg.
B. IgG anti-HBsAg.
C. IgG anti-HAV.
D. IgM anti-HAV.
E. IgM anti-HBsAg.

Question 14: Which of the following antibodies is protective?

A. Anti-HIV-1/2.
B. Anti-HTLV-I/II.
C. Anti-HCV.
D. Anti-HBsAg.
E. Anti-HBc.

Question 15: A blood donor who was not previously immunized was vaccinated for HBV 3 days before donation. Which of the following routine blood donor tests would most likely become positive because of this vaccination?

A. Anti-HBc.
B. Anti-HBsAg.
C. Anti-HIV-1/2.
D. Anti-HCV.
E. HBsAg.

Question 16: According to federal regulations, requalification (reentry) of a donor is available for which of the following test results?

A. Positive anti-HIV-1/2 EIA with an indeterminate Western blot.
B. Positive HBsAg that is neutralizable.
C. Positive anti-HCV EIA with a negative RIBA.
D. Positive HIV-1 p24 antigen that is neutralizable.
E. Positive anti-HBc on two separate donations.

Question 17: Which of the following statements concerning HCV and transfusion is *true*?

A. It is currently the most common cause of transfusion-transmitted hepatitis.
B. Twenty-five percent of recipients of an HCV-infected blood component will develop chronic hepatitis.
C. Donors with a positive HCV EIA and an indeterminate HCV RIBA are eligible to donate.
D. Eighty percent of patients with posttransfusion HCV will develop chronic hepatitis.
E. Eighty percent of donors infected with HCV have no identifiable risk factors.

Question 18: Which of the following is most likely to occur?

A. Donor is repeat reactive with HTLV-I/II ELISA.
B. Donor is repeat reactive with HBsAg.
C. Donor is repeat reactive with anti-HBc.

D. Donor is repeat reactive with HIV-1 p24 antigen.
E. Donor is repeat reactive with HIV-1/2 EIA.

Question 19: For the prevention of transfusion-transmitted CMV infection, the use of CMV-seronegative or leukocyte-reduced blood components are indicated for which of the following patient groups?

A. Recipients of intrauterine transfusion (IUT).
B. Seronegative low-birthweight neonates born to seronegative mothers.
C. Seronegative patients infected with HIV.
D. Seronegative pregnant patients.
E. All of the above.

Question 20: CMV can be effectively transmitted by which of the following components?

A. Non-leukocyte-reduced Red Blood Cells (RBCs).
B. FFP.
C. Cryoprecipitated AHF.
D. Apheresis Platelets Leukocytes Reduced.
E. Deglycerolized RBCs.

Question 21: Which one of the following infectious agents can lyse erythroblasts in the marrow of a patient with chronic hemolytic anemia resulting in a sudden onset aplastic crisis?

A. *Babesia microti*.
B. *Borrelia burgdorferi*.
C. Colorado tick fever virus.
D. Parvovirus B19.
E. Encephalitis virus.

Question 22: Which of the following conditions is *not* a cause for the permanent deferral of a prospective donor?

A. Syphilis.
B. Babesiosis.
C. Kaposi's sarcoma.
D. Chagas' disease.
E. Viral hepatitis after age 11.

Question 23: Blood donations are currently screened by serologic methods for syphilis. Which of the following statements concerning syphilis and transfusion is *true*?

A. Numerous cases of transfusion-transmitted syphilis have been reported since 1980.
B. Syphilis screening is an effective surrogate marker for HIV infection.
C. Transfusion-transmitted syphilis presents as acute, fulminant secondary syphilis.
D. *T. pallidum* is stabile at 4 C and, therefore, is easily transmitted by red cells.
E. *T. pallidum* prefers an environment rich in oxygen and, therefore, is easily transmitted by platelet products.

Question 24: Which of the following is *true* concerning the testing of donors for syphilis?

A. Examples of nontreponemal tests include the RPR and the microhemagglutination assay-*T. pallidum* (MHA-TP).
B. Treponemal tests have higher sensitivity than nontreponemal tests.
C. Nontreponemal tests have lower specificity than treponemal tests.
D. A donor with positive nontreponemal and treponemal test results and a negative nontreponemal test result 12 months later is not eligible to donate.

E. A donor with a positive nontreponemal test and no follow-up testing should be deferred for 6 months.

Question 25: A donor emigrated from a malaria-endemic area 15 years ago. He has a history of malaria, with the last symptoms experienced 5 years before emigration. The donor has not visited any malaria-endemic countries since emigrating. Infection with which of the following *Plasmodium* species would be most likely to cause transfusion transmission from blood from this donor?

A. *P. ovale.*
B. *P. vivax.*
C. *P. malariae.*
D. *P. falciparum.*

Question 26: City X is located in a malaria risk area according to the Centers for Disease Control and Prevention (CDC). Which of the following donors is eligible to donate?

A. Visited City X and returned 3 months ago. Did not take malaria prophylaxis.
B. Visited City X and returned 11 months ago. Did take malaria prophylaxis.
C. Visited City X and returned 13 months ago. Did not take malaria prophylaxis.
D. Visited City X and returned 3 months ago. Did take malaria prophylaxis. Did not go out at dusk.
E. Visited City X and returned 3 months ago. Did take malaria prophylaxis. Did go out at dusk.

Question 27: AABB *Standards for Blood Banks and Transfusion Services (Standards)* addresses donor infection with all of the following protozoan parasites *except*:

A. *P. vivax.*

B. *P. falciparum.*
C. *Leishmania donovani.*
D. *Trypanosoma cruzi.*
E. *Babesia microti.*

Question 28: Which one of the following statements is *true* about Creutzfeldt-Jakob disease (CJD)?

A. It is a viral disease.
B. Blood relatives of affected individuals are not eligible to donate blood.
C. Numerous cases of transfusion transmission have been reported.
D. It has been transmitted to individuals through clotting factor concentrates.
E. It has not been transmitted to individuals receiving dura mater grafts.

Question 29: Which of the following statements concerning variant CJD (vCJD) is *true*?

A. The average age of diagnosis is similar to that of classic CJD.
B. Donors spending more than 6 weeks in Great Britain since 1980 are permanently deferred.
C. It is thought to represent a human form of bovine spongiform encephalopathy.
D. Animal models have not demonstrated transfusion transmission.
E. Leukocyte reduction of blood components has been shown to prevent its transmission.

Question 30: Which of the following statements concerning WNV is *true*?

A. Twenty percent of infected individuals are asymptomatic.
B. Infected humans can transmit the virus to mosquitoes, completing the virus's life-cycle.

C. One out of 150 individuals who develop West Nile fever (WNF) will experience severe neurologic consequences.
D. The main reservoir for the virus is rodents.
E. A chronic carrier state develops in 7% of infected individuals.

Question 31: Which of the following statements concerning the transfusion transmission of WNV and related testing is *true*?

A. Despite the implementation of NAT, the frequency of transfusion transmission has remained steady.
B. Individual NAT has offered no benefit over pooled NAT.
C. Testing for IgM antibodies to WNV is an effective alternative to NAT.
D. Immunosuppressed individuals have a 40-fold increased risk of developing severe neurologic disease from transfusion-transmitted WNV.
E. A donor with a diagnosis of WNF or a positive NAT is deferred for 30 days following the diagnosis or positive test result.

Question 32: Which of the following statements about *Trypanosoma cruzi* is *true*?

A. *T. cruzi* is transmitted by the bite of the phlebotomine sandfly.
B. *T. cruzi* can be transmitted vertically from mother to child.
C. Infection is usually self-limited, resolving within 3 to 4 years.
D. The symptoms of acute infection include esophageal and colonic dysfunction.
E. The seroprevalence of *T. cruzi* infection is decreasing in the United States.

Question 33: Which of the following statements about transfusion-transmitted *T. cruzi* and testing for *T. cruzi* is *true*?

A. The most common blood component reported to transmit *T. cruzi* is platelets.

B. In North America, 250 cases of transfusion transmission have been reported.
C. The Center for Biologics Evaluation and Research (CBER) has licensed a *T. cruzi* NAT for the detection of the parasite.
D. *T. cruzi* is not a concern for peripheral blood progenitor cell products as it does not survive freezing in 5% dimethyl sulfoxide (DMSO).
E. The Food and Drug Administration (FDA)-licensed confirmatory assay is a xenodiagnostic assay where reduviid bugs feed on the individual and then attempts are made to transmit the infection to guinea pigs.

Question 34: Look-back refers to the situation when a donor is found to be infected with a transfusion-transmitted virus or to have positive screening and supplemental test results on a donation. For which of the following diseases has the CBER-mandated notification of the recipient and, if the recipient is no longer alive, their next of kin?

A. HCV.
B. HIV.
C. HTLV.
D. HBV.
E. Syphillis.

Question 35: In a look-back case, who has the final responsibility for performing the recipient notification?

A. The physician who ordered the transfusion.
B. The medical director of the blood center that collected the transfused component.
C. The medical director of the transfusion service that issued the component.
D. The primary care physician who routinely cares for the patient.
E. The hospital legal department.

ANSWERS

Question 1: C

Explanation:

- The estimated risk of transfusion-transmitted viral disease is shown in Table 11-1.
- Despite the use of highly sensitive laboratory testing, it is likely that there will *always* be a risk of transfusion-transmitted viral disease. This is because of "window period" disease transmission (ie, the time between onset of infection in the donor and laboratory detection of infection).

Table 11-1.

Virus	Per-Unit Risk
HCV	1:2,000,000
HBV	1:250,000 to 1:500,000
HTLV	1:3,000,000
HIV	1:2,000,000
WNV	1:7,000,000

Question 2: D

Explanation:

- Implemented in early 1999, NAT has reduced the window period for HCV detection by 50 to 60 days.
- Table 11-2 summarizes NAT for HCV and HIV in the United States and Canada.
- NAT is now licensed for routine blood donor testing.
- Pool size: 16 or 24 donations depending on the test manufacturer.

Table 11-2.

	HCV	HIV
Window period (days): serologic testing	70 to 75	16 to 21
Window period reduction (days): nucleic acid testing	50 to 60	5 to 9
Donations screened (millions) between 1999 and 2003	20	20
Yield of window period cases	74	5

Question 3: C

Explanation:

- Leukocyte-associated viruses that may be transmitted by transfusion of blood components include HTLV-I, HTLV-II, Epstein-Barr virus, human herpesvirus-8, and CMV. For these agents, leukocyte reduction may reduce/eliminate infectivity of blood components. For most of these agents, however, this has not been studied. The exception is CMV, where numerous studies in different high-risk populations have demonstrated the equivalence of CMV-seronegative and leukocyte-reduced blood components.
- Transfusion transmission of syphilis is exceedingly rare because spirochetes remain viable in blood stored at 4 C for no more than 4 days.
- The transmission of infectious agents by blood constituents and plasma is described in Table 11-3.

Table 11-3.

Agents	Class	Location within Blood Component	Disease
Babesia microti/ divergens*	Intra-erythrocytic protozoan parasites	Red cells	Babesiosis
Plasmodium malariae Plasmodium falciparum Plasmodium ovale Plasmodium vivax	Intra-erythrocytic protozoan parasites	Red cells	Malaria
HTLV-I	Virus	Infected viable CD4+ lymphocytes	1. ATL[†] 2. HAM[‡]
HTLV-II	Virus	Infected viable CD4+ lymphocytes	HAM-like illness
Epstein-Barr virus	Human herpesvirus-4	B lymphocytes	1. Infectious mononucleosis 2. Burkitt's lymphoma 3. Nasopharyngeal carcinoma
HHV-8	Human herpesvirus-8	White cells	1. Kaposi's sarcoma 2. Body cavity B-cell lymphoma 3. Multicentric Castleman's disease
Cytomegalovirus	Human herpesvirus-5	White cells	CMV infection
Toxoplasma gondii	Protozoan parasite	White cells	Toxoplasmosis
Parvovirus B19	Virus	Plasma	Parvovirus B19 infection
Hepatitis B virus	Hepatitis virus	Plasma	HBV infection
Hepatitis C virus	Hepatitis virus	Plasma	HCV infection
Treponema pallidum	Spirochete	Plasma	Syphilis
Hepatitis A virus	Virus	Plasma	HAV infection

* *Babesia microti* is the causative agent of babesiosis in the United States; *Babesia divergens* is the causative agent of babesiosis in Europe.
[†]ATL = adult T-cell leukemia/lymphoma.
[‡]HAM = HTLV-associated myelopathy (tropical spastic paraparesis).

Question 4: D

Explanation:

- The estimated risk of bacterial contamination of blood components (shown in Table 11-4) exceeds the risk of HIV, HBV, HCV, and HTLV contamination combined.

Table 11-4.

	Bacterial Contamination of Blood Products	
	Platelets	**RBCs**
Incidence of bacterial contamination	1 in 5,000 units	1 in 31,385 units
Risk of clinically relevant septic reaction	1 in 74,807 units	1 in 500,000 units
Risk of fatal septic reaction	1 in 498,711 units	1 in 10 million units

- The most common bacterial flora isolated from platelets:
    - Coagulase-negative *Staphylococci*.
    - *Serratia marcescens*.
    - *Streptococci*.
- Factors contributing to bacterial contamination of platelets:
    - Storage: 22 to 24 C for 5 days.
    - Because contamination usually results from skin cores during phlebotomy, pooled products (6 to 10 needle sticks) have a higher risk of contamination than apheresis platelet products (one needle stick).
- *Y. enterocolitica* accounts for >50% of sepsis cases resulting from red cell transfusion.
- Factors contributing to *Y. enterocolitica* contamination of red cells:

- Grows at 4 C (cryophilic or psychrophilic organism).
- Calcium-free environment of anticoagulated blood.
- Iron-rich environment of blood favors growth.
- Potent endotoxin is formed during storage.
- Chance of sepsis increases after 21 days of storage.
- Donors harboring the organism are asymptomatic or have nonspecific complaints. Donor selection procedures, history, and physical examination may not rule out donors harboring *Y. enterocolitica*.
- AABB *Standards* requires bacteria detection or inactivation in platelet components.

Question 5: D

Explanation:

- HIV donor testing consists of a screening test, either an HIV-1/2 combination EIA or separate HIV-1 and HIV-2 EIAs. HIV NAT has been licensed by the Food and Drug Administration's Center for Biologics Evaluation and Research (CBER) but is not required at the time of this writing. It is the standard of care, however. HIV-1 p24 antigen is a required test *if* a licensed HIV NAT is not performed.
- Because of the widespread adoption of HIV NAT, most centers have eliminated testing for p24 antigen. In fact, test kits for p24 antigen are not routinely available.
- If the EIA is repeatedly reactive, then supplemental testing is performed, consisting of either an HIV Western blot or an HIV IFA. If these results are positive or indeterminate, then the donor is deferred. If the supplemental test results are negative, then requalification is allowed.
- HIV requalification is shown in Fig 11-5.
- While HIV NAT is licensed by the FDA, final guidance concerning reentry of donors with positive test results and the use of HIV NAT in the context of reentering donors with positive serologic test results has not been published, though a draft guidance was published in July 2005.

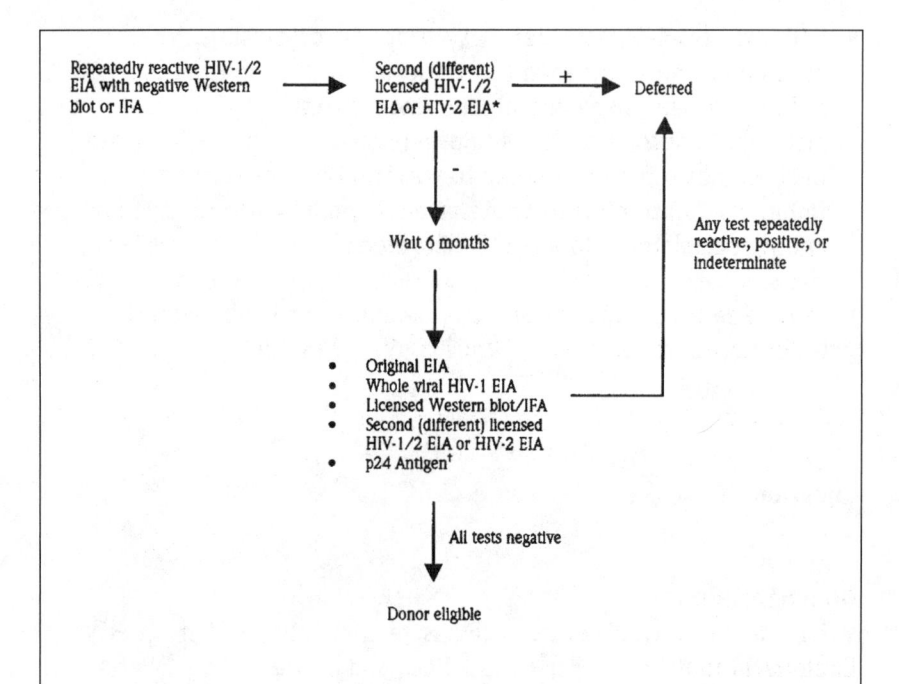

```
Repeatedly reactive HIV-1/2          Second (different)
EIA with negative Western    ──▶    licensed HIV-1/2        ──+──▶  Deferred
blot or IFA                          EIA or HIV-2 EIA*
                                            │                          ▲
                                            │ −                        │
                                            ▼                   Any test repeatedly
                                       Wait 6 months            reactive, positive, or
                                            │                   indeterminate
                                            ▼
                                    • Original EIA
                                    • Whole viral HIV-1 EIA
                                    • Licensed Western blot/IFA  ──────┘
                                    • Second (different) licensed
                                      HIV-1/2 EIA or HIV-2 EIA
                                    • p24 Antigen†
                                            │
                                            ▼ All tests negative

                                       Donor eligible
```

*The HIV-2 component of an HIV-1/2 EIA must be different from the HIV-2 component of the original HIV-1/2 EIA. This step is to demonstrate that the Western blot or IFA is not negative due to infection with HIV-2, the cause of the positive HIV-1/2 EIA.

†A 1992 FDA memorandum states that if "other licensed screening tests are performed" they must be negative. 1995 and 1996 FDA memoranda dealing with HIV-1 p24 antigen do not address the role of HIV-1 p24 antigen testing in re-entry. Also, 2004 FDA guidance on HCV and HIV NAT does not address the use of NAT in requalification.

Figure 11-5.

Question 6: A

Explanation:

- The Western blot identifies antibodies directed against the individual structural proteins of the HIV virus.

- HIV viral lysate is separated by electrophoresis. The viral antigen bands are then transferred to nitrocellulose, which is incubated with serum, washed, and incubated with antihuman IgG labeled with a marker. This is washed, and the substrate for the marker is added. The nitrocellulose is then examined for bands. The banding pattern is interpreted according to Centers for Disease Control and Prevention and Association of State and Territorial Public Health Directors criteria:
  - Negative: no bands present.
  - Positive: at least two bands from p24, gp41, or gp 120/160 present.
  - Indeterminate: presence of bands, but they do not fulfill the criteria for a positive determination.

Question 7: D

Explanation:

- HIV-1 p24 antigen testing began in 1996. It was estimated to decrease the window period by 6 days. From 1996 to 2001, eight p24-antigen-positive, HIV-EIA-negative donations were identified.
- If the HIV-1 p24 antigen testing is repeatedly reactive, it is confirmed through a neutralization assay. If the test neutralizes, the donor is deferred. If it is nonneutralizable, additional testing is required to determine the donor's eligibility.
- Figure 11-7 shows reentry of donors with HIV p24-antigen-positive screens.
- Because HIV RNA is detected before or simultaneously with p24 antigen, HIV-1 p24 antigen testing does not offer additional safety in the setting of NAT for HIV. Because CBER does not require p24 antigen testing if a licensed HIV NAT is used for screening, most centers no longer use this assay.
- HIV-1 p24 antigen levels fluctuate throughout the course of HIV infection, depending on the degree of viremia as well as the antibody response of the infected individual. Consequently, p24 antigen may not be detected despite the presence of infection.

Figure 11-7.

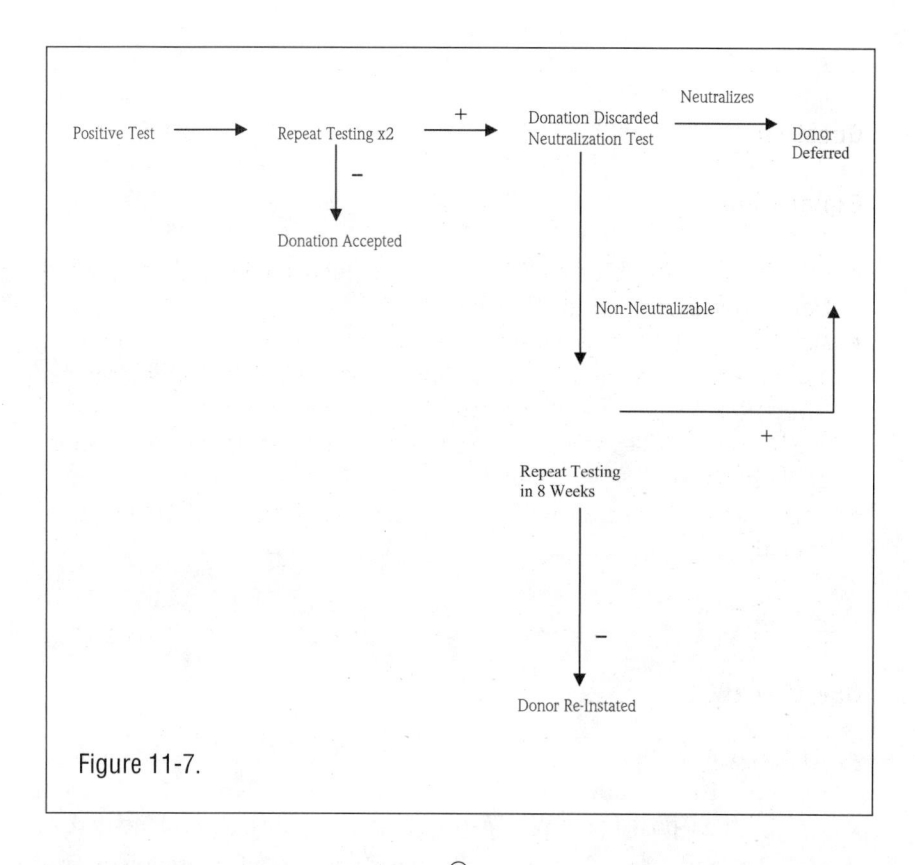

Question 8: B

Explanation:

- Implemented in early 1999, NAT has reduced the window period for HIV detection by 11 to 15 days, compared to HIV antibody testing, and 5 to 9 days compared to p24 antigen testing.
- Table 11-2 summarizes NAT for HCV and HIV in the United States and Canada.
- NAT is now licensed for routine blood donor testing.
- Final guidance concerning reentry of donors with positive test results and the use of HIV NAT in the context of reentering donors with positive serologic test results has not been published, though a draft guidance was published in July 2005.
- Pool size: 16 or 24 donations depending on the test manufacturer.

Question 9: A

Explanation:

- FFP and Cryoprecipitated AHF have not been implicated in cases of transfusion-transmitted HTLV infection.
- Male-to-female sexual intercourse, breast feeding, intravenous drug abuse, and transfusion (whole blood, red cells, and platelets) can transmit HTLV-I/II. After storage for 10 days or more, red cells are much less likely to transmit HTLV-I/II, as compared to other modes of transmission.
- HTLV-I and -II are transmitted by lymphocytes present in blood components.

Question 10: C

Explanation:

- HTLV-I is endemic in Central and West Africa, southern Japan, and the Caribbean basin, where the primary routes of transmission are through sexual contact and vertical transmission. HTLV-II has been reported to occur mainly in intravenous drug users and has been found in a number of countries in Europe, North and South America, and Asia.
- HTLV-I infection is associated with the development of both ATL and TSP or HAM. The lifetime risk of developing TSP is 0.25%, and the risk of developing ATL is 2% to 5%. HTLV-II infection has been described as a cause of rare cases of atypical hairy cell leukemia and has been detected in some patients with spastic myelopathy similar to that described with HTLV-I.
- HTLV-I and -II are highly cell-associated and therefore would theoretically be removed by leukocyte reduction. In addition, the viruses are not stabile during blood storage. In one study, antibodies were detected in 79% of recipients receiving non-leukocyte-reduced blood stored for 1 to 5 days compared to 55% receiving blood stored for 11 to 16 days.

Question 11: A

Explanation:

- The algorithm for testing for transfusion-transmissible diseases is to perform a screening test followed by a supplemental test. FDA-approved supplemental tests are not available for anti-HBc or HTLV-I/II. Anti-HBc has poor specificity, while HTLV-I/II is associated with a high false-positive rate in the donor population because of the low prevalence of infection. As a result, a donor must be repeatedly reactive on two separate occasions before he or she is deferred. These occasions do not need to be consecutive. In other words, if a donor is positive on his or her first donation, negative on the next 10, and positive on the 12th donation, he or she is deferred. An anti-HTLV-I/II testing algorithm is shown in Fig 11-11A. An algorithm for anti-HBc testing is shown in Fig 11-11B.

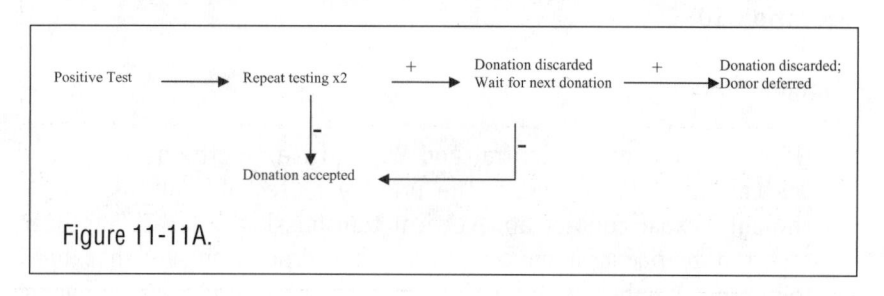

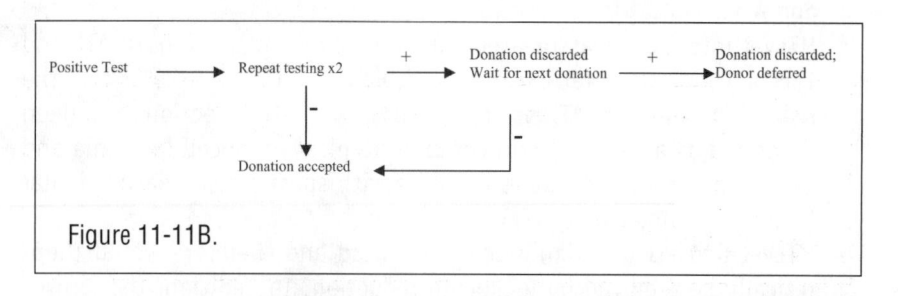

Figure 11-11A.

Figure 11-11B.

- A donor with a positive nontreponemal test for syphilis (RPR, Venereal Disease Research Laboratory) and a positive treponemal test [FTA, microhemagglutination assay-*T. Pallidum* (MHA-TP)] is not eligible to donate for 12 months. Figure 11-11C shows an algorithm for syphilis testing.

INFECTIOUS COMPLICATIONS 411

Figure 11-11C.

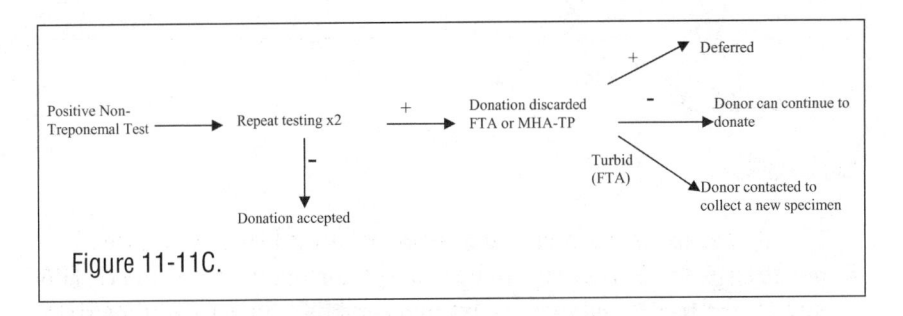

- Donors with a neutralizable HBsAg are positive for HBV and are not eligible to donate. Figure 11-11D shows an algorithm for HBsAg testing.

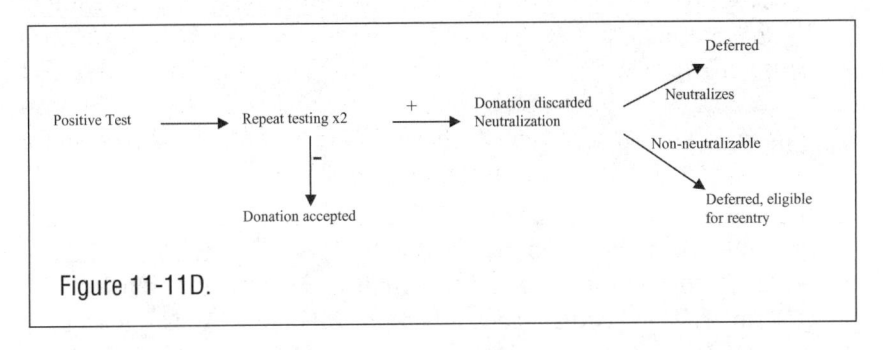

Figure 11-11D.

- Donors with a positive HCV EIA and an indeterminate RIBA are not eligible to donate. An algorithm for anti-HCV testing is shown in Fig 11-11E.

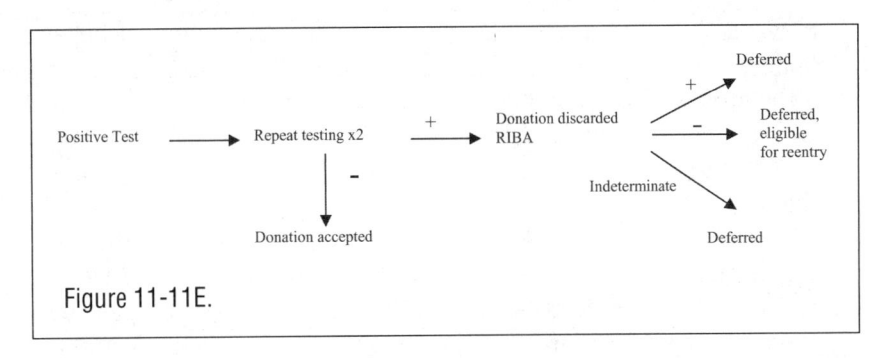

Figure 11-11E.

Question 12: B

Explanation:

- The HBV genome is a partially double-stranded DNA molecule.
- Hepatitis G virus (HGV) is an RNA virus. Transmission by blood transfusion has been demonstrated; however, the clinical significance is not firmly established. It has not been demonstrated to cause hepatitis. The designation of HGV as a hepatitis virus may be premature.

Question 13: D

Explanation:

- The patient has developed mild, self-limiting hepatitis probably caused by HAV. The incubation period for HAV is short: 15 to 45 days. The most common mode of transmission is the fecal-oral route.
- IgM anti-HAV indicates recent infection. IgM anti-HAV is replaced by IgG anti-HAV after a few months. IgG anti-HAV persists for years and offers protective immunity against all strains of HAV.
- HAV is not associated with a chronic carrier state, and complete recovery usually occurs.
- HAV-associated mortality is 0.1% and is caused by fulminant hepatic failure.
- Although transfusion-associated HAV is rare, it can occur when blood is collected from individuals with a high-titer viremia. This typically occurs during the asymptomatic viremic state, 7 to 28 days before the onset of clinical illness.
- HBsAg and IgM anti-HBsAg are markers for HBV infection. HBV has a long incubation period, from 6 to 8 weeks (range = 4 to 26 weeks), and most often is acquired parenterally. IgG anti-HBsAg could be a marker for past HBV infection, immunization, or passive immunity.
- IgG anti-HAV, IgG anti-HBsAg, IgG anti-HDV, and IgG anti-HGV offer protective immunity for years, perhaps for life.
- IgG anti-HCV does not offer protective immunity against reinfection. HCV RNA may persist in the circulation despite the presence of the neutralizing antibody.

Question 14: D

Explanation:

- HIV-1/2 antibody and HTLV-I/II antibody indicate a continuing infectious state.
- High percentages (80%) of those who test positive for HCV antibody also continue to be infected with the virus. Anti-HCV, in the absence of HCV RNA, may not offer protection from subsequent reinfection.
- Donors with positive tests for the above antibodies are permanently deferred from future donations.
- IgG anti-HBsAg is a protective, immune antibody. Active immunity for HBV is acquired by:
  - Previous exposure and clearance of HBsAg.
  - Vaccination with inactive HBsAg.
  - Vaccination with a recombinant DNA product synthesized in yeast.
- Protective, immune IgG anti-HBsAg develops in 80% to 97% of subjects receiving a full HBV vaccination course. The protection conferred appears to last 15 years or more in most, though in some it may not last longer than 2 to 5 years.
- Between 80% and 97% of subjects will respond to the HBV vaccine. In the group that does not, there is an increased frequency of certain HLA haplotypes (eg, HLA-B8, -DR3, -B44, and -DR7) in nonresponders.
- Passive immunity is acquired by treatment with Hepatitis B Immune Globulin (HBIG).
- Donors who have received HBIG are deferred for 12 months because they have been exposed to HBV, the reason for the HBIG administration. The 12 months is to allow them to develop serologic evidence of infection that would be detected at the time of future donations.

Question 15: E

Explanation:

- Because of the extreme sensitivity of the HBsAg assay, the amount of HBsAg in a dose of HBV vaccine was found to be detectable for up to 5 days following immunization. As this represents "real" HBsAg, it would be neutralizable. It is not a false-positive test result in the usual sense.
- Although the vaccine is given to induce anti-HBsAg, this test is *not* a routine donor screening test. Also, in a donor who is receiving a first dose of HBV vaccine, a primary immune response, requiring 14 days before antibody is detectable, is what would be expected.
- HBV vaccine contains *only* HBsAg. Anti-HBc does not result from HBV immunization.
- Interestingly, HBV immunization has been listed as a cause for false-positive HIV-1/2 EIA results, but this is rare.

Question 16: C

Explanation:

- Requalification (reentry) is available for individuals who have a positive HCV EIA with a negative RIBA. These donors most likely have a false-positive HCV EIA. The presence of a positive or indeterminate supplemental test (eg, Western blot), or an antigen detection test that neutralizes, excludes requalification.
- For requalification algorithms, see the explanations for Question 5 for HIV requalification and Question 8 for p24 requalification.
- An HBsAg reentry algorithm is shown in Fig 11-16A.
- HCV requalification is shown in Fig 11-16B.

Figure 11-16A.

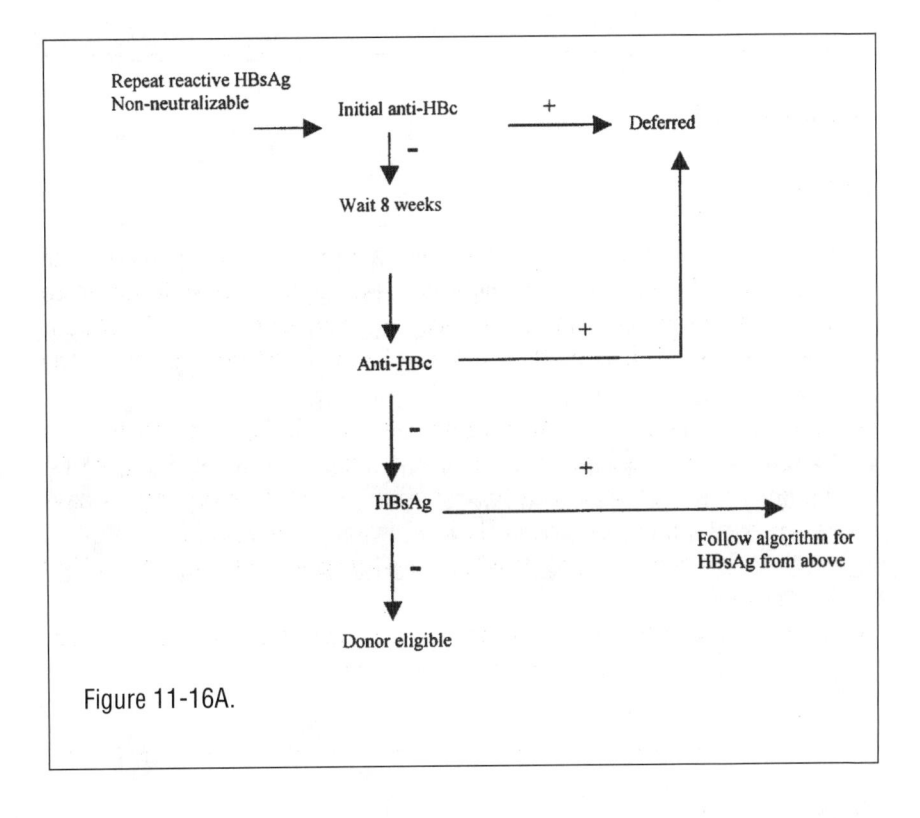

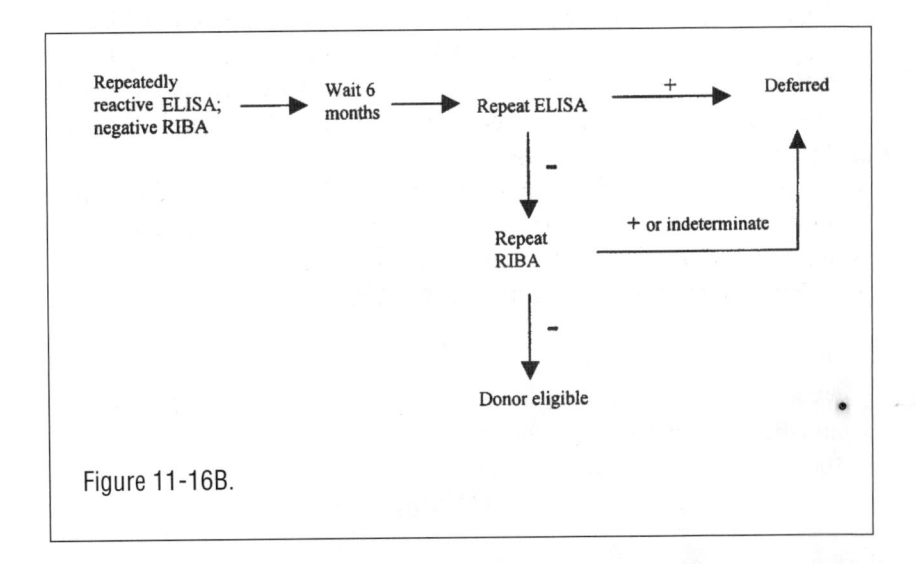

Figure 11-16B.

Question 17: D

Explanation:

- Up to 80% of patients with posttransfusion HCV infection will develop chronic hepatitis with 50% progressing to cirrhosis, 5% developing hepatocellular carcinoma, and 20% dying of HCV-related complications.
- Approximately 20% of individuals infected with HCV have no identifiable risk factors.
- Transfusion-associated HBV infection is more common (1:250,000 to 500,000) than HCV (<1:2,000,000).
- The algorithm for HCV testing is shown in Fig 11-17.

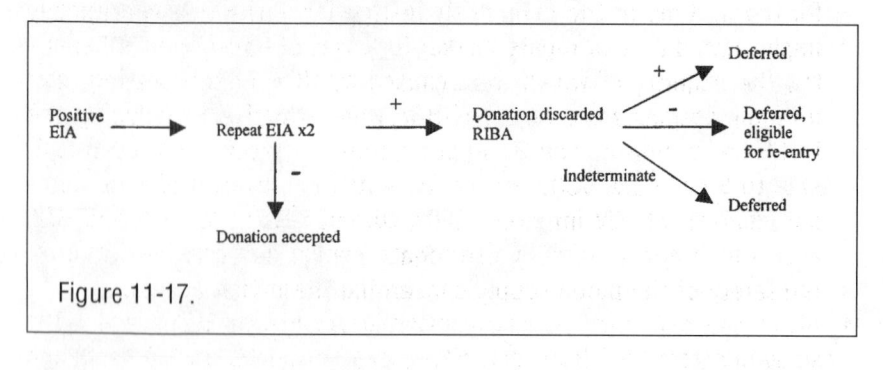

Figure 11-17.

Question 18: C

Explanation:

- Unfortunately, assays for anti-HBc are problematic when applied to donor screening. In these assays, a solid-phase reagent that consists of recombinant HBc antigen is incubated with donor serum. A labeled anti-HBc probe is then added and competes with any anti-HBc in the donor serum for antigen sites. The solid-phase reagent is washed, and the substrate for the indicator is added. The presence of anti-HBc in the donor serum results in a low signal, as it has bound to the HBc substrate with the result being the binding of less labeled anti-HBc. In the absence of anti-HBc in the donor's serum, more

labeled anti-HBc binds, resulting in a higher signal. Competitive assays of this type are sensitive to operator error. In addition, because there is not a clear differentiation between positive and negative populations, numerous false-positive results are generated. In one report, anti-HBc testing resulted in more repeat-reactive donations (0.62%) than all of the remaining serologic tests for viral infection combined (0.47%).
- Anti-HBc can detect a small number of patients who are in the "window period" for HBsAg. During an acute infection with HBV, HBsAg declines over a period of weeks as anti-HBsAg titers rise. During this period, donors would still be infectious despite the absence of detectable HBsAg. Anti-HBc is present during this period and would identify these donors.
- Anti-HBc is the first antibody to appear after infection with HBV. The antibody appears shortly after the appearance of HBsAg and persists for the lifetime of the individual. Testing for anti-HBc was originally implemented as a surrogate marker for cases of non-A, non-B hepatitis, the majority of which were caused by HCV. In this setting, alanine aminotransferase and anti-HBc were effective in reducing the incidence of non-A, non-B hepatitis from 20 cases per 1000 recipients to 5 cases per 1000 recipients. Anti-HBc also served as a surrogate marker for HIV infection. With current testing for HCV and HIV, anti-HBc is not an effective surrogate marker and does not improve the safety of the blood supply concerning these viral agents.
- All of the remaining assays mentioned are EIA or ELISA tests. The screening test for HBsAg and HIV-1 p24 antigen is an EIA test, and the confirmatory test is a neutralization assay.

Question 19: E

Explanation:

- CMV is a cell-associated virus and its DNA can be found within the white cells of most people who have been infected by the virus.
- Several categories of immunocompromised patients should be protected from transfusion-transmitted CMV infection by transfusing CMV-seronegative or leukocyte-reduced blood components. Components containing $<5 \times 10^6$ white cells are at reduced risk of transmitting CMV and are generally felt to be equivalent to CMV-seronegative

components. Categories of patients for whom CMV-reduced-risk components should be considered include:
- Recipients of IUT.
- Seronegative pregnant patients.
- Seronegative low-birthweight neonates (birthweight less than 1200 g) or infants born at ≤30 weeks of gestation to seronegative mothers.
- Seronegative patients infected with HIV, and AIDS patients.
- Seronegative patients who are candidates for or recipients of marrow or progenitor cell transplants.
- Seronegative solid organ transplant recipients who receive a seronegative solid organ.

- CMV seronegative units are *not* indicated for the routine transfusion of immunocompetent patients.
- The incidence of transfusion-associated CMV infection in at-risk patients receiving either leukocyte-reduced or CMV-seronegative blood components is 1% to 4%.
- CMV infection in pregnancy is associated with neonatal jaundice, thrombocytopenia, cerebral calcifications, motor disability, mental retardation, deafness, and death.

Question 20: A

Explanation:

- Leukocyte-reduced cellular blood components with less than 5×10^6 white cells/component are considered equivalent to CMV-seronegative units with regard to the transmission of CMV. Because of the presence of white cells, non-leukoctye-reduced RBCs can transmit CMV infection.
- FFP, Cryoprecipitated AHF, Deglycerolized RBCs, and Apheresis Platelets Leukocytes Reduced (at the source) are CMV-reduced-risk components as they do not contain sufficient white cells for CMV transmission.

Question 21: D

Explanation:

- Parvovirus B19 can cause a variety of clinical syndromes.
- Table 11-21 lists the various syndromes associated with parvovirus B19 infection.

Table 11-21.

Age	Clinical Condition	Clinical Significance
Fetus	Anemia and hydrops fetalis	Severe
Children and adults	Erythema infectiosum or Fifth disease	Mild and insignificant
Children and adults with chronic hemolytic anemia	Acute aplastic crisis with hypoplastic anemia	Severe
Immunocompromised adults	Pancytopenia	Severe

- Documented modes of transmission of parvovirus B19:
  - Respiratory (major).
  - Transfusion of clotting factor concentrates of Factors VIII and IX.
  - Blood component transfusion (rare).
- Dividing erythropoietic cells and fetal myocardial cells are affected by fetal parvovirus B19 infections.
- Anti-parvovirus B19 IgG antibody is protective.
- Persistent infection with anemia can occur in immunosuppressed individuals, but in immunocompetent individuals, parvovirus B19 is a self-limited infection.
- Parvovirus B19 binds to the P antigen of the globoside collection.
- The prevalence of antibodies to parvovirus B19 in the donor population is 30% to 60%. The prevalence of viremia in the blood donor

population has been found to be 1 in 35,000 donors but can increase during epidemics of Fifth disease (1 in 4,000).
- Intravenous immune globulin contains antibodies to parvovirus B19 and can be used to treat persistent B19 infections.

Question 22: A

Explanation:

- Prospective donors with a history of babesiosis and Chagas' disease (American trypanosomiasis) are permanently deferred as chronic infection with minimal symptoms and circulating parasitemia can exist even after recovery from acute infection.
- Kaposi's sarcoma and CMV retinitis are two of the 26 AIDS-defining clinical conditions defined by the CDC.
- Prospective donors with clinical or laboratory evidence of HIV must be permanently deferred.
- Prospective donors with a history of viral hepatitis after the 11th birthday must be permanently deferred.
- See the explanation for Question 24 for syphilis deferral criteria.

Question 23: C

Explanation:

- The transmission of syphilis by transfusion is exceedingly rare, with the last reported cases occurring approximately in 1965. The reasons postulated to explain the rarity of this transfusion complication include the following:
    - A lower incidence rate of the disease, not only in blood donors but also in the general population, when compared to the periods when transmission occurred by transfusion.
    - The switch from paid donors to volunteer donors.
    - Deferral of donors with high-risk behaviors through the donor history questionnaire.
    - Serologic testing of donors.

INFECTIOUS COMPLICATIONS   421

- ○ Poor viability of the organism at 4 C (red cells) and at high oxygen concentrations (platelets).
- Serologic testing for syphilis has been suggested as a surrogate marker for HIV infection. One study has shown, however, that very few cases of window-period HIV infections would be deferred based on syphilis testing (0.2 cases avoided between 1992 and 1994). In addition, this study was performed before the implementation of either HIV-1 p24 antigen testing or NAT, further reducing syphilis testing's value as a surrogate for HIV.
- Transfusion-transmitted syphilis presents as acute, fulminant secondary syphilis. This is characterized by spirochetemia with deposition of the organisms in all organs of the body. The characteristic finding is a mucocutaneous rash caused by deposition of the organisms within the skin.

---- ○ ----

Question 24: C

Explanation:

- Tests for syphilis are described in Table 11-24.

Table 11-24.

TP/Non-TP	Tests	Antigen	Specificity	Sensitivity	ST/CT
TP	1. FTA 2. MHA-TP	Treponemal cellular antigens	94% to 100%	69% to 100%	CT
Non-TP	1. ART 2. RPR 3. VDRL	Cardiolipin	Lower (depends on assay used)	77% to 100%	ST

TP = Treponemal tests; Non-TP = Nontreponemal tests; FTA = Fluorescent treponemal absorption test; MHA-TP = Microhemagglutination assay-*T. pallidum*; ART = Automated reagin test; RPR = Rapid plasma reagin; VDRL = Veneral Disease Research Laboratory; CT = Confirmatory test; ST = Screening test.

- Nontreponemal tests are serologic tests for syphilis (STS) that detect reagin antibodies toward cardiolipin, a lipid hapten found in spirochetes as well as in many human tissues.
- Nontreponemal tests are screening tests because they have high sensitivity but lower specificity.
- Unfortunately, large numbers of false-positive results may occur, especially in a low-prevalence population such as blood donors. Causes of false-positive results include the following:
  - Pregnancy, immunizations, bacterial and viral infections (STS may be temporarily positive).
  - Autoimmune diseases—eg, systemic lupus erythematosus and rheumatoid arthritis (STS may be permanently positive).
- Treponemal tests are confirmatory tests because they have a lower sensitivity but a higher specificity compared to nontreponemal tests.
- The algorithm for syphilis testing is given in the explanation for Question 11.
- According to AABB *Standards*, as well as FDA memoranda and guidance documents, prospective donors are deferred for 12 months for the following:
  - History and treatment of syphilis and gonorrhea.
  - Positive screening test result for syphilis with a positive confirmatory test result.
  - Positive screening test result with no confirmatory testing performed.
- Prospective donors with a positive STS are deferred because these donors may be at greater risk for transmission of other transfusion-related diseases. STS is considered a surrogate marker.
- If there is a history of treatment for syphilis, the deferral period may start from the date of diagnosis. Following the 12-month deferral (because of a history of syphilis or a positive screening test without confirmatory testing), the donor is eligible to donate if he or she has a negative screening test result. If the donor had both a positive screening test result and a positive confirmatory test result, the donor must have a negative screening test result and have documented evidence of treatment for syphilis in order to be eligible to donate.

Question 25: C

Explanation:

- The majority of transfusion-transmitted cases that have been reported have occurred because of a failure to identify at-risk individuals. Most of these cases would have been prevented had the donors answered questions appropriately or criteria been applied appropriately.
- *P. malariae* can persist in the blood as an asymptomatic infection for the life of an individual, but asymptomatic infections can persist for all organisms beyond the 12-month and 3-year deferrals.
- *P. ovale*, *P. vivax*, and *P. falciparum* can persist for shorter periods (see Table 11-25).

Table 11-25.

Incubation Period (Days)	*Plasmodium* Species	Persistence of Asymptomatic Infection
15	*P. ovale*	7 years
15	*P. vivax*	5 years
12	*P. falciparum*	5 years
30	*P. malariae*	life

- For all species, persistence of asymptomatic infection beyond 3 years is uncommon.
- AABB *Standards* related to donor selection criteria for malaria:
  - Asymptomatic donors from a low-prevalence (nonendemic) area traveling to an area where malaria is endemic are deferred for 1 year after their return to a low-prevalence area.
  - Asymptomatic donors from an endemic area are deferred for 3 years upon their arrival in a low-prevalence area.
  - Donors with a history of malaria are deferred for 3 years after becoming asymptomatic.

Question 26: C

Explanation:

- Federal regulations and AABB *Standards* state that the CDC determines malaria-endemic areas. The criteria for malaria deferrals do not include consideration for prophylaxis, time of day of exposure, or altitude of area visited. The acceptable and unacceptable areas are defined by the CDC in its publication "Health Information for International Travelers" and are also available on its Web site (see references).
- The deferrals for malaria are summarized in the explanation for Question 25.

Question 27: C

Explanation:

- Donors with a history of malaria are deferred for 3 years after becoming asymptomatic, whereas those infected with *T. cruzi* or *B. microti* are permanently deferred. AABB *Standards* does not state what should be done with regard to other protozoal infections such as *T. gondii* or *Leishmania* species. As a result, decisions concerning the status of donors with infections with these organisms are determined by the medical director of the collecting facility, either on a case-by-case basis or through standard operating procedures (SOPs).
- *T. gondii* circulates in the blood as an intracellular parasite. Transfusion-transmitted toxoplasmosis has been reported to have occurred only in the setting of granulocyte transfusions to immunosuppressed individuals.
- *Leishmania* species circulate in the blood within mononuclear cells and granulocytes. Cases of transfusion transmission have occurred. In 1991 and 2003, 12-month deferrals were implemented by the US Department of Defense for personnel stationed in endemic areas in Iraq.
- Table 11-27 describes transfusion-transmitted protozoan parasitic disease.

Table 11-27.

Species	Mode of Transmission	Disease	Deferral
Plasmodium species	Bite of female *Anopheles* mosquito	Malaria	3 years (AABB *Standards*)
Toxoplasma gondii	Ingestion of undercooked meat or food contaminated with cat feces	Toxoplasmosis	Determined by the medical director of the collection facility
Leishmania species	Bite of sandfly	Leishmaniasis	Determined by the medical director of the collection facility. 1 year deferral for personnel serving in Iraq.
Trypanosoma cruzi	Bite of reduviid bug	Trypanosomiasis (Chagas' disease)	Permanent deferral because of persistence of low-level parasitemia (AABB *Standards*)
Babesia microti	Tick bite	Babesiosis	Permanent deferral because of persistence of low-level parasitemia (AABB *Standards*)

Question 28: B

Explanation:

- CJD is not a viral disease. The infectious agent is an abnormal variant of an evolutionarily conserved protein, PrP. In CJD, an abnormal structural form (PrP^{Sc}) catalyzes the alteration of the normal form into the pathologic form. This form results in neuronal death and dropout, leading to the characteristic spongiform change in the central nervous system.
- The majority of cases of CJD are sporadic (85%), with 10% to 15% being familial.
- Documented modes of iatrogenic transmission of CJD:
  - Corneal transplantation.
  - Growth hormone derived from cadaveric human pituitary gland.
  - Allogeneic human dura mater graft.
  - Implantation of contaminated intracerebral electrodes.
- Transmission of CJD through blood transfusion has not been reported and studies of at-risk populations have failed to demonstrate an increased frequency of CJD.
- Prospective donors with blood relatives who have CJD are permanently deferred (AABB *Standards*).
- Recipients of growth hormone derived from human pituitary gland and allogeneic human dura mater grafts are permanently deferred (AABB *Standards*).
- Recombinant human growth hormone, available since 1985, is not associated with CJD.
- CJD statistics:
  - Worldwide incidence: one per million population.
  - Incubation period: decades.
  - Pathology: spongiform encephalopathy.
  - Clinical presentation: rapidly progressive dementia, often with myoclonus.
  - Prognosis: fatal; average duration of life is 7 months after diagnosis.

INFECTIOUS COMPLICATIONS 427

Question 29: C

Explanation:

- vCJD is a spongiform encephalopathy of which approximately 100 cases have been identified in Great Britain, with a handful of cases being diagnosed in other countries. Like CJD, it is characterized by dementia, but it differs in that the average age of diagnosis is younger (29 vs 65). It also has a longer duration after diagnosis (14 vs 4.5 months), it lacks the characteristic electroencephalograph pattern of CJD, and the brain lesion demonstrates amyloid plaque formation in addition to spongiform change. It is thought to represent a prion disease that has jumped from one species (cattle) to humans.
- Four cases of possible transfusion transmission of vCJD have been documented. In addition, an animal model involving the collection and transfusion of blood from sheep fed bovine spongiform encephalopathy (BSE)-infected nervous tissue has shown transmission.
- Permanent deferral criteria for vCJD include the following:
  - Residence in Great Britain (England, Wales, Scotland, Northern Ireland, the Isle of Man, Channel Islands, Gibraltar, Falkland Islands) for 3 months or more between 1980 and 1996.
  - Receipt of bovine insulin since 1980 produced from cattle from a country in which BSE is endemic.
  - Transfusion of blood or blood components in the United Kingdom or France between 1980 and the present.
  - Cumulative residence or travel in France for 5 years or more since 1980.
  - Cumulative residence or travel in Europe for 5 years or more since 1980.
  - Residence of US military personnel, civilian employees, or their dependents at US military bases in Northern Europe (Germany, United Kingdom, Belgium, and the Netherlands) for 6 months or more between 1980 and 1990.
  - Residence of US military personnel, civilian employees, or their dependents at US military bases in Southern Europe (Greece, Turkey, Spain, Portugal, Italy) for 6 months or more between 1980 and 1996.

Question 30: C

Explanation:

- WNV is a flaviviridae. It is transmitted by the bite of infected mosquitoes. The main reservoir for the virus is birds, with humans and other animals representing dead-end hosts, incapable of completing the viral life-cycle.
- Eighty percent of infected individuals are asymptomatic.
- Twenty percent develop WNF, characterized by fever, malaise, anorexia, nausea, vomiting, eye pain, headache, myalgias, rash, and lymphadenopathy.
- One out of 150 people with WNF develop meningitis, encephalitis, or a syndrome of flaccid paralysis mimicking acute inflammatory demyelinating polyneuropathy (Guillain-Barré syndrome).
- WNV infection is a self-limited infection characterized by the development of permanent immunity.
- Individuals at either age extreme, the young or the elderly, are at greatest risk for WNF and neurologic complications.
- Mortality rate among those hospitalized with WNF is 4% to 14%.

Question 31: D

Explanation:

- In 2002, before the implementation of NAT, there were 23 cases of transfusion-transmitted WNV. With the implementation of NAT in 2003, this decreased to 6 cases, with fewer than 10 cases since.
- Because of breakthrough transmissions resulting from failure of pooled NAT to detect low-level viremia, in 2007 AABB required rules for the implementation of individual NAT when certain frequencies of WNV are detected in the donor population of a geographic area. CBER has issued draft guidance for comment as well. There were no transfusion-transmitted cases in 2007.
- IgM antibodies to WNV appear early but persist for up to 512 days. As viremia is cleared within 104 days, the use of IgM testing would

result in the deferral of donors and discard of products that were not viremic.
- A donor diagnosed with WNF or with a positive NAT is deferred for 120 days from onset of symptoms/diagnosis or the positive NAT.

Question 32: B

Explanation:

- *T. cruzi* is a parasite transmitted by the reduviid (triatomine) bug. The bite itself does not transmit infection. When it takes a meal, the bug defecates. If this is rubbed into the bite or conjunctiva, infection occurs.
- Reduviid bugs are found living in the walls and roofs of mud brick and thatched roof housing in Central and South America. They are nocturnal, feeding at night.
- Acute infection is characterized by fever, anorexia, lymphadenopathy, mild hepatosplenomegaly, and myocarditis. This syndrome lasts for 4 to 8 weeks. Treatment at this stage can cure infection. Infants, young children, and the immunocompromised can develop myocarditis or meningoencephalitis.
- Following the acute infection, chronic infection, which is incurable, occurs. Thirty percent of chronically infected individuals develop dementia, megacolon, megaesophagus, or cardiac failure. These result from destruction of neurons within the brain and myenteric plexus by the parasite.
- Additional routes of infection include vertical transmission from mother to child as well as by transfusion. The former is important as it is possible for an infected individual to never have visited an endemic area. In fact, reports of cases have been published where the maternal family members of infected individuals had not been in endemic areas for three generations.
- As a result of changing demographics, with increased emigration from Central and South America, the seroprevalence has been found to be increasing.

Question 33: A

Explanation:

- *T. cruzi* has been transmitted by platelets and red cells. Platelet transfusion has been the most common route involved in 5 of the 6 cases identified in North America.
- Only 6 cases of transfusion-transmitted *T. cruzi* have been reported in North America.
- Currently, the only CBER-licensed assay for blood donors is an ELISA-based assay. The supplemental test is a radioimmunoprecipitation assay (RIPA). It uses radiolabeled parasites to detect the presence of antibodies to *T. cruzi*. It is offered only by a limited number of laboratories.
- A xenodiagnostic assay involving the transmission from humans to guinea pigs is available but is not FDA licensed.
- The organisms can survive liquid-nitrogen freezing in 5% DMSO. This is the method used to preserve them for study. Although no cases of transmission by progenitor cells have been reported, it is a theoretical risk.

Question 34: B

Explanation

- According to federal regulations, look-back is required for HIV, HCV, HBV, and HTLV.
- For HCV, the recipient(s) of blood components from 12 months before the last negative blood donation from the recently discovered donor is (are) to be notified and counseled. If the recipient is dead, nothing further is done.
- For HIV, the recipient(s) of blood components from 12 months before the last negative blood donation from the recently discovered donor is (are) to be notified, but if they have died, the legal representative or relative is to be notified.

- For HBV and HTLV, look-back consists of identification and discard of in-date components from the donor. (This is also performed with regard to HCV and HIV.)
- Look-back has not been defined for syphilis.

Question 35: C

Explanation:

- Regulations require that the transfusion service that issued the component have final responsibility for notification. Because of the doctor-patient relationship that exists between the patient and other physicians, and because of the questions that arise from the patient concerning the appropriateness of transfusion, many transfusion services have the physician who ordered the transfusion contact the patient. If the physician refuses, however, it is the transfusion service's legal responsibility.

REFERENCES

1. Fiebig EW, Busch MP. Infectious disease screening. In: Roback JD, Combs MR, Grossman BJ, Hillyer CD, eds. Technical manual. 16th ed. Bethesda, Maryland: AABB, 2008:241-82.
2. Food and Drug Administration. Guidance for industry: Use of nucleic acid tests on pooled and individual samples from donors of whole blood and blood components (including source plasma and source leukocytes) to adequately and appropriately reduce the risk of transmission of HIV-1 and HCV. (October 2004) Rockville, MD: CBER Office of Communication, Training, and Manufacturers Assistance, 2004.*
3. Food and Drug Administration. Memorandum: Clarification of FDA recommendations for donor deferral and product distribution based on the results of syphilis testing. (December 12, 1991) Rockville, MD: CBER Office of Communication, Training, and Manufacturers Assistance, 1991.
4. Food and Drug Administration. Guidance for Industry: Donor screening for antibodies to HTLV-II. (August 1997) Rockville, MD: CBER Office of Communication, Training, and Manufacturers Assistance, 1997.

5. Code of federal regulations. Title 21, CFR Part 610.41(a). Washington, DC: US Government Printing Office, 2009 (revised annually).
6. Food and Drug Administration. Memorandum: Revised recommendations for the prevention of human immunodeficiency (HIV) transmission by blood and blood products. (April 23, 1992) Rockville, MD: CBER Office of Communication, Training, and Manufacturers Assistance, 1992.
7. Food and Drug Administration. Memorandum: Recommendations for donor screening with a licensed test for HIV-1 antigen. (August 8, 1995) Rockville, MD: CBER Office of Communication, Training, and Manufacturers Assistance, 1995.
8. Food and Drug Administration. Memorandum: Additional recommendations for donor screening with a licensed test for HIV-1 antigen. (March 14, 1996) Rockville, MD: CBER Office of Communication, Training, and Manufacturers Assistance, 1996.
9. Food and Drug Administration. Memorandum: Recommendations for the management of donor and units that are initially reactive for hepatitis B surface antigen (HBsAg). (December 2, 1987) Rockville, MD: CBER Office of Communication, Training, and Manufacturers Assistance, 1987.
10. Food and Drug Administration. Memorandum: Revised recommendations for testing whole blood, blood components, source plasma, and source leukocytes for antibody to hepatitis C virus encoded antigen (anti-HCV). (August 5, 1993) Rockville, MD: CBER Office of Communication, Training, and Manufacturers Assistance, 1993.
11. Food and Drug Administration. Memorandum: Recommendations for deferral of donors for malaria risk. (July 26, 1994) Rockville, MD: CBER Office of Communication, Training, and Manufacturers Assistance, 1994.
12. Price TH, ed. Standards for blood banks and transfusion services. 26th ed. Bethesda, MD: AABB, 2009.
13. Food and Drug Administration. Draft guidance for industry: Nucleic acid testing (NAT) for human immunodeficiency virus type 1 (HIV-1) and hepatitis C virus (HCV): Testing, product disposition, and donor deferral and reentry. (July 19, 2005) Rockville, MD: CBER Office of Communication, Training, and Manufacturers Assistance, 2005.
14. Centers for Disease Control and Prevention. Malaria map application. Atlanta, GA: CDC, 2006. [Available at http://www.cdc.gov/malaria/risk_map (accessed May 11, 2009).]
15. Food and Drug Administration. Guidance for industry: "Lookback" for hepatitis C virus (HCV): Product quarantine, consignee notification, further testing, product disposition, and notification of transfusion recipients based on donor test results indicating infection with HCV. (August 2007) Rockville, MD: CBER Office of Communication, Training, and Manufacturers Assistance, 2007.
16. Food and Drug Administration. Memorandum: Recommendations for the quarantine and disposition of units from prior collections from donors with repeatedly reactive screening tests for hepatitis B virus (HBV), hep-

atitis C virus (HCV), and human T-lymphotrophic virus type I (HTLV-I). (July 19, 1996) Rockville, MD: CBER Office of Communication, Training, and Manufacturers Assistance, 1996.

17. Code of federal regulations. Title 21, CFR Part 610.46. Washington, DC: US Government Printing Office, 2008 (revised annually).
18. Code of federal regulations. Title 21, CFR Part 610.47. Washington, DC: US Government Printing Office, 2008 (revised annually).

---

*Food and Drug Administration draft guidances, final guidances, and memoranda can be accessed at http://www.fda.gov/BiologicsBloodVaccines/ResourcesforYou/Industry/default.htm

12

Coagulation

QUESTIONS

Question 1: Which of the following proteins and/or prostaglandins is *not* localized or synthesized in the platelet?

A. Thromboxane synthetase.
B. Arachidonic acid.
C. Thromboxane A_2.
D. Prostacyclin.
E. Cyclo-oxygenase.

Question 2: Regarding thrombin and prothrombin, which of the following is *true*?

A. The primary physiologic method of thrombin generation is via the intrinsic system.
B. Factor Va is the protease that cleaves prothombin to thrombin.
C. Thrombin generation is the major route of platelet activation.
D. Prothrombin is synthesized in endothelial cells.
E. Thrombin is a cofactor for protein C activation.

Question 3: Which of the following statements concerning Factor XII (Hageman factor) is *true*?

A. Its activation triggers the extrinsic pathway of coagulation.
B. It is an important determinant of in-vitro hemostasis but is not a determinant of physiologic hemostasis.
C. Deficiency of Factor XII is associated with a mild bleeding disorder.
D. Deficiency of Factor XII causes a marked prolongation of the prothrombin time (PT).
E. Factor XII deficiency has a prevalence of about 1 in 500,000.

Question 4: Which of the following statements regarding the thrombin and reptilase times is *true*?

A. They both measure the conversion of prothrombin to thrombin.
B. Thrombin time (TT) is prolonged by the addition of protamine.
C. Reptilase time (RT) is prolonged in the presence of heparin.
D. Both are prolonged in the presence of an abnormal fibrinogen.
E. Both will be prolonged by vitamin K deficiency.

Question 5: The activated partial thromboplastin time (aPTT) is normal in patients with *severe* deficiencies of which of the following clotting factors?

A. Factor VIII:C.
B. Factor IX:C.
C. Factor XIII.
D. Factor V.
E. von Willebrand factor (vWF).

Question 6: Which of the following plasma coagulation factors is found in Cryoprecipitated AHF?

A. Factor VII.
B. Factor II.
C. Factor IX.
D. Fibrinogen.
E. Factor XI.

Question 7: The differentiation of type IIB von Willebrand disease (vWD) from all other subtypes depends on which of the following laboratory tests?

A. Bleeding time.
B. Low-strength ristocetin platelet aggregation.
C. Full-strength ristocetin platelet aggregation.
D. Multimeric assay of Factor VIII.
E. Ristocetin cofactor assay.

Question 8: Which of the following is an appropriate screening test for the presence of lupus anticoagulant (LA)?

A. Reptilase time.
B. Dilute aPTT.
C. Prothrombin level.
D. Fibrinogen level.
E. Protein S level.

Question 9: An elevated level of D-dimer is specific for:

A. Disseminated intravascular coagulation (DIC).
B. Primary fibrinolysis.
C. Both.
D. Neither.

Question 10: Primary fibrinolysis is *most* suggested by which of the following sets of results?

A. Short euglobulin lysis time and decreased Factor I.
B. Low levels of all clotting factors and positive monochloroacetic acid (MCA) lysis.

C. Thrombocytopenia, low levels of all clotting factors, short euglobulin lysis time, and elevated fibrin degradation products (FDPs).
D. Elevated levels of plasminogen and fibrin degradation products.
E. None of the above.

Question 11: Which of the following is the *best* test to monitor the therapy of thrombotic thrombocytopenic purpura?

A. Platelet count.
B. aPTT.
C. Fibrinogen level.
D. Platelet aggregation with ristocetin.
E. ADAMTS13 activity.

Question 12: Which of the following statements concerning acquired Factor VIII inhibitors in nonhemophiliacs is *true*?

A. Occur more commonly than LAs.
B. Are usually IgG.
C. Are usually of little clinical significance with regard to bleeding.
D. Are best treated with plasma exchange.
E. Hemorrhages are usually treated with high doses of Cryoprecipitated AHF.

Question 13: Which *one* of the following test results *rules out* the diagnosis of a lupus anticoagulant?

A. Normal aPTT.
B. Negative antiphospholipid antibody.
C. Negative anticardiolipin antibody.
D. Normal tissue thromboplastin inhibition index.
E. No single test has yet been identified that effectively rules out the presence of an LA.

Question 14: Vitamin K deficiency affects the function of which of the following proteins?

A. Protein S.
B. Factor V.
C. Fibrinogen.
D. Factor XII.
E. Antithrombin.

Question 15: Which of the following abnormalities has been associated with an abnormal activated protein C resistance test?

A. Defective release of thrombomodulin.
B. A mutation in the Factor V gene.
C. Decreased thrombin ability to bind thrombomodulin.
D. A genetic defect in the Factor VIII gene.
E. A genetic defect in the inactive precursor molecule of protein C.

Question 16: A 60-year-old woman presents to her physician with complaints of unexplained bruising. She has no other complaints. Multiple ecchymoses are seen on her arms and legs. She has a history of uncomplicated cholecystectomy, hysterectomy, and vaginal deliveries (three). Her medical history is otherwise unremarkable, and she is not currently on any medications. The complete blood count is normal, as is the PT. The aPTT is prolonged. The prolongation is not corrected by mixing with normal plasma. The most likely explanation for the patient's findings is:

A. Type I vWD.
B. LA.
C. Acquired Factor IX inhibitor.
D. Acquired Factor V inhibitor.
E. Acquired Factor VIII inhibitor.

Question 17: Which of the following is *true* regarding the international normalized ratio (INR)?

A. It is useful for comparing the PT and aPTT results with those of different laboratories.
B. It is calculated as {patient PT ÷ control PT}^{ISI} where PT = prothrombin time, and ISI = sensitivity index for thromboplastin used in test.
C. It is recommended for monitoring warfarin during the first few days of therapy.
D. It Is useful for monitoring patients receiving heparin therapy.
E. It is most sensitive to Factor II levels.

Question 18: Elevation of fibrin degradation products (FDPs) may be caused by:

A. Recent thrombosis.
B. Renal and liver disease.
C. Recent surgery.
D. Primary fibrinolysis.
E. All of the above.

Question 19: Which of the following is *not* true regarding heparin-induced thrombocytopenia (HIT)?

A. Typically occurs 3 to 14 days after heparin administration.
B. Can be associated with heparin flushes.
C. Is more commonly associated with porcine than bovine heparin.
D. Largely remains a clinical rather than a laboratory diagnosis.
E. Is associated with thrombosis.

Question 20: Regarding low-molecular-weight heparin (LMWH), which of the following is *true*?

A. Exerts its major effect against thrombin in an action similar to that of heparin.
B. Response is monitored by the aPTT assay.
C. Is not associated with risk of HIT.
D. Is associated with a significant reduction in deep vein thrombosis and pulmonary embolus when given postoperatively to patients undergoing elective hip replacement.
E. Is reversed with plasma transfusion.

Question 21: Which of the following statements concerning DIC is *true*?

A. Decreased levels of antithrombin III are associated with increased mortality.
B. Protein C and protein S activity are increased.
C. The presence of thrombocytopenia makes the diagnosis of DIC highly likely.
D. Factor VIII:C levels are increased in most patients with DIC.
E. Absence of a low fibrinogen makes the diagnosis of DIC highly unlikely.

Question 22: The aPTT is not sensitive to:

A. Factor II.
B. Factor V.
C. Factor VII.
D. Factor IX.
E. Factor X.

Question 23: The factor with the shortest half-life is:

A. Factor II.
B. Factor V.
C. Factor VII.
D. Factor IX.
E. Factor X.

Question 24: The PT is a screening test for all the following *except:*

A. Factor II.
B. Factor V.
C. Factor VII.
D. Factor IX.
E. Factor X.

Question 25: A mild hemophiliac weighs 50 kg and has a Factor VIII activity of 10% and a hematocrit of 40%. He is scheduled to have a minor surgery. How many units of Factor VIII would be required to raise the patient's Factor VIII level to 50%?

A. 350.
B. 840.
C. 1050.
D. 2100.
E. 3500.

Question 26: The in-vivo half-life of Factor VIII is:

A. 6 hours.
B. 12 hours.
C. 24 hours.
D. 36 hours.
E. 48 hours.

Question 27: The pattern of inheritance of hemophilia A is:

A. Autosomal recessive.
B. X-linked dominant.
C. Autosomal dominant.

D. X-linked recessive.
E. X-linked codominant.

Question 28: A 64-year-old female presents with a history of cough, fever, and right chest pain. After the appropriate workup, a diagnosis of deep right femoral vein thrombosis with pulmonary embolism is made. Symptoms resolve with bed rest and heparin anticoagulation. Long-term anticoagulation with warfarin is instituted and heparin is discontinued. Six months later, the patient is brought to the emergency room unresponsive. A computed tomography scan shows an intracerebral hemorrhage. Her INR is 9. The most effective immediate treatment is:

A. Intramuscular (IM) vitamin K.
B. Prothrombin complex concentrate (PCC).
C. Fresh Frozen Plasma (FFP).
D. Intravenous (IV) vitamin K.
E. Cryoprecipitated Antihemophilic Factor (AHF).

Question 29: With regard to agratroban and fondaparinux, which of the following is *true*?

A. They are direct thrombin inhibitors.
B. They are indirect Factor Xa inhibitors.
C. They are reversed by recombinant Factor VIIa (rFVIIa).
D. They are reversed by PCCs.
E. Agratroban is a direct thrombin inhibitor; fondapirinux is an indirect Xa inhibitor.

Question 30: A 42-year-old male is brought to the emergency department with acute chest pain with S-T segment elevations on electrocardiogram. An emergency cardiac catherization reveals a single high-grade obstruction of the left anterior descending artery. An attempt at angioplasty is made but is unsuccessful. Abciximab was administered during the attempted angioplasty. The patient is now taken for emergent coronary bypass surgery. Regarding the administration of abciximab, which is *true*?

A. Abciximab is a coagulation factor inhibitor; therefore, FFP should be transfused to reverse the anticoagulation.
B. The patient should be transfused with 2 units of Platelets before surgery.
C. The patient should undergo dialysis to remove free abciximab from the plasma.
D. Platelets should be made available for surgery and transfused if there is evidence of excessive bleeding.
E. The patient will likely need Cryoprecipitated AHF transfusion during surgery.

ANSWERS

Question 1: D

Explanation:

- Prostacyclin, a platelet aggregation inhibitor, is produced in the vascular endothelium.
- Arachidonic acid is cleaved from the platelet membrane by phospholipases.
- Cyclo-oxygenase is located in the dense tubular system of the platelet. It metabolizes arachidonic acid to an intermediate substance, which thromboxane synthetase converts to thromboxane A_2.

Question 2: C

Explanation:

- Thrombin is a stronger platelet agonist than collagen, adenosine diphosphate (ADP), or thromboxane A2. Tissue factor/Factor VIIa (TF-VIIa)-mediated generation of thrombin is the major route of platelet activation.
- The physiologic mechanism for initiating thrombin generation is via the extrinsic system through the interaction of Factor VIIa with tissue factor. Although thrombin formation is initiated by the TF-FVIIa interaction, Factors VIIIa and IXa are necessary to generate hemostatic levels of thrombin.
- The TF-FVIIa complex activates Factor X to Xa. Xa combined with Va, Ca^{++}, and platelet membrane phospholipids constitute the extrinsic system prothrombinase that cleaves prothombin to thrombin. Xa is the protease and Factor Va is the cofactor.
- The TF-FVIIa complex is also critical for the formation of the intrinsic system tenase. TF-FVIIa directly converts IX to IXa, which in combination with Factor VIIIa, Ca^{++}, and phospholipid as cofactors, cleaves X to Xa.
- Once low levels of thrombin are generated, thrombin amplifies more thrombin generation by activating Factors XIa, VIIIa, and Va.

- Antithrombin is a natural anticoagulant that inactivates thrombin. Antithrombin-mediated inactivation of thrombin is enhanced by the binding of heparin.
- Congenital deficiency of antithrombin is inherited as an autosomal dominant trait.
  - A deficiency of antithrombin may cause thrombosis.
  - High levels have not been associated with bleeding.

Question 3: B

Explanation:

- In the classic depiction of hemostasis, Factor XII is a component of the intrinsic system.
- Factor XII (Hageman factor), prekallikrein (Fletcher factor), and Factor XI are protein zymogens that are known as the "contact system" because of the autoactivation of Factor XII when it comes in contact with negatively charged surfaces, eg, glass tubes.
- Although important for in-vitro measurement of coagulation, Factor XII is not physiologically necessary for coagulation, as evidenced by the finding that individuals with Factor XII deficiency do not exhibit a bleeding disorder. In-vitro, homozygous deficiency of Factor XII will cause a marked prolongation of the activated partial thromboplastin time (aPTT; ~200 seconds). Heterozygous deficiency prolongs the aPTT to a less significant degree.
- Factor XII does participate in other physiologic functions, including fibrinolysis, complement activation, inflammation, and chemotaxis. Its importance in these functions remains largely undetermined.
- Some studies have reported a higher incidence of thrombosis in patients with Factor XII deficiency, and others have refuted this association. There is no consensus on whether Factor XII deficiency imposes a tendency towards thrombosis.
- The prevalence of homozygous Factor XII deficiency is about 1 per million. Heterozygous Factor XII deficiency is more common and is often detected as an otherwise unexplained prolongation of the aPTT.

Question 4: D

Explanation:

- The TT measures the conversion of fibrinogen to fibrin. Bovine or human thrombin is added to the patient's citrated plasma sample, then time to clot formation is measured in seconds. Normal range varies with the laboratory but should be somewhere within 15 to 25 seconds. The TT is prolonged with the following:
    - Heparin or direct thrombin inhibitors.
    - Hypofibrinogenemia or hyperfibrinogenemia.
    - Dysfibrinogenemia.
    - Elevated fibrin degradation products.
    - Markedly elevated plasma proteins.
- Reptilase is an enzyme derived from snake venom. Like thrombin, it splits fibrinogen to fibrin and generates fibrinopeptide A. Unlike thrombin it does not split fibrinopeptide B from fibrin.
    - Reptilase is not inhibited by heparin; therefore, an RT will help distinguish elevation in TT due to heparin from other causes of elevated TT.
    - The RT is otherwise prolonged by all of the same causes of TT prolongation.
- Because the TT and RT measure conversion of fibrinogen to fibrin after addition of exogenous thrombin or reptilase, it is not affected by deficiency in vitamin K, which affects the function of Factors II, VII, IX, and X, as well as inhibitors of coagulation proteins C, S, and Z.
- Protamine neutralizes the effect of heparin and may be added to specimens suspected of containing heparin as a means of demonstrating that a TT prolongation is attributable to heparin. Protamine will not prolong the TT.

Question 5: C

Explanation:

- The aPTT is a measure of the function of the intrinsic pathway (contact factors and Factors XI, IX, and VIII) and common pathways (Factors X, V, and II and fibrinogen) of coagulation. To perform the test, calcium is added to citrated plasma, to which thromboplastin and kaolin or another negatively charged substance have been previously added. The endpoint is the time to clot formation, measured in seconds.
- Factor XIII is responsible for crosslinking fibrin and stabilizing the formed clot; its activity is not measured by the aPTT.
- von Willebrand disease (vWD) patients may have a prolonged aPTT as a result of the decrease in Factor VIII:C which accompanies vWD abnormalities. While the prolongation of the aPTT may be minimal or absent in mild cases, in severe type III vWD, the Factor VIII:C is markedly reduced, and the aPTT is prolonged.

Question 6: D

Explanation:

- Cryoprecipitated AHF is the cold, insoluble fraction of plasma that precipitates when Fresh Frozen Plasma (FFP) is thawed at 1 to 6 C. Cryoprecipitated AHF contains concentrated forms of Factor VIII, vWF, fribrinogen, and fibronection.
- The most common indication for Cryoprecipitated AHF use is hypofibrinogenemia caused by consumption (eg, DIC) or loss (eg, massive bleeding).
- Other indications include the following:
  - Management of hereditary dysfibrinogenemia.
  - Bleeding associated with uremia.
    - A functional defect in the vWF-platelet interaction is thought to contribute to platelet dysfunction in uremia. Administration of Cryoprecipitated AHF has been shown to shorten the bleeding time in some patients with uremia. Results are highly vari-

able, but when effective, a response in bleeding time is seen within 4 to 12 hours, with some responses as early as within 1 hour.
- Cryoprecipitated AHF administration in uremia is typically reserved for patients undergoing surgical procedures or experiencing difficult-to-control bleeding.
- Historically, Cryoprecipitated AHF was developed for the treatment of hemophilia and vWD. Pathogen-safe factor concentrates are now available for management of these bleeding disorders and should be used when factor replacement is necessary.
- Cryoprecipitated AHF is still recommended for Factor XIII deficiency.

Question 7: B

Explanation:

- vWD is categorized into three major types. Types I and III are characterized by a quantitative defect in vWF. Type II is characterized by a qualitative difference in vWF. In brief:
  - Type I (~75%)—partial quantitative deficiency of vWF.
    - Bleeding symptoms are usually mild to moderate; some cases may be asymptomatic until a hemostatic challenge.
  - Type II (~20%)—functionally deficient.
    - Type IIA—decrease in the intermediate and high-molecular-weight vWF multimers that are necessary for hemostasis.
    - Type IIB—vWF has an increased ability to bind to the platelet receptor glycoprotein 1b (GP1b).
      - High-molecular-weight multimers readily bind to platelets and are lost from circulation.
      - May also cause clearance of platelets from circulation because of agglutination.
      - Use of desmopressin (DDAVP) may increase platelet clearance and produce thrombocytopenia. DDAVP is contraindicated for management.
      - Distinct from platelet-type vWD.
    - Type IIM (uncommon).
      - Reduced binding to GPIb.
      - Bleeding may be significant.

- Type IIN (uncommon).
  - vWF has an abnormal Factor VIII binding site.
  - Rapid clearance of Factor VIII.
  - Hemophilia-type bleeding.
- Platelet-type (or pseudo vWD).
  - Abnormal GPIb.
  - vWF is normal.
  - Clinical features are similar to type IIB.
- Type III (rare).
  - Complete absence of vWF.
  - vWF is the carrier protein for Factor VIII; therefore, Factor VIII is rapidly cleared from circulation, and Factor VIII levels are <10%.
  - Severe bleeding disorder, exhibiting both mucosal (platelet-type) and soft tissue and joint (hemophilia-type) bleeding.
- The most commonly used tests for the diagnosis of vWD can be divided into tests that answer the following questions:
  1. How much vWF antigen is present?
  2. How much vWF activity is present?
  3. Is the quality of the vWF interaction with platelets normal?
  4. Is the multimeric composition of the vWF normal?
  5. Is Factor VIII activity normal?
  - Plasma vWF antigen (**vWF:Ag**) is a quantitative measure of the amount of vWF antigen in the circulation. vWF:Ag is reduced when vWF production is decreased.
  - Plasma vWF activity (ristocetin cofactor activity, or **vWF:Rco**) is a measure of the ability of vWF to interact with platelet GPIb. vWD types characterized by a qualitative difference in vWF will have a low vWF:Rco relative to vWF:Ag.
  - Ristocetin binds to platelet GPIb and to vWF. Platelets with bound vWF will aggregate in the presence of ristocetin. Ristocetin-induced platelet aggregation (**RIPA**) is a measure of the affinity with which vWF binds to GPIb. Ristocetin is added to aliquots of patient platelet-rich plasma at various concentrations. The vWF of type IIB vWD readily binds GPIb; therefore, ristocetin will induce aggregation at lower concentration than is seen with normal individuals or other forms of vWD.
  - **vWF multimer distribution** is a gel electrophoresis test used to qualitatively assess the quantity and molecular weight distribution of the patient's vWF multimers. It provides a visual estimate of the amount of vWF present and whether it is compositionally normal.

- **Factor VIII activity** is a coagulation factor assay. Factor VIII activity is reduced when the amount of vWF is reduced, or when there is a defect in the vWF binding site for Factor VIII.
- Bleeding time and other tests for assessing platelet plug formation may also be included in the assessment of vWD.

Question 8: B

Explanation:

- Phospholipid antibodies are directed at phospholipids and phospholipid-binding proteins such as cardiolipin and β_2-glycoprotein.
- LA is the term applied to phospholipid antibodies that interfere with the function of coagulation and anticoagulation factors.
- The in-vivo interaction of lupus anticoagulants with their antigen is a prothrombotic event. In vitro, the LA is manifested as an inhibition of coagulation.
- The aPTT is prolonged in only approximately 50% of patients with LA. When LA is strongly suspected, coagulation testing should be performed by methods that are more sensitive to phospholipid levels.
- The dilute PT, dilute aPTT, and the dilute Russel viper venom test are low-phospholipid-concentration clotting tests that respectively evaluate the extrinsic, intrinsic, and final common pathways and are recommended for the initial detection of LA. In the presence of LA, the phospholipid in these tests is not sufficient to support coagulation. Other low-phospholipid tests include the colloidal silica clotting time and the kaolin clotting time.
- If there is prolongation of a phospholipid-dependent test, the next step is to determine if a 1:1 mixing test corrects the prolongation.
- If the prolongation does not correct, the presence of LA is confirmed by demonstrating that addition of excess phospholipid or platelets shortens or corrects the prolonged coagulation test.
- The RT, fibrinogen level, protein S levels, and prothrombin levels are typically normal in the presence of LA.

Question 9: D

Explanation:

- The presence of soluable D-dimer indicates that the sequence of coagulation, crosslinking of fibrin, and fibrinolysis has occurred. The D-dimer assay detects a specific fibrin degradation product and is an indicator of fibrinolysis of any cause. It is not an indicator of fibrinogenolysis because D-dimer elaboration depends on the crosslinking of fibrin monomers, followed by plasmin lysis.
- D-dimers are elevated in DIC but they are not specific to DIC.
- D-dimers are elevated with deep vein thrombosis; pulmonary emboli; sepsis; pregnancy, especially when preeclampsia is present; following surgery; or with large hematomas.

Question 10: A

Explanation:

- Primary fibrinolysis may be caused by an increase in plasminogen activators (tissue-type or urokinase-type plasminogen activators), a decrease in plasmin inhibitors (α-2 antiplasmin, thrombin-activatable fibrinolysis inhibitor), or decreased inhibition of plasminogen activators (plasminogen activator inhibitors 1 and 2).
- In addition to congenital abnormalities of the fibrinolytic system, primary fibrinolysis occurs in association with many common clinical settings, including cardiopulmonary bypass, severe liver disease, hepatic resection or transplantation, genitourinary tract surgery (associated with urokinase-type plasminogen activator release), oral surgery, cardiac bypass surgery, trauma, and malignancy.
- If direct lysis of fibrinogen (as well as fibrin) occurs, it is called fibrinogenolysis, which is always pathologic.
- The euglobulin fraction refers to fibrinogen, plasminogen, tissue plasminogen activator, and other proteins that precipitate when citrated plasma is diluted at low pH and low ionic strength. The precipitated euglobulins are resuspended in buffer and then clotted by the addition of thrombin. The time to lysis of that clot is a measure of

fibrinolytic activity and is reported as the euglobulin lysis time. A shortened euglobulin lysis time combined with a disproportionate decrease in fibrinogen (Factor I) is suggestive of primary fibrinolysis.
- An important distinction between primary hyperfibrinolysis and secondary hyperfibrinolysis as seen with DIC is that with primary fibrinolysis there is a disproportionate consumption of fibrinogen and plasminogen relative to consumption of coagulation factors. Consumption of coagulation factors and platelets in the presence of a short euglobulin time is supportive of DIC. FDPs are elevated with both.
- Plasminogen and antiplasmin levels may be useful for confirming the presence of fibrinolysis, but their levels decrease rather than increase because of consumption.
- In DIC, fibrinogen is decreased in proportion to other clotting factors.
- The MCA lysis test is a screening test for Factor XIII deficiency. In the absence of Factor XIII, MCA will solubilize the patient's clotted plasma. Factor levels of 1% to 2% are sufficient to prevent solubilization.

Question 11: A

Explanation:

- The platelet count is the most consistently abnormal test in thrombotic thrombocytopenic purpura (TTP), and platelets play a clear role in the pathologic process, resulting in renal and neurologic dysfunction. While some may use lactate dehydrogenase levels and creatinine levels to monitor a patient with TTP, the platelet count is the best indicator of response to therapy.
- Although always associated with a decreased platelet count, TTP is not a primary platelet disorder but, rather, one in which platelet activation and microthombi development is secondary to another underlying defect. The presence of abnormal, unusually large von Willebrand factor (ULvWF) multimers and endothelial injury are the two most commonly implicated mechanisms of platelet activation in TTP.
- ADAMTS13 is a metalloproteinase necessary for the cleavage of ULvWF multimers. Deficiency of ADAMTS13 because of either congen-

ital mutations or development of autoantibodies is one mechanism by which ULvWF may accumulate in the circulation.
- ADAMTS13 levels are not always decreased in TTP, and although decreased levels of ADAMTS13 (<5% of normal) are highly specific for TTP, severe decreases have also been reported with sepsis and DIC.
- ADAMTS13 levels may remain persistently low even in the presence of excellent clinical responses to therapy; therefore, levels are not used to monitor response to therapy.
- The PT, aPTT, and fibrinogen levels are typically within normal range in patients with TTP.

Question 12: B

Explanation:

- Inhibitors to Factor VIII are rare autoantibodies, typically IgG4, that are often associated with life-threatening bleeding. They occur in association with pregnancy or the postpartum period, autoimmune disorders, and malignancy, and in some cases as drug reactions. Nearly half of all cases are idiopathic.
- Factor VIII inhibitors occur more commonly in women than men, and in older (>64) rather than younger individuals (pregnancy-associated cases excluded).
- Prednisone followed by cyclophosphamide for nonresponders is commonly recommended as the therapy of choice. However, intravenous immune globulin is also used as initial therapy. Plasma exchange is now infrequently used for management of Factor VIII inhibitors.
- High doses of Factor VIII concentrates may be used to treat hemorrhages in patients with low inhibitor levels (<5 Bethesda units), but for those with strong inhibitors, recombinant activated Factor VII (rFVIIa, Novoseven, Novo Nordisk, Bagsvaerd, Denmark) therapy is preferred. Cryoprecipitated AHF is not appropriate for management of these patients.

COAGULATION 455

Question 13: E

Explanation:

- No single currently available test effectively rules out the diagnosis of LA.
- At a minimum, two tests should be used to screen for LA. Recommended screening tests are those that use low levels of phospholipids in the assay as discussed in Question 8 (see explanation).

Question 14: A

Explanation:

- Coagulation Factors II (prothrombin), VII, IX, and X, as well as anticoagulation proteins C, S, and Z, are vitamin K dependent.
- Vitamin K is a necessary cofactor for γ-carboxylation of glutamic acid residues on vitamin-K-dependent coagulation proteins. Carboxylation of glutamic acid residues leads to chelation of Ca^{++} and allows these proteins to bind phospholipids and cell membranes by means of protein-Ca^{++}-phospholipid bridges. In the absence of carboxylation, the complexes necessary for coagulation proteins to effectively interact are not formed, rendering the proteins functionally inactive.
- Warfarin inhibits vitamin K reductase (vitamin K 2,3-epoxide reductase) and blocks the regeneration of the active form of vitamin K.

Question 15: B

Explanation:

- Addition of activated protein C prolongs the aPTT in normal patients. Absence of prolongation indicates resistance to the action of protein C. Recent reports show that abnormal resistance test results may occur in 40% of patients with otherwise unexplained thrombosis. In

addition, 95% of those with abnormal resistance test results have been found to have Factor V Leiden.
- Protein C is activated by thrombin complexed with thrombomodulin. Activated protein C inactivates Factor Va by sequentially cleaving Va in three locations. The first proteolytic cleavage is at the Arg506 residue and is necessary for cleavage at the other two sites.
- The Factor V Leiden gene has a guanine-to-adenine point mutation at nucleotide 1691 that results in a glutamine in place of an arginine at position 506 of the protein. Factor V Leiden is not susceptible to protein C cleavage at position 506; therefore, inactivation of Va is delayed. Factor V Leiden heterozygotes and homozygotes both have thrombophilia; however, the risk of thrombotic events is greater for homozygotes.
- Activated protein C in combination with deactivated Factor V and protein S plays a role in the deactivation of Factor VIIIa, but this is also dependent on the prior cleavage of Va at residue 506.
- Thrombin and thrombomodulin are necessary to generate activated protein C, but the activated protein C resistance test assesses defects downstream of protein C generation.

Question 16: E

Explanation:

- LAs are antibodies that result in prolongation of coagulation assays in vitro but clinically are associated with thrombosis, not hemorrhage.
- New onset of bleeding in the absence of a history of bleeding, despite multiple challenges, is indicative of an acquired, not congenital, bleeding disorder.
- Antibodies to specific coagulation factors may occur as alloantibodies in patients with congenital coagulation factor deficiency, or as autoantibodies in people with previously normal coagulation.
- The most common acquired coagulation factor autoantibodies are antibodies to Factor VIII. Autoantibodies to other coagulation factors are rare.
- Acquired Factor VIII inhibitors are seen with a frequency of about 1 per 1.5 million population per year. They occur more commonly in

women than men and are more common in those over age 50, unless associated with pregnancy.
- The clinical course is marked by bleeding (ecchymosis, intramuscular hematomas, and gastrointestinal, genitourinary, and mucosal bleeding), often severe, and often a medical emergency. Intracranial hemorrhage is uncommon.
  - Factor VIII inhibitor should always be suspected when there is onset of unexplained skin and soft tissue bleeding in older patients without a history of bleeding disorder, particularly if they have a prolonged aPTT.
- Acquired inhibitors to thrombin and Factor V are usually associated with exposure to bovine thrombin and Factor V with use of topical fibrin glue.

Question 17: B

Explanation:

- The INR prevents confusion arising from the use of different PT assays in different laboratories by correcting for the sensitivity of the thromboplastin used in each assay compared to an international standard. Therefore, an INR from one laboratory can be directly compared to an INR from another without knowing a control value for the PT and without concern for the type of assay either laboratory uses.
- For most clinical situations the recommended range for the INR is between 2.0 and 3.0. Patients with mechanical cardiac valves are an exception and should have an INR between 2.5 and 3.5.
- The INR is most sensitive to the inhibition of Factor VII because it has the shortest half-life (4-6 hours) of any of the vitamin-K-dependent factors.
- The INR should not be routinely used to follow patients with liver disease or vitamin K deficiency, and is not accurate in the early phases of warfarin therapy. In these cases, the PT should be used.
- The INR is not relevant to the aPTT assay.

Question 18: E

Explanation:

- FDPs form whenever plasmin cleaves soluable fibrin monomers formed as a result of clotting. Fibrinogen degradation products form as a result of plasmin's action on fibrinogen. D-dimer is a specific type of fibrin degradation product formed when plasmin acts on crosslinked fibrin; it is an indication that both coagulation and fibrinolysis have occurred.
- Any disorder associated with increased coagulation or increased generation of plasminogen activator may result in the formation of FDPs.
- Fibrin degradation products cause feedback inhibition of thrombin and reptilase and may prolong the TT and RT. Therefore, they have clot inhibitory properties. This is not usually clinically significant except in a situation such as DIC, where degradation products are sometimes grossly elevated and may contribute to the already abnormal hemostatic state.

Question 19: C

Explanation:

- Heparin-induced thrombocytopenia (HIT) occurs in about 2% to 5% of patients receiving unfractionated heparin (UFH) for more than 4 days. It usually appears 3 to 14 days after the start of heparin administration and may occur with minute doses, including heparin flushes. Onset of HIT may be very rapid in those with previous exposure to heparin.
- The risk of developing HIT is greatest with use of UFH, with surgical rather than medical patients, and in females. More cases have been associated with bovine (85%) than porcine (15%) heparin.
- The diagnosis of HIT should be considered when there is an otherwise unexplained drop in platelet count (even if still above normal range) of 50% within 3 to 14 days after heparin therapy.
- Thrombocytopenia without thrombosis is the most frequent presentation of HIT. The thrombocytopenia is usually not severe, with median

platelet counts remaining in the 60,000/μL range. There is rarely need to consider platelet transfusion, and because of the risk of thrombosis, prophylactic platelet transfusion is contraindicated. In contrast, posttransfusion purpura and immune thrombocytopenic purpura, which are often included in the differential, are associated with platelet counts below 20,000/μL.
- HIT is associated with a high risk of thrombosis. Thrombotic events may precede the development of thrombocytopenia; therefore, HIT should be considered as a cause of otherwise unexplained thrombosis. The risk of thrombosis in patients managed by heparin discontinuation alone is the range of 20% to 50%. Venous thrombosis is by far more common than arterial thrombosis, but arterial thrombosis is seen frequently enough to have garnered HIT the synonym *white clot syndrome*.
- HIT is an immune-mediated disorder caused by antibodies directed at an epitope of platelet factor 4 (PF4) that is only available when heparin is complexed with PF4. The PF4-heparin complexes attach to platelets and induce activation.
- Diagnostic assays for HIT either directly detect heparin-dependent antibodies or look for functional evidence of the antibodies.
  - Enzyme-linked immunosorbent assays use PF4 complexed with heparin (or similar anionic molecules) affixed to microtiter wells as a target for detecting antibodies in patient serum. This is a highly sensitive but not very specific assay, as many patients without HIT may have demonstrable antibodies. A negative result is strong evidence against the diagnosis of HIT, but a positive result may be misleading.
  - Functional assays include serotonin release and heparin-induced platelet aggregation. These assays evaluate whether heparin at therapeutic levels enables the patient's plasma to activate platelets.
    - The serotonin release assay being both highly sensitive and specific is the "gold standard" for laboratory diagnosis of HIT. However, this assay is not always easily available.
    - Platelet aggregation assays are specific but not sensitive.
- Diagnostic tests or their results may not be readily available, nor are all available tests equally sensitive; therefore, the diagnosis of HIT remains largely clinical.
- Once a clinical diagnosis of HIT has been made, nonheparin, rapidly acting anticoagulation therapy should be promptly initiated. Discontinuation of heparin therapy is not sufficient for protecting the

patient from thrombotic complications, as the highest risk for thrombosis appears to be during the first few days after stopping heparin.
- In the presence of HIT, warfarin should not be started without other rapidly acting anticoagulants because of an increased risk of warfarin-induced skin necrosis.

Question 20: D

Explanation:

- Because of its short size, LMWH is largely unable to simultanenously bind antithrombin and thrombin to exert a direct effect on thrombin. LMWH exerts its major action against Factor Xa. The aPTT is not usually prolonged by LMWH; response to therapy is monitored by measuring anti-Xa activity. Advantages of LMWH include the following:
  - Response is correlated to body weight; therefore, fixed dosing is possible.
  - Ongoing monitoring is not required for most patients. Pediatric, obese, and renal failure patients may require more frequent monitoring.
  - May be administered in the outpatient setting.
  - Is less likely to induce heparin-associated antibodies. However, patients with established HIT will respond to LMWH administration in the same manner as heparin. It has no role in the management of HIT.
- LMWH is at least equally effective as UFH for deep vein thrombosis prophylaxis, and anticoagulation before warfarin therapy in patients with mechanical valve replacement. LMWH is also indicated for the prevention of deep vein thrombosis and pulmonary emboli in patients undergoing hip replacement.
- It is not currently recommended for the therapy of formed clots.
- LMWH is reversed by protamine sulfate, but not as efficiently as heparin is reversed.

Question 21: A

Explanation:

- The critical step in the pathogenesis of acute DIC is the formation of thrombin at sites of endothelial injury by the action of the TF-FVIIa system. Massive generation of thrombin triggers systemic coagulation which overwhelms anticoagulation and fibrinolytic pathways.
- In addition to consumption, impaired synthesis/regulation of antithrombin, protein C, and protein S contribute to the low levels of these proteins seen in DIC. Low antithrombin levels in DIC are associated with increased mortality.
- Although both coagulation and fibrinolysis are activated in DIC, activation of coagulation is disproportional to activation of fibrinolysis. End-organ damage in DIC is attributable to widespread fibrin deposition and tissue ischemia.
- The platelet count is a sensitive test in DIC, particularly if it dramatically drops over a short interval of time. About 95% of patients with DIC have thrombocytopenia. However, low or decreasing platelet counts may be associated with a variety of disorders, including bleeding. A normal platelet count is strong evidence against this diagnosis.
- Fibrinogen is an acute phase reactant; therefore, fibrinogen levels alone are not a very sensitive test for DIC. Fibrinogen levels are decreased in less than 50% of patients with DIC and are lowest in patients with severe acute uncompensated DIC.
- No single test or combination of tests is specific or sensitive enough to give a definitive diagnosis of DIC. Routinely available tests that are of value in the diagnosis include those described below:
  - FDPs and D-dimers should both be elevated in DIC (see explanation for Question 19).
  - Soluable fibrin monomers are increased.
  - PT and aPTT are elevated as a result of consumption of coagulation factors.
  - Fibrinogen may be decreased.
  - TT and RT are prolonged.
  - Platelets are decreased.
  - Antithrombin levels are decreased.
  - Factor V and Factor VIII levels may be decreased in acute DIC. Factor VIII levels are variable because, like fibrinogen, Factor VIII is an acute-phase reactant.

Question 22 C

Explanation:

- The aPTT is a screening test for all coagulation factors except Factors VII and XIII. The aPTT is less sensitive to the proteins of the common pathway than is the PT.
- Also see explanation for Question 3.

Question 23: C

Explanation:

- The half-life of Factor VII is 4 to 6 hours (coagulation factor with the shortest half-life).
- The half-life of Factor XIII is 144 hours (coagulation factor with the longest half-life).

Question 24: D

Explanation:

- The PT is a screening test for Factors I, II, V, VII, and X (extrinsic and common pathway).

Question 25: B

Explanation:

- The initial dosage to achieve the desired plasma level of Factor VIII (% activity) is calculated as follows:
  - Blood volume (mL) = weight (kg) × 70; 50 × 70 = 3500 mL
  - Plasma volume (mL) = blood volume (mL) × (1 − Hct); 3500 × (1 − 0.4) = 2100

- Factor VIII requirement = plasma volume × (desired Factor VIII level % − pretransfusion Factor VIII level %); 2100 × (0.5 − 0.1) = 840
- The subsequent dosage is administered every 8 to 12 hours depending upon the clinical status of the patient.

Question 26: B

Explanation:

- Half-life of Factor VIII: 8 to 12 hours.
- Half-life of Factor IX: 18 to 24 hours.

Question 27: D

Explanation:

The pattern of inheritance of hemophilia A and hemophilia B is X-linked recessive, as shown in Table 12-27.

Table 12-27.

	Hemophilia A	Hemophilia B
Synonyms	Factor VIII deficiency	Factor IX deficiency Christmas disease PTC deficiency
Incidence	1:5000 to 10,000	1:30,000 to 50,000 Increased incidence in Jews
Diagnosis	Factor VIII:C assay	Factor IX assay
Treatments of choice	Recombinant Factor VIII	Recombinant Factor IX

PTC = plasma thromboplastin cofactor.

Question 28: B

Explanation:

- The choice of method for warfarin reversal is dependent on the urgency of the situation and the thrombotic risk consequent to interrupting anticoagulation.
- When there is major life-threatening bleeding such as intracranial hemorrhage, the goal is to effect rapid and complete reversal of warfarin. PCCs or recombinant Factor VIIa (rFVIIa), in combination with intravenous vitamin K, will reverse warfarin within 10 to 15 minutes. If PCCs or rFVIIa are not available, FFP may be used, but the response will be less effective.
- In situations where bleeding is serious but not life threatening, and fast warfarin reversal is needed, FFP may be used in combination with intravenous vitamin K. Some guidelines recommend against using FFP for reversal of warfarin because the reversal is incomplete, and the volumes of plasma needed for an adult (upwards of 2 liters) pose a risk of transfusion-associated circulatory overload.
- In the absence of bleeding or with only minor bleeding, a decision must be made about whether to simply discontinue warfarin or to discontinue warfarin and administer vitamin K. Generally speaking, vitamin K administration is usually not necessary when the INR is <5, may be necessary when the is INR >5<9, and is frequently necessary when the INR is >9. When making the decision to withhold or administer vitamin K, careful attention must be given to the balance of bleeding and thrombotic risks.
- Vitamin K may be administered via IV, IM, and oral routes.
  - IM administration is not recommended because of the risk of IM hemorrhage, variable absorption, and the possibility of a residual effect on warfarin reinstatement.
  - IV vitamin K will have an effect within 4 to 6 hours and is not adequate as a sole source of reversing warfarin with severe bleeding. Recommended dosing is 5 to 10 mg for life-threatening bleeding. Doses of 1 mg are appropriate for marked elevations in INR (>9) in the absence of bleeding.
  - Oral vitamin K takes effect within 24 hours. Doses are generally 1 to 2 mg orally, unless the INR is markedly elevated, in which case doses may be in the 2- to 5-mg range.

- In all cases of warfarin intoxication, warfarin should be discontinued until it is safe to resume.
- Cryoprecipitated AHF does not have a role in warfarin reversal.

Question 29: E

Explanation:

- Until recently, anticoagulation therapy has been based on UHF, LMWH, and vitamin K antagonists. A high risk of adverse consequences and difficulty of use have driven a search for alternative agents.
- Alternatives currently available or in the process of clinical evaluation include drugs targeted at the inhibition of thrombin, activated Factor X, and the TF-FVIIa complex.
- Argatroban, lepirudin, and bivalirudin are direct thrombin inhibitors that are administered intravenously and monitored using the aPTT. The Food and Drug Administration (FDA) has approved their use for HIT and percutaneous coronary interventions.
- Reversal of direct thrombin inhibitors:
  - Direct thrombin inhibitors have short half-lives and are administered as continuous infusions. Reversal is primarily dependent on stopping the infusion. If rapid reversal is required, activated PCCs have been reported to be more effective than rFVIIa.
- Fondaparinux is an indirect Xa inhibitor that is FDA approved for the prevention and treatment of venous thromboembolism. It is a pentasaccharide that binds to antithrombin, inducing a conformational change that increases the natural Xa inhibitory effect of antithrombin 300-fold. Upon antithrombin binding to Xa, fondaparinux is released and is available to act upon other free antithrombin molecules. Bound Xa-antithrombin complexes are cleared from the circulation.
- Reversal of Fondaparinux:
  - Fondaparinux is not reversed by administration of FFP, PCCs, or protamine.
  - rFVIIa has been shown to reverse fondaparinux.

Question 30: D

Explanation

- Platelet-mediated coronary thrombosis is the primary pathophysiologic mechanism of acute coronary syndromes and acute ischemic complications of percutaneous interventions. Inhibition of platelet aggregation is an essential therapeutic intervention in the management of acute coronary syndromes.
- **GPIIb/IIIa inhibitors:**
  - Abciximab (ReoPro, Centocor BV, Leiden, the Netherlands) is a GPIIb/IIIa receptor antagonist. Two other GPIIb/IIIa antagonists are available for use: tirofiban (Aggrastat, Medicure Pharma, Somerset, NJ) and eptifibatide (Integrelin, Schering-Plough, Kenilworth, NJ).
    - Abciximab is a monoclonal antibody with a strong affinity for the GPIIb/IIIa receptor.
    - Although the serum half-life is only 15 to 30 minutes, it takes approximately 48 hours to return to 50% of baseline platelet function.
- Eptifibitide and tirofiban are drugs that have weaker affinity for the GPIIb/IIIa receptor.
  - Their half-lives are 2.5 and 2 to 2.5 hours, respectively.
  - After discontinuation of infusion, platelet aggregation returns to baseline within 4 to 8 hours.
  - Patients who require emergency cardiac surgery following attempted angioplasty are likely to have received a GPIIb/IIIa inhibitor, and are at increased risk of bleeding during surgery.
    - Whenever possible, the drug should be discontinued at least 12 hours before surgery.
    - The risk of bleeding with abciximab is directly related to the dose of heparin used for coronary artery bypass graft (CABG). At low doses of heparin, the incidence of major hemorrhage with abciximab is comparable to that of patients who did not receive abciximab.
    - Because there is little free abciximab in the plasma, platelet infusion replenishes the number of GPIIb/IIIa receptors available for interacting with fibrinongen.

- When surgery cannot be delayed, platelet transfusion should be administered to those patients who demonstrate unexpected bleeding. Evidence to support the routine administration of platelets to all patients on abciximab is lacking.
- Tirofiban and eptifibatide do circulate free in the plasma. Because they undergo significant renal elimination, platelet function returns to baseline within 4 to 8 hours of discontinuation.
    - The drugs should be discontinued a minimum of 4 hours before surgery.
    - If immediate reversal is necessary, the presence of free drug makes platelet transfusion much less effective.

- **Clopidogrel:**
    - Clopidogrel is an irreversible inhibitor of ADP-induced platelet aggregation and the subsequent ADP-mediated activation of the GPIIb/IIIa complex.
    - Clopidogrel is used in combination with aspirin in the management of acute coronary syndromes. Patients on clopidogrel are at higher risk of excessive bleeding during CABG.
        - The half-life is 8 hours.
        - Whenever possible, the drug should be discontinued at least 5 to 7 days before surgery.
        - In an emergency, it is desirable to wait at least 6 hours after a dose of clopidogrel.
        - Platelets may be administered for reversal of clopidogrel. The efficacy of this therapy, or the number of doses required, has not been formally studied.

- **Aspirin:**
    - Aspirin irreversibly inhibits platelet cyclooxygennase-reducing synthesis of thromboxane A2, a potent platelet aggregator and vasoconstrictor.
        - Doses of 75 mg/day achieve complete blockage of platelet cyclooxygenase.
        - As new platelets enter the circulation, platelet response to aggregating agents is restored.
            - Aspirinated platelets are capable of participating in adhesion and aggregation with nonaspirinated platelets.
        - Aspirin inhibiton of platelets does not usually necessitate platelet transfusion.

REFERENCES

1. Levi M, de Jonge E, Meijers J. The diagnosis of disseminated intravascular coagulation. Blood Rev 2002;16:217-23.
2. Greinacher A, Warkentin TE. Recognition, treatment, and prevention of heparin-induced thrombocytopenia: Review and update. Thromb Res 2006;118:165-76.
3. Schulman S, Bijstervel N. Anticoagulants and their reversal. Transfus Med Rev 2007;21:37-48.
4. Hanley JP. Warfarin reversal. J Clin Pathol 2004;57:1132-9.
5. Bauer K. New anticoagulants. Curr Opin Hematol 2008;15:509-15.
6. Leung L. Overview of hemostasis. In: Basow DS, ed. UpToDate. Waltham, MA, 2008.
7. Leung L. Clinical features, diagnosis, and treatment of disseminated intravascular coagulation in adults. In: Basow DS, ed. UpToDate, Waltham, MA, 2008.
8. Zehnder JL. Clinical use of coagulation tests. In: Basow DS, ed. UpToDate. Waltham, MA, 2008.
9. Drews RE. Approach to the patients with a bleeding diathesis. In: Basow DS, ed. UpToDate. Waltham, MA, 2008.
10. Rick ME. Clinical presentation and diagnosis of von Willebrand disease. In: Basow DS, ed. UpToDate. Waltham, MA, 2008.
11. Coutre S. Heparin-induced thrombocytopenia. In: Basow DS, ed. UpToDate. Waltham, MA, 2008.
12. Bermas ML, Schur PH, Pathogenesis of the antiphospholipid syndrome. In: Basow DS, ed. UpToDate. Waltham, MA, 2008.
13. Coutre S. Acquired inhibitors of coagulation. In: Basow DS, ed. UpToDate. Waltham, MA, 2008.
14. Bermas BL, Erkan D, Schur PH. Clinical manifestations of the antiphospholipid syndrome. In: Basow DS, ed. UpToDate. Waltham, MA, 2008.
15. Fay W. Thrombotic and hemorrhagic disorders due to abnormal fibrinolysis. In: Basow DS, ed. UpToDate. Waltham, MA, 2008.
16. Schmaier H, Thornburg CD, Pipe SW. Hemostasis and thrombosis. In: McPherson RA, Pincus MR, eds. Henry's clinical diagnosis and management by laboratory methods. 21st ed. Philadelphia: Saunders Elsevier, 2006. [Retrieved from http://www.mdconsult.com (accessed September 14, 2008).]
17. Marlar RA, Fink LM, Miller JL. Laboratory approach to thrombotic risk. In: McPherson RA, Pincus MR, eds. Henry's clinical diagnosis and management by laboratory methods. 21st ed. Philadelphia: Saunders Elsevier, 2006. [Retrieved from http://www.mdconsult.com (accessed September 14, 2008).]

13

Hemapheresis

QUESTIONS

Question 1: During the process of apheresis, using centrifugation to separate blood components, which component is located the farthest from the axis of rotation?

A. Plasma.
B. Platelets.
C. Lymphocytes.
D. Red cells.
E. Granulocytes.

Question 2: Which of the following statements is *true* for intermittent flow centrifugation separators?

A. Blood is processed continuously, with individual layers being removed and retained or returned to the patient/donor.
B. They have a lower rate of citrate toxicity than continuous flow centrifugation separators.
C. All instruments that perform single-needle apheresis procedures are intermittent flow centrifugation separators.
D. Procedures performed on intermittent flow centrifugation separators tend to take longer than those using continuous flow centrifugation separators when processing the same amount of blood.

E. Most modern centrifugation separators are intermittent flow separators.

Question 3: In therapeutic plasma exchange, what percentage of a pathologic substance found only in the intravascular compartment would be present after a 1.5 plasma volume exchange?

A. 70%.
B. 30%.
C. 50%.
D. 25%.
E. 90%.

Question 4: The American Society for Apheresis (ASFA) classifies diseases/disorders treated by apheresis in order to assist in determining the appropriateness of treating a patient with this modality. Which of the following categories is defined as follows: "There is a suggestion of benefit for which existing evidence is insufficient, either to establish the efficacy of therapeutic apheresis or to clarify the risk/benefit (or sometimes cost/benefit) ratio associated with therapeutic apheresis. Included are disorders in which controlled trials have produced conflicting results or for which anecdotal reports are too few or too variable to support adequate consensus"?

A. Category I.
B. Category II.
C. Category III.
D. Category IV.
E. Category P.

Question 5: Which of the following statements about thrombocytapheresis (therapeutic plateletpheresis) is *true*?

A. Thrombocytapheresis should be performed when the patient's platelet count is 500×10^9/L.

B. Primary causes of thrombocytosis are more commonly associated with complications than secondary disorders.
C. Chemotherapeutic agents should be started only if thrombocytapheresis cannot control the thrombocytosis.
D. A 3-hour therapeutic platelet procedure would be expected to reduce the patient's platelet count by approximately 90%.
E. Thrombosis is the only indication for thrombocytapheresis in a patient with thrombocytosis.

Question 6: Which of the following statements concerning leukocytapheresis (therapeutic leukapheresis) is *true*?

A. It may be used instead of chemotherapy to treat all patients with chronic myelogenous leukemia (CML).
B. It can be used to prevent tumor lysis syndrome in patients with acute myelogenous leukemia (AML).
C. It is associated with improved long-term survival in patients with AML.
D. It is most often performed in the setting of acute lymphoblastic leukemia (ALL).
E. It results in reductions of the circulating white cell count between 20% and 30%.

Question 7: Which of the following statements about therapeutic erythrocytapheresis (red cell exchange) is *true*?

A. It is routinely used to treat uncomplicated malaria.
B. It is routinely used to treat uncomplicated babesiosis.
C. It has fewer long-term complications than surgery when used to treat priapism in sickle cell disease.
D. It is used instead of transfusion for the treatment of painful crises in sickle cell disease.
E. Transfusion is superior to erythrocytapheresis in the treatment of acute chest syndrome in sickle cell disease.

Question 8: Which of the following statements concerning the performance of erythrocytapheresis for complications of sickle cell disease is *true*?

A. The fraction of cells remaining (FCR) should be 70%.
B. Postprocedure hemoglobin S should be 30% or less.
C. It is unnecessary to screen the replacement red cells for hemoglobin S.
D. The final hematocrit target at the end of the procedure should be 45%.
E. The red cells should be phenotypically matched for all known red cell antigens.

Question 9: Which of the following statements about the pathophysiology of thrombotic thrombocytopenic purpura (TTP) is *true*?

A. A normal distribution of von Willebrand factor (vWF) multimers is present in the plasma during active disease
B. Episodes of disease are regularly associated with decreased levels of the largest vWF multimers.
C. The thrombi in the microvasculature consist of platelets, fibrin, and other activated coagulation factors.
D. Activity of ADAMTS13, a metalloproteinase that cleaves multimers of vWF, is deficient in many cases of TTP.
E. An autoantibody that decreases ADAMTS13 activity is present in all cases of congenital TTP (Upshaw-Schulman syndrome).

Question 10: Which of the statements concerning the use of therapeutic plasma exchange in the treatment of TTP is *true*?

A. The standard volume treated is 0.75 plasma volumes.
B. Plasma exchange is performed every other day for 7 treatments.
C. Plasma exchange is discontinued only when schistocytes are absent.

D. Tapering of plasma exchange has been shown to be superior to abrupt withdrawal when response criteria are reached.
E. The use of Plasma Cryoprecipitate Reduced (also called cryosupernatant plasma or cryopoor plasma) as the replacement solution appears to be superior to Fresh Frozen Plasma (FFP) in refractory patients.

Question 11: Therapeutic plasma exchange requires that a replacement fluid be used to replace the volume of plasma removed. For which of the following disorders is FFP indicated as a replacement fluid?

A. Myasthenia gravis.
B. Acute inflammatory demyelinating polyneuropathy.
C. TTP.
D. Refsum's syndrome.
E. All of the above.

Question 12: Myasthenia gravis (MG) is considered a Category I indication for therapeutic plasma exchange. Which of the following is *true* with regard to the characteristics of myasthenia gravis and its treatment?

A. The major cause of death is cardiac failure.
B. It is associated with other autoimmune phenomena and thymic abnormalities such as thymoma.
C. The disorder is caused by autoantibodies directed toward acetylcholine esterase.
D. Patients lacking detectable autoantibodies do not respond to plasma exchange.
E. Concurrent immunosuppressive therapy is not indicated and may interfere with the effect of plasma exchange.

Question 13: Acute inflammatory demyelinating polyneuropathy [Guillain-Barré syndrome (GBS)] is a Category I indication for plasma exchange. Which of the following statements concerning this disorder and its treatment are *true*?

A. Females are more frequently affected than males.
B. It is caused by autoantibodies toward calcium channels on the neuron terminal.
C. Intravenous immune globulin (IVIG) is less effective than plasma exchange.
D. Plasma exchange is associated with a greater likelihood of recovery of function.
E. Corticosteroids are an effective therapy.

Question 14: Chronic inflammatory demyelinating polyradiculopathy (CIDP) is a Category I indication for plasma exchange. Which of the following statements is *true* of CIDP and its treatment?

A. Plasma exchange is superior to the other treatment modalities of steroids and IVIG.
B. Results from inflammatory demyelination of the central nervous system.
C. Has a characteristic presentation and clinical course.
D. Response to plasma exchange lasts for 10 to 14 days.
E. A standard schedule of 7 consecutive daily plasma exchanges is indicated for all patients.

Question 15: Hyperviscosity syndrome may occur in patients with markedly elevated plasma protein levels. Which of the following statements is *true* of hyperviscosity syndrome and its treatment?

A. It more commonly occurs with multiple myeloma than with Waldenström's macroglobulinemia.
B. It is commonly seen with polyclonal increases in immunoglobulins.
C. The decision to institute plasma exchange should be based on serum viscosity levels.

D. Waldenström's macroglobulinemia resistant to chemotherapy therapy has been reported to be effectively treated with plasma exchange for extended periods of time.
E. Concurrent therapy with chemotherapeutic agents is not indicated when initiating plasma exchange for hyperviscosity.

Question 16: Anti-basement membrane antibody syndrome is characterized by pulmonary and renal hemorrhage. Which of the following statements is *true* of this disorder and its treatment?

A. The disorder usually presents with pulmonary hemorrhage only.
B. Plasma exchange should be implemented only after the failure of cytotoxic and immunosuppressive therapy.
C. Plasma exchange should be instituted only when the patient is dialysis dependent.
D. In a patient with no hope of renal recovery, plasma exchange is indicated if pulmonary hemorrhage occurs.
E. Plasma exchange for longer than 6 months after onset is common.

Question 17: Familial hypercholesterolemia (FH) is characterized by markedly elevated low-density lipoprotein (LDL) cholesterol levels and accelerated atherosclerosis. Which of the following statements concerning FH and its treatment is *true*?

A. Hypercholesterolemia unresponsive to medical management is a Category I indication for plasma exchange.
B. Selective removal of LDL cholesterol can be performed by LDL apheresis but offers no advantages over plasma exchange.
C. LDL apheresis is a first-line therapy for hypercholesterolemia.
D. Plasma exchange has been associated with improved survival of patients with hypercholesterolemia.
E. Plasma exchange has not been associated with the disappearance of xanthomas and regression of coronary artery lesions.

Question 18: A 30-year-old woman is donating platelets by apheresis. Near the end of the collection, the donor complains of light-headedness and nausea. The donor subsequently vomits. Following this, she relates that her hands feel funny. The most likely cause for her complaints is:

A. Hypotension caused by a vasovagal reaction.
B. Hypotension caused by hypovolemia as a result of a large extracorporeal volume.
C. Allergic reaction to ethylene oxide used to sterilize the disposable kit.
D. Presence of a low ionized calcium due to anticoagulation.
E. Presence of an underlying viral illness not detected during donor screening.

Question 19: Which of the following is a risk factor for developing citrate toxicity during an apheresis procedure?

A. Hypoventilation.
B. Acid-citrate-dextrose formula B (ACD-B) as the anticoagulant as compared to ACD-A.
C. Use of FFP as a replacement fluid.
D. Slow rate of infusion.
E. Use of a continuous flow centrifugation instrument.

Question 20: Which of the following would be appropriate therapy for the treatment of perioral paresthesias caused by citrate?

A. Ignore the symptoms because they are mild and occur commonly.
B. Discontinue the procedure and restart the procedure without any anticoagulant.
C. Give the donor or patient intravenous (IV) magnesium.
D. Increase the whole-blood-to-citrate ratio.
E. Increase the rate of reinfusion.

Question 21: A 45-year-old male with MG is undergoing a therapeutic plasma exchange procedure. Normal serum albumin is used as the replacement fluid. Approximately 5 minutes into the procedure, the patient experiences hypotension, shortness of breath, and flushing. Which of the following could be responsible for this reaction?

A. Ethylene oxide used to sterilize the disposable kit.
B. Angiotensin-converting enzyme (ACE) inhibitor taken the morning of the procedure.
C. Sodium caprylate used as a preservative in the albumin.
D. Albumin.
E. All of the above.

Question 22: An anxious first-time platelet donor experiences hypotension during an apheresis donation. The reaction occurs 2 minutes into the procedure. The donor's preprocedure vital signs and the vital signs at the time of the reaction are given in Table 13-22. The most likely explanation for the reaction, based on the information given, is:

Table 13-22.

	Blood Pressure (mm Hg)	Pulse (bpm)	Respiratory Rate (breath cycles per minute)	Temperature
Preprocedure	125/70	80	18	37 C
Reaction	80/50	50	20	37 C

A. Hypotension caused by hypovolemia.
B. Hypotension caused by a vasovagal reaction.
C. Hypotension caused by an allergic reaction to ethylene oxide.
D. Hypotension caused by an air embolus.
E. Hypotension caused by a citrate reaction.

Question 23: The appropriate treatment of the donor in Question 22 includes:

A. Reassuring the donor.
B. Giving the donor a bolus of saline.
C. Applying cold compresses to the donor's forehead and/or neck.
D. Placing the donor in the Trendelenburg position.
E. All of the above.

Question 24: For which of the following diseases is extracorporeal photopheresis a "standard and acceptable primary therapy based upon a broad non-controversial base of published experience"?

A. Erythrodermic cutaneous T-cell lymphoma.
B. Scleroderma.
C. Nephrogenic systemic fibrosis.
D. Pemphigus vulgaris.
E. Cutaneous graft-versus-host disease (GVHD).

Question 25: Which of the following statements about extracorporeal photopheresis is *true*?

A. The product collected and treated in the procedure is plasma.
B. The hematocrit of the product must be greater than 7%.
C. The photoactivation chamber exposes the product to ultraviolet B light.
D. 8-methoxypsoralen is the sensitizing agent used in the procedure.
E. The instrument used for the procedure is a continuous flow apheresis instrument.

Question 26: The infusion of citrate as an anticoagulant results in hypocalcemia. Which of the following electrolyte and acid/base abnormalities is also produced by citrate infusion?

A. Metabolic acidosis.
B. Hypokalemia.
C. Hypermagnesemia.
D. Hyponatremia.
E. All of the above.

ANSWERS

Question 1: D

Explanation:

- Centrifugal force separates the various components of blood according to their specific gravity (density). The densest components collect the farthest from the axis of rotation, while the least dense layer collects the closest.
- The order of the layers of separation from the axis of rotation outward is plasma, platelets, lymphocytes, granulocytes, and red cells.
- Red cells and granulocytes have an overlap in densities, resulting in poor separation. This is why granulocyte products contain large numbers of red cells. Greater separation can be achieved by the addition of hydroxyethyl starch. This aggregates the red cells, resulting in their having a greater density than the granulocytes.

Question 2: D

Explanation:

- In intermittent flow centrifugation separators, blood is pumped into the separation chamber. When it is filled, the chamber is spun in order to separate the various components into layers. The component of interest is removed and the centrifuge is stopped and the remainder of its contents is returned to the patient/donor. Blood is processed in batches.
- In continuous flow centrifugation separators, blood is pumped into a spinning separation chamber continuously, with the layers being removed and retained or returned to the patient/donor. As blood leaves the separation chamber, it is continuously replaced with fresh whole blood.
- In intermittent flow centrifugation separators, processing occurs in batches, with a large bolus of anticoagulated blood being returned to the patient/donor as opposed to a continuous infusion. Citrate toxicity occurs more frequently with intermittent instruments. In addi-

tion, the extracorporeal blood volume tends to be larger and a higher incidence of hypotensive reactions is seen.
- Because the separation chambers must fill and empty and there is not a continuous flow of blood from the patient, intermittent flow instruments tend to take longer than continuous flow instruments to process the same amount of blood.
- Continuous flow centrifugation separators can be used in single-needle procedures. In these, blood fills a reservoir that then feeds the separation chamber. The blood from the reservoir flows into the separation chamber, replacing blood being returned to the patient/donor. The machine does have to refill the reservoir but the separation chamber does not empty completely as in an intermittent instrument. Because of the presence of the reservoir and the resulting larger extracorporeal volume, when using a single-needle kit, there is the possibility of a greater frequency of hypotensive reactions. When a two-needle kit is used with a continuous flow instrument, the extracorporeal volumes are usually smaller than those seen in intermittent flow instruments.
- Most instruments currently used are continuous flow centrifuge separators.

Question 3: B

Explanation:

- The removal of substances located within the intravascular compartment is defined by the equation $Y/Y_0 = e^{-x}$ where Y = final concentration of the substance, Y_0 = the initial concentration of the substance, and x = the number of times a patient's plasma volume is exchanged. This equation shows that the relationship is an exponential, rather than linear, one (see Fig 13-3).
- As plasma is removed, it is replaced with a replacement fluid such as albumin. This further dilutes the amount of substance of interest that is left. In other words, with each plasma volume processed, a fixed percentage of the substance of interest remaining is removed. This results in "diminishing returns" on the "investment" of time and resources and is why most therapeutic plasma exchange procedures process only 1 to 1.5 plasma volumes.

Figure 13-3.

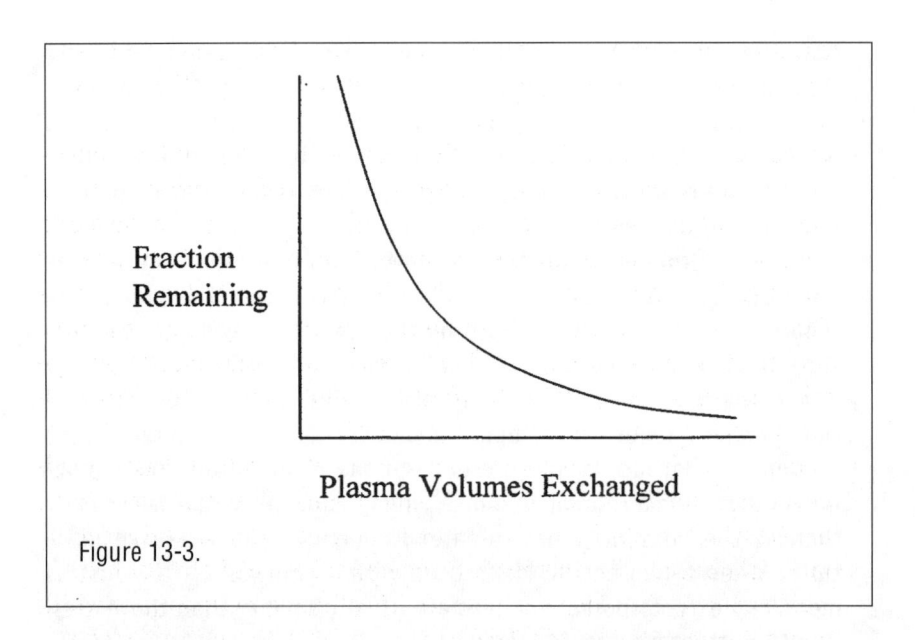

- It is important to remember that plasma exchange is nonselective. Both undesired (eg, LDL cholesterol, autoantibodies) and desirable solutes [eg, high-density lipoprotein (HDL) cholesterol, coagulation factors, normal antibodies, some drugs] are removed.

Question 4: C

Explanation:

- Unfortunately, most diseases treated by apheresis are "orphan diseases" that have a limited incidence. As a result, large, randomized, placebo, controlled trials are uncommon. This means that the available literature consists most often of cases, case series, and trials with historical controls. Because of the quality of the literature, the ASFA Clinical Application Committee reviews the medical literature on all diseases reported to be treated by apheresis every 3 years. The committee categorizes the disorders into one of five categories on the basis of the evidence in the literature.
- Category I: Therapeutic apheresis is standard and acceptable, either as a primary or a valuable first-line adjunct therapy. The perception of efficacy is usually based on well-designed randomized, controlled

trials or on a broad noncontroversial base of published experience [eg, thrombotic thrombocytopenic purpura (TTP), myasthenia gravis, anti-basement membrane syndrome].
- Category II: Therapeutic apheresis is generally accepted but considered to be supportive or adjunctive to other, more definitive treatments rather than a primary first-line therapy. Randomized, controlled trials are available for some, but for others the literature contains only case series or informative case reports (eg, Lambert-Eaton syndrome, acute central nervous system demyelination refractory to steroids, antineutrophil cytoplasmic antibody-associated rapidly progressive glomerulonephritis, conditioning for ABO or crossmatch-incompatible renal transplant).
- Category III: There is a suggestion of benefit for which existing evidence is insufficient, either to establish the efficacy of therapeutic apheresis or to clarify the risk/benefit (or sometimes cost/benefit) ratio associated with therapeutic apheresis. Included are disorders in which controlled trials have produced conflicting results or for which anecdotal reports are too few or too variable to support adequate consensus (eg, catastrophic antiphospholipid antibody syndrome, red cell aplasia, warm autoimmune hemolytic anemia, sepsis).
- Category IV: Controlled trials have not shown benefit, or anecdotal reports have been discouraging. Therapeutic apheresis should be discouraged and carried out only in the context of an institutional review board-approved clinical trial (eg, psoriasis, schizophrenia).
- Category P: Disease that can be treated by therapeutic apheresis using devices that are not available in the United States and/or do not have Food and Drug Administration (FDA) clearance. Generally, these devices are being studied in Phase III trials in the United States (eg, dilated cardiomyopathy, inflammatory bowel disease, age-related macular degeneration).
- It should be mentioned that third-party payers will usually reimburse for Category I and II disorders and will almost never reimburse for Category IV diseases. Category III disorders may or may not be reimbursed and may require communication between the apheresis physician and the appropriate physician for the payer. This is not a trivial concern, given the cost of providing these procedures and the potential adverse consequences to patients and their families caused by repeated, expensive therapeutic interventions.
- Not all disease have been categorized. Whether to treat a patient with an uncategorized disease is a decision to be made after reviewing the pertinent medical literature, discussing options with the

requesting physician, and discussing risks and benefits with the patient and the patient's family.

Question 5: B

Explanation:

- The initiation of thrombocytapheresis should be determined by the presence of symptoms in the patient. These symptoms may represent either thrombosis or bleeding, as the latter can also be seen with markedly elevated platelet counts. Although platelet counts of $\geq 1{,}500 \times 10^9/L$ are associated with complications, thrombosis or bleeding may occur at lower counts. The variability seen is caused by patient risk factors such as age and a previous history of thrombotic events. As a result, patient symptoms should be used to determine when to start or stop treatment.
- Although thrombocytapheresis will reduce the platelet count by approximately 45%, this effect will be temporary because more platelets will be produced. As a result, medical treatment, usually with chemotherapeutic agents such as hydroxyurea, should be implemented around the time of thrombocytapheresis. Thrombocytapheresis by itself will not be effective in controlling a patient's platelet count.
- Secondary causes of thrombocytosis include splenectomy, acute hemorrhage, iron deficiency, chronic inflammation, and rebound after myelosuppression. These accounted for only 18% of cases of thrombocytosis in one study (see Buss, 1994, in Winters, 2006). Complications in the setting of secondary thrombocytosis are uncommon, occurring in only 4% of these patients. Primary thrombocytosis includes essential thrombocytosis, agnogenic myeloid metaplasia, polycythemia vera, and chronic myelogenous leukemia (CML). These account for 82% of cases of thrombocytosis. Complications occur in 56% of these patients.

Question 6: B

Explanation:

- As with thrombocytapheresis, leukocytapheresis is indicated when patients become symptomatic from their high white cell counts. These symptoms usually result from hyperviscosity of blood caused by the elevated white cell counts or leukostasis with the leukemic blasts "clogging" the microvasculature. This takes the form of either neurologic symptoms (eg, transient ischemic attack, stroke, etc) or poor oxygenation associated with chest pain (pulmonary leukostasis). In addition, removal of large numbers of white cells before the start of chemotherapy can prevent disseminated intravascular coagulation (DIC) and renal damage from uric acid and phosphate that can result from the death of these cells when chemotherapy is begun (ie, tumor lysis syndrome).
- Prophylactic leukocytapheresis (ie, leukocytapheresis in the absence of symptoms) is indicated for counts >100 $\times 10^9$/L in AML and, due to the lower incidence of complications, ≥400 $\times 10^9$/L in ALL. At these counts, there is a greater frequency of complications, primarily central nervous system (CNS) infarction and hemorrhage. Leukocytapheresis is usually not indicated in CLL or chronic phase CML. The exception is in the setting of CML in pregnant women. Leukocytapheresis has been used to avoid chemotherapy in women with chronic phase CML until the child has been delivered.
- In studies of patients with AML, a white cell count >100 $\times 10^9$/L at presentation has been found to be associated with a greater frequency of CNS infarction and hemorrhage as well as pulmonary complications when compared with those with counts <50 $\times 10^9$/L. Three studies have demonstrated that the use of leukocytapheresis in those with white counts >100 $\times 10^9$/L is associated with improved 2- to 3-week mortality (see Porcu, 1997; Thiébaut, 2000; and Giles, 2001, in Winters, 2008, Chapter 2). Long-term survival is *not* improved, being determined by the prognostic factors of the AML and the patient.
- As with thrombocytapheresis, chemotherapy should begin around the time that apheresis is started in order to prevent further production of cells. Leukocytapheresis will result in a decrease in white cell count of 50% to 85%, but this will be temporary unless other therapies are initiated.

- Hyperviscosity syndrome, in the setting of leukemia, most commonly occurs in the setting of AML. This results from the larger size of the cells, greater complexity of their cytoplasm, and, most importantly, the expression of adhesion molecules on these cells, which results in adherence to endothelium. With ALL, this is not the case.

Question 7: C

Explanation:

- Eyrthrocytapheresis can be performed using either manual or automated methods. The automated method allows for better control of how much of the patient's own red cells are left at the end of the procedure, and, as a result, it is more effective.
- Erythrocytapheresis has been used to treat both babesiosis and malaria. In the case of *Babesia* infection, it is used to treat an erythrocyte parasitemia >10% in symptomatic disease or in an asplenic individual. The latter patient population is at great risk for rapid deterioration. It is not routinely used in uncomplicated cases of babesiosis. In malaria, it is most commonly used to treat infections with *Plasmodium falciparum*, as they are most frequently associated with symptomatic hyperparasitemia. It is indicated when the erythrocyte parasitemia is >10% or if the patient has severe malaria manifested by altered mental status, nonvolume overload pulmonary edema, or renal complications.
- Erythrocytapheresis is also used to treat threatened end-organ damage in sickle cell disease. In this setting, hemoglobin-S-containing red cells are removed and replaced with normal red cells, thereby improving blood flow and tissue oxygenation. It allows for the operator to determine the fraction of hemoglobin-S-containing cells to be left at the end of the procedure while maintaining a selected hematocrit. It has the benefit over simple transfusion in that it does not result in an increase in hematocrit with an accompanying increase in blood viscosity.
- Erythrocytapheresis is indicated in sickle cell disease for the treatment of acute chest syndrome, priapism, cerebrovascular accident, retinal artery vaso-occlusion, hepatic failure, and septic shock. The use of red cell exchange in preparation for surgery is somewhat controversial in that studies have shown no benefit over simple transfusion.

- Red cell exchange is not indicated for the routine treatment of painful crises. In these cases, therapy consists of hydration, oxygenation, and pain medications.
- Pharmacologic intervention, such as instillation of alpha-agonists, is used as first-line therapy. Surgery may be required for unresponsive cases. Erythrocytapheresis may be used in an attempt to avoid surgical intervention, which is associated with a high-frequency of erectile dysfunction.

Queistion 8: B

Explanation:

- The goal of erythrocytapheresis is to reduce the amount of hemoglobin-S-containing red cells below 30%.
- The FCR is the desired number of the patient's red cells remaining after the completion of the procedure. A procedure treating 1 red cell volume (RCV) will remove 70% of the patient's red cells, resulting in an FCR of 30%. If a patient with sickle cell anemia has not been transfused recently, the amount of hemoglobin S remaining would reach the 30% goal after the exchange of 1 RCV. If the patient has been transfused, the percentage of red cells containing hemoglobin S will be less than 100%, and as a result a smaller RCV will need to be exchanged. A hemoglobin electropheresis can be used to determine the starting hemoglobin S level and used to adjust the FCR accordingly.
- Because the goal is to reduce the hemoglobin S levels below 30%, it is necessary to use hemoglobin-S-negative red cells in performing the procedure. The replacement red cells should be screened for hemoglobin S.
- It is undesirable to increase the final hematocrit above 30% in sickle cell disease patients. Their endothelium is abnormally "sticky" and a "normal" hematocrit can result in increased viscosity and the potential for triggering sickling by producing hypoxia caused by poor perfusion.
- It would be impossible to match for all red cell antigens. It has been suggested that red cell units be matched for C, E, and K1 as well as ABO and D. Additionally, the products should be leukocyte reduced and, in order to maximize the time of survival, as fresh as possible.

Question 9: D

Explanation:

- The pathophysiology of TTP includes the following facets:
  - Abnormal vWF multimer patterns with unusually large forms (ie, >10,000,000 kD) are detected in the plasma of patients with chronic relapsing TTP during symptom-free intervals. These unusually large vWF multimers are considered potential important mediators of the platelet aggregation that underlies the clinical manifestations of this disease.
  - Unusually large vWF multimers are produced by human endothelial cells (in Weibel-Palade bodies) and platelets (in α-granules). These multimers are most effective in aggregating platelets under high shear stress situations and in vitro in response to ristocetin.
  - Somewhat paradoxically, episodes of disease are regularly associated with decreased levels of the unusually large forms. This is thought to be the result of their use in the formation of intravascular platelet aggregates.
  - The abnormal release of unusually large vWF multimers and/or their inability to undergo appropriate processing into smaller forms leads to abnormal platelet aggregation and endothelial adhesion in the microcirculation, with resulting thrombosis and microangiopathic hemolysis.
  - ADAMTS13 (A Disintegrin And Metalloprotease with Thrombospondin type I motifs 13), a metalloproteinase that cleaves multimers of vWF, is deficient in many cases of TTP. A genetic deficiency in enzyme production is the cause of the congenital Upshaw-Schulman syndrome.
  - It has been shown that in patients with idiopathic or sporadic TTP, an autoantibody is present that decreases ADAMTS13 activity by inhibiting the enzyme and/or resulting in its rapid clearance.
  - Platelet aggregates in TTP consist of platelets and vWF. They do not contain activated coagulation factors. In contrast to the thromboses of DIC, the intravascular thrombi formed during episodes of TTP stain strongly for vWF antigen, but only weakly for fibrinogen.

Question 10: E

Explanation:

- There is variability in the treatment of TTP.
- The standard therapeutic prescription according to ASFA is a 1- to 1.5-plasma-volume exchange daily until treatment goals are reached.
- The standard treatment goals as outlined by ASFA are a platelet count of $150 \times 10^9/L$, a lactate dehydrogenase near normal, and resolution of neurologic symptoms for 2 to 3 days.
- The presence of schistocytes on peripheral smear at the time of discontinuation of plasma exchange has been shown to not be associated with relapse. If the goals described above are reached, the presence of schistocytes does not warrant continued plasma exchange.
- Once treatment goals are reached, plasma exchange can be discontinued abruptly or weaned. There have been *no* trials comparing one form of discontinuation with the other and one cannot be said to be superior to the other.
- A study by the Canadian Apheresis Study Group suggested superiority of Plasma Cryoprecipitate Reduced (official component name; also called cryosupernatant plasma or cryopoor plasma), the waste product left-over from the manufacture of Cryoprecipitated AHF, compared to FFP in TTP patients who failed to respond to plasma exchange with FFP. Randomized trials comparing the use of FFP and Plasma Cryoprecipitate Reduced as replacement fluid at presentation in sporadic TTP patients who were not refractory demonstrated equivalency between the two replacement fluids (see Zeigler, 2001, and Rock, 2005, in Winters, 2008, Chapter 3).

Question 11: C

Explanation:

- FFP can transmit viral infections and is associated with a number of transfusion reactions, including allergic reactions (both simple and anaphylactic), febrile reactions, posttransfusion purpura, and trans-

fusion-related acute lung injury (TRALI). As a result, the use of FFP as a standard replacement fluid is limited to only a few diseases.
- Most procedures use a combination of albumin and/or saline as replacement fluids because of the greater safety of these products. Those disorders in which FFP is indicated are ones in which FFP serves to replace a factor missing in the patient's plasma. These disorders include the following:
  - TTP—replaces ADAMTS13.
  - Hemolytic uremic syndrome (HUS)—replaces ADAMTS13, which may also be involved in this disorder as well.
  - Factor XI deficiency—replaces Factor XI, for which a concentrate is currently not available.
- FFP may also be used to replace coagulation factors lost during the nonselective removal of plasma components in patients at risk for bleeding, such as those with recent biopsies or planned surgical procedures. In this setting, partial FFP replacement—for example, 4 units of FFP with the remaining replacement consisting of albumin—can be given at the end of the procedure. The timing of this is important. If the FFP is given at the beginning of the procedure, then the coagulation factors will be removed as part of the procedure itself. Some monitor fibrinogen levels in patients, providing FFP as part of the replacement if the levels fall below 150 mg/dL.
- Thawed plasma and 24-hour plasma can also be used as replacement fluid in TTP.
- Plasma Cryoprecipitate Reduced is that fraction of plasma remaining after the removal of cryoprecipitable proteins (ie, cryoprecipitate). This component contains approximately half of the fibrinogen, Factor VIII, and fibronectin found in FFP. It is depleted of the largest multimers of vWF. Additional facts regarding Plasma Cryoprecipitate Reduced:
  - Used to treat TTP, either initially or following a trial of FFP.
  - TTP is the only disease for which Plasma Cryoprecipitate Reduced is specifically used as a therapeutic modality.
  - Refractory TTP is the only FDA-approved indication for Plasma Cryoprecipitate Reduced.
  - Recent trials suggest the equivalence of FFP and Plasma Cryoprecipitate Reduced in the initial treatment of TTP.

Question 12: B

Explanation:

- MG is an autoimmune disorder caused by autoantibodies directed against the acetylcholine receptor on the motor endplate. These autoantibodies increase receptor turnover, block the binding of acetylcholine, and fix complement with degradation of the receptor.
- Clinically, MG is characterized by weakness of voluntary muscle groups. It may involve only the extraocular muscles or it may be generalized. Bulbar muscle weakness can lead to aspiration in the setting of a weakened diaphragm, resulting in severe respiratory compromise. This was the major cause of death in these patients in the past. MG can be seen in association with other autoimmune phenomena and is associated with thymic abnormalities, including thymoma.
- The treatment of MG is directed toward increasing the amount of acetylcholine at the motor endplate through the use of acetylcholine esterase inhibitors as well as decreasing the antibody production through immunosuppression. Intravenous immune globulin (IVIG) has also been used to treat MG and has been found to produce effects similar to plasma exchange.
- Plasma exchange is performed to lower the level of acetylcholine receptor antibody, although it has also been reported to be successful in the 10% to 15% of patients with symptoms of MG who do not have detectable antibody.
- Intensive courses of plasma exchange are recommended for those patients with MG who have severe disease (impaired respiratory function, swallowing, and locomotion) unresponsive to maximal pharmacologic therapy. It is also used to prepare patients for thymectomy or other surgical procedures. Patients with stable chronic disease, who experience mild exacerbation, can be treated with shorter, intermittent courses of plasma exchange.

Question 13: D

Explanation:

- GBS is the most frequently encountered paralytic disorder and affects males more frequently than females.
- GBS is an autoimmune disorder caused by antibody-mediated damage to peripheral nerve myelin followed by an inflammatory response. Complement-fixing antibodies to peripheral myelin have been identified in some patients.
- GBS is characterized initially by leg weakness, which progresses proximally to involve the arm, face, and oropharyngeal muscles. Sensory loss is minimal, but paresthesias may be present. Disease progression stops by the third week of the illness, and then improves after a variable period of stability.
- The titers of antibodies to peripheral nerve myelin correlate with the clinical course of disease as well as the response to plasma exchange and relapse following plasma exchange. Treatment of GBS consists of supportive care. IVIG is also beneficial in the treatment of GBS and, in randomized controlled trials, has been found to be as effective as plasma exchange. Corticosteroids have not proven to be effective and may actually interfere with the response to plasma exchange.
- Plasma exchange is associated with improvement in disability, greater likelihood of recovering function, and a shortened course. Patients requiring ventilatory support for several days before the initiation of plasma exchange are less likely to benefit from the procedure. However, ventilator-dependent patients have been found to have a shorter course of ventilator dependency when treated with plasma exchange. Plasma exchange should be initiated as early in the course of the disorder as possible.
- Lambert-Eaton myasthenic syndrome is the disorder characterized by antibodies directed against voltage-gated calcium channels on the neuron terminus.

Question 14: D

Explanation:

- CIDP is a chronic neurologic condition characterized by sensorimotor neuropathy with pain and weakness involving the upper and lower extremities. It has a variable course that may be progressive or relapsing and remitting.
- It is an inflammatory demyelinating neuropathy of peripheral nerves, possibly caused by autoantibodies.
- Treatment consists of steroids, IVIG, or plasma exchange. All of these treatments have been found to be equivalent, and the choice depends on costs, complications, availability, and patient response.
- Initial plasma exchange therapy consists of 2 to 3 plasma exchanges using albumin as the replacement fluid until response is achieved. After cessation of plasma exchange, the effect of the treatment lasts for 10 to 14 days, after which the patient may need further treatment with plasma exchange or one of the other modalities.
- Because patient response is variable and the duration of response is variable, the treatment plan needs to be individualized. Patients may require intermittent chronic plasma exchange to control symptoms.

Question 15: D

Explanation:

- Hyperviscosity syndrome results from the presence of large concentrations of paraprotein that increases blood viscosity by causing sludging of the red cells. It results in occlusion of the microcirculation with organ ischemia. Symptoms usually occur when the viscosity increases to 4 to 6 Ostwald units (normal blood viscosity is 1.5 to 1.8 Ostwald units), but patients may be asymptomatic at very high protein concentrations and viscosity levels (8 to 10 Ostwald units) or symptomatic at low levels (3 to 4 Ostwald units).
- Hyperviscosity syndrome is characterized by mental status changes, a bleeding diathesis, retinopathy, and hypervolemia with congestive heart failure. It occurs in less than 5% of multiple myeloma patients

but in as many as 70% of patients with Waldenström's macroglobulinemia. It is only rarely seen with polyclonal increases in immunoglobulin.
- The treatment of hyperviscosity syndrome is directed at decreasing paraprotein production with chemotherapy and improving blood flow by acutely decreasing paraprotein levels. This second goal can be achieved with plasma exchange.
- In hyperviscosity syndrome caused by an IgM monoclonal protein, 1 to 2 plasma exchanges may be sufficient to remove enough protein to improve viscosity, as IgM is located almost entirely within the intravascular space. With IgG or IgA paraproteins, the immunoglobulin is also present within the extravascular space, and more procedures may be necessary to decrease paraprotein levels. The primary goal of therapy should be relief of symptoms, with subsequent frequency tailored to the needs of the patient.
- In instances of Waldenström's macroglobulinemia resistant to therapy, repeated plasma exchange alone has been used to control hyperviscosity for extended periods, as long as 17 years.

Question 16: D

Explanation:

- Anti-basement membrane antibody disease is a rare disorder characterized by the combination of pulmonary hemorrhage and renal hemorrhage (nephritic syndrome). When both occur together, it is referred to as Goodpasture syndrome or anti-basement antibody syndrome. It more commonly affects men and is most frequent between 18 and 35 years of age.
- This disorder is autoimmune, caused by a transient autoantibody directed against the 3 chain of type IV collagen found in glomerular and pulmonary basement membranes. The autoantibody appears to be triggered by damage to the respiratory system. Anti-basement membrane antibody syndrome frequently presents with pulmonary symptoms of cough, hemoptysis, and dyspnea with laboratory evidence of renal failure and renal inflammation. The mortality rate may be as high as 50%.

THERAPEUTIC HEMAPHERESIS   495

- Treatment is focused on suppressing antibody production and inflammation with immunosuppressive and cytotoxic agents as well as removing the antibody with plasma exchange.
- Plasma exchange is usually performed daily with concurrent immunosuppression. Because the antibody is transient, treatment longer than 6 months is uncommon.
- Plasma exchange should be initiated early in the course of therapy for this disorder, as recovery of renal function is unlikely once scarring and atrophy of glomeruli and tubules occur. In patients with severe renal disease (defined by oliguria, dialysis dependency, or a serum creatinine >6.8 mg/dL), plasma exchange should be reserved for concomitant pulmonary hemorrhage because the recovery of renal function is unlikely.

Question 17: D

Explanation:

- FH, or hyperlipoproteinemia type II, is an autosomal dominant disorder characterized by abnormalities in the LDL receptor within the liver. This results in the inability to remove LDL cholesterol and lipoprotein a [Lp(a)]. The presence of these lipoproteins leads to accelerated atherosclerosis and tissue deposition of cholesterol in the form of xanthomas. Individuals homozygous for the gene have cholesterol levels of 650 to 1000 mg/dL and have xanthomas within the first 4 years of life. Death from coronary artery disease usually occurs by age 20. Heterozygotes have cholesterol levels of 350 to 550 mg/dL with xanthomas by age 20 and atherosclerosis by age 30. Heterozygotes for FH are common, occurring at a frequency of 1 in 500, whereas homozygotes are rare, with a frequency of 1 in 1,000,000.
- The primary treatment for FH is medical management. The combination of 3-hydroxy-3-methylglutaryl-coenzyme A reductase inhibitors, bile acid binding resins, nicotinic acid, and dietary modification can result in significant reductions of cholesterol in heterozygotes. Unfortunately, all homozygotes and some heterozygotes are unresponsive to such therapies. In these cases, surgical approaches are considered (eg, distal ileal bypass, portacaval shunts, liver transplantation).

- Plasma exchange has been used to treat FH in homozygotes as well as heterozygotes unresponsive to drug therapy. Comparison of the life expectancy of patients treated with this therapy and their untreated siblings as well as series and case reports of treated patients have been described. Significant reductions in cholesterol, disappearance of xanthomas, disappearance of electrocardiogram abnormalities, regression of coronary artery lesions, improvement in exercise tolerance, and prolongation of life span have been reported.
- A number of selective removal systems have been developed that remove LDL and Lp(a) predominantly while leaving most of the HDL, immunoglobulins, and other plasma proteins behind. Comparisons of these systems with plasma exchange have shown superior reductions in LDL cholesterol (70% vs 50% reduction), Lp(a), and fibrinogen but significantly less removal of HDL and immunoglobulins. Also, LDL apheresis does *not* expose the patient to albumin or other replacement fluids. Published studies of these systems have demonstrated clinical effects such as regression of atherosclerotic coronary artery lesions and prevention of progression. Because of the selective nature of these systems, they are considered superior to plasma exchange. LDL apheresis using these systems is considered a Category I indication, whereas the use of plasma exchange is considered a Category II indication. Plasma exchange is used predominantly at institutions where the more specialized LDL apheresis equipment is not available or to treat pediatric patients because of the extremely large extracorporeal volume of these instruments.
- Criteria for the initiation of apheresis treatments for hypercholesterolemia have been published. One criterion reflects the understanding that heterozygous patients should be treated with maximally tolerated drug therapy before apheresis procedures are considered. Because of the relatively slow production of cholesterol, patients are treated every other week.

Question 18: D

Explanation:

- Citrate is used as the primary anticoagulant in both donor and therapeutic apheresis procedures because it effectively prevents coagulation and is short acting and easily reversible, unlike heparin. Citrate

chelates calcium ions, producing a soluble complex, making them unavailable for biologic reactions (eg, coagulation).
- Within the apheresis instrument, plasma citrate concentrations reach 15 to 24 mmol/L, lowering the calcium ion concentration below 0.2 to 0.3 mmol/L, the level necessary for coagulation. This level of anticoagulation requires the infusion of approximately 500 mL of acid-citrate-dextrose formula A (ACD-A) solution. It would be expected that the infusion of this volume of solution into the donor or patient would result in a calcium ion concentration of 0.2 mmol/L, a level incompatible with life. This does not occur, however.
- Upon return of the blood from the apheresis instrument to the donor or patient, the citrate is diluted throughout the total extracellular fluid. In addition, the liver, kidneys, and muscles rapidly metabolize citrate, releasing the bound calcium. Finally, the body also responds to the decrease in ionized calcium by increasing parathyroid hormone levels with a mobilization of calcium from skeletal stores as well as increased absorption by the kidneys.
- In therapeutic plasma exchange procedures using either FFP or Plasma Cryoprecipitate Reduced as replacement fluids, an additional source of citrate is infused in the form of the anticoagulant present in these solutions. Again, the effects of this citrate load are minimized as described above.
- Despite compensatory mechanisms, citrate infusion can result in a decrease in ionized calcium levels to a point where symptoms develop in the patient. These result from a decrease in ionized calcium to levels where the excitability of nerve membranes increases until spontaneous depolarization can occur.
- The signs and symptoms of citrate toxicity include circumoral paresthesias, acral paresthesias, shivering, light-headedness, twitching, and tremors. In addition, some patients experience nausea and vomiting. As the ionized calcium levels fall further, these symptoms may progress to carpopedal spasm, tetany, and seizure.
- It is important to elicit the presence of the early symptoms of citrate toxicity from the patient so that interventions can occur before the more severe symptoms. In addition to the symptoms described above, prolongation of the QT interval on electrocardiograms as well as depressed myocardial contractility have been seen, and fatal arrhythmias have been reported.

Question 19: C

Explanation:

- Factors that have been found to influence the rate of citrate reactions in donor and therapeutic apheresis include the following:
  - Alkalosis caused by hyperventilation (decreases ionized calcium).
  - The type of anticoagulant solution used, with ACD-A having more reactions than ACD-B (half the concentration of citrate compared to ACD-A solution).
  - Rapid rate of infusion of the anticoagulant solution.
  - The amount of citrate infused, including the infusion of replacement fluids, such as FFP, which contain citrate.
  - Low serum albumin (less albumin-bound calcium to buffer the fall).
  - Hypomagnesemia (inhibits parathyroid hormone release and action).
- Intermittent flow hemapheresis procedures tend to have a greater frequency of citrate reactions because there is a higher rate of citrate infusion when the separation chamber is emptied, as compared with continuous apheresis procedures.

Question 20: D

Explanation:

- Hypocalcemia caused by citrate toxicity is characterized by perioral and acral paresthesias, shivering, lightheadedness, twitching, tremors, nausea, and hypotension. If not treated, these can progress to carpopedal spasm, tetany, and seizure activity. Mild symptoms should not be ignored because they may progress to severe symptoms.
- The treatment of citrate reactions includes slowing the reinfusion rate to allow for dilution of citrate and metabolism of the calcium-citrate complex, increasing the blood-to-citrate ratio to decrease the amount of citrate infused; giving oral calcium in the form of calcium antacids; and giving intravenous calcium gluconate or calcium chloride.

- Calcium gluconate or chloride infusions are usually not necessary in donor procedures but may be required with therapeutic procedures and hematopoietic progenitor cell collections. This is especially true when plasma products (anticoagulated with citrate) are used as replacement fluids or when lengthy procedures are instituted.
- Citrate can cause hypomagnesemia because it will bind magnesium, a divalent cation. Hypomagnesemia is less common than hypocalcemia. It can present as hypocalcemic symptoms that fail to respond to calcium infusion and should be considered in this clinical situation.
- Studies have demonstrated limitations in the use of oral calcium supplementation. While increasing ionized calcium levels and reducing severity of paresthesias, it did not prevent symptom development. Administration of intravenous solutions before the procedure or at the time of symptoms has been found in some studies not to be effective. Finally, studies have suggested that continuous infusions result in fewer reactions and higher ionized calcium levels.
- In most cases, anticoagulation is required to perform an apheresis procedure. Attempts to perform procedures without citrate or heparin anticoagulation will result in thrombosis of the extracorporeal circuit.

Question 21: E

Explanation:

- Allergic, anaphylactoid, and anaphylactic reactions can occur in both donors and patients undergoing apheresis procedures. Causes of allergic reactions include the following:
  - Antibodies generated toward ethylene oxide used to sterilize disposable kits. This occurs after repeated procedures or donations where ethylene oxide in the kit binds to plasma proteins, inducing an immune response. Some studies of platelet donors have reported an incidence of 1%.
  - Antibodies have been found against sodium caprylate used as a preservative in albumin. In addition, aggregates in albumin preparations can trigger allergic-like reactions. Finally, the processing of the albumin may modify the molecule such that it appears foreign and is capable of eliciting an immune response.

- Hydroxyethyl starch, used as a colloidal replacement fluid or to enhance separation of red cells from white cells, can activate complement and produce allergic-like phenomena.
- In IgA-deficient individuals, antibodies to IgA can cause allergic reactions, ranging from hives to anaphylaxis. These reactions are most commonly seen in procedures using plasma products as replacement fluids, but IgA may be present in normal serum albumin as well.
- ACE inhibitors inactivate kinase I and II. These enzymes normally inactivate bradykinin. During plasma exchange, prekallikrein-activating factor present in the albumin preparation can result in the production of bradykinin. In selective removal systems, such as LDL apheresis, the negatively charged columns can also cause bradykinin generation. Bradykinin is normally rapidly inactivated upon reinfusion of the blood. Individuals taking ACE inhibitors cannot do this, however, and may experience flushing, hypotension, bradycardia, and dyspnea. Patients or donors should discontinue ACE inhibitors a minimum of 24 to 48 hours before apheresis procedures. Longer lengths of time may be required for ACE inhibitors with longer half-lives.

Question 22: B

Explanation:

- Allergic, anaphylactoid, and anaphylactic reactions are associated with hypotension.
- An air embolus can cause hypotension. In this reaction, air enters the venous system through a leak in the extracorporeal circuit. If a large enough quantity enters, it can obstruct right ventricular output by causing pulmonary artery vasospasm and by obstructing the outflow tract. Dyspnea, tachypnea, tachycardia, cyanosis, and hypotension may result. Air embolism is extremely rare because all modern apheresis instruments have sensors that will stop the instrument if air is detected within the circuit.
- More common causes of hypotension are hypovolemia and vasovagal reactions. In the first, hypotension results from intravascular volume depletion as a result of the volume of blood present within the extracorporeal circuit. Such reactions are characterized by both increased vascular tone and an increased cardiac output as the sympathetic nervous system attempts to compensate for the hypovolemia.

Increases in both heart rate and contractility produce the increase in cardiac output.
- Hypotensive reactions caused by hypovolemia are not common among hemapheresis donors because the volume of the extracorporeal circuit is limited to 10.5 mL/kg (see AABB *Standards for Blood Banks and Transfusion Services*, Reference Standard 5.4.1A). In addition, donors must fulfill stringent health and weight requirements. In therapeutic procedures, the patient has an underlying disease that may make hypovolemia more likely. For example, the presence of hypotension is more common in patients with neurologic diseases.
- Vasovagal reactions are also characterized by hypotension and may occur during apheresis procedures. In these reactions, hypovolemia results in a decrease in blood pressure. As stated above, the normal compensatory response is to increase cardiac output and vascular tone. In contrast, during a vasovagal reaction, parasympathetic output increases, resulting in a slowing of the heart rate and decreased vascular tone. This results in an exacerbation and prolongation of the hypotensive state. Factors associated with vasovagal reactions in whole blood donors include a younger age, a lower weight, first-time donation, and an inattentive staff.

Question 23: E

Explanation:

- Hypovolemic and vasovagal reactions are treated in a similar manner. The procedure should be temporarily interrupted, and a fluid bolus should be infused. If the reaction is caused by hypovolemia, the blood pressure should increase and the pulse rate should decrease in response to this intervention. If the reaction is caused by a vasovagal reaction, this may not occur.
- Additional treatments for vasovagal reactions include placing the person in the Trendelenburg position (head down), applying cold compresses to the forehead and neck, and providing reassurance.

Question 24: A

Explanation:

- The following description defines Category I indications for apheresis: ". . . standard and acceptable, either as a primary or a valuable first-line adjunct therapy. The perception of efficacy is usually based on well-designed randomized controlled trials or on a broad non-controversial base of published experience."
- Erythrodermic cutaneous T-cell lymphoma (also called mycosis fungoides) is a Category I indication for extracorporeal photoperesis (commonly referred to as photopheresis). This disorder is a skin-based T-cell lymphoma characterized by a long premalignant phase of eczematous skin rash. Following this, it can progress to a tumor phase, characterized by cutaneous masses, and a leukemic phase called Sezary's syndrome. Treatment of the cutaneous erythrodermic phase with photopheresis is associated with longer survival in patients with this disorder than chemotherapy (60 months vs 31 months). Treatment of later stages of the disease (eg, tumor phase) is not associated with response and is considered a Category IV indication.
- Scleroderma, progressive systemic sclerosis, is an autoimmune condition characterized by an accumulation of collagen in the skin and other organs. It is a Category IV indication for photopheresis because three randomized trials have failed to show statistically significant improvement in skin and joint involvement compared with standard therapy.
- Nephrogenic systemic fibrosis is a recently identified disorder thought to represent an inflammatory response to gadolinium contrast agent in patients with chronic renal failure. It is characterized by progressive fibrosis of subcutaneous tissues as well as organ involvement. Case series have reported some benefit but it is currently *not* categorized.
- Pemphigus vulgaris is an autoimmune blistering skin disease that can be potentially fatal. It is a Category III indication because of limited supporting evidence.
- Cutaneous GVHD is a Category II indication for photopheresis. Between 60% and 80% of patients with steroid refractory chronic GVHD will respond to photopheresis.

- Another Category I indication for photopheresis is the prevention of heart transplant rejection. Randomized, controlled multicenter trials have demonstrated a decreased frequency of rejection, a reduction in the frequency of HLA antibodies, and reduced coronary artery wall thickness in those prophylactically treated with photopheresis.

Question 25: D

Explanation:

- In extracorporeal photopheresis, a buffy coat consisting of mononuclear cells suspended in plasma is generated using an intermittent flow centrifugation device [UVAR XTS (Therakos, Exton, PA)]. A photoactivation compound, 8-methoxypsoralen (8-MOP) is added to this and incubated. The buffy coat is then passed through a photoactivation chamber where it is exposed to ultraviolet A (UVA) light. After treatment, the buffy coat is reinfused into the patient.
- The buffy coat must have a hematocrit <7% as the red cells will block the UVA light. Also, too much plasma can be collected, which can dilute the white cells and result in insufficient exposure to the UVA light.
- The mechanism of photopheresis has not been completely elucidated. It is thought to modulate the immune system by resulting in the generation of antigen-loaded dendritic cells, which, when reinfused, home to lymph nodes and induce a T-cell response.

Question 26: B

Explanation:

- Citrate is metabolized through the Kreb's cycle, resulting in the generation of bicarbonate. The result is that most donors and patients will experience a slight metabolic alkalosis. It usually produces no symptoms and resolves with time. In patients with severe renal dysfunction (eg, systemic lupus erythematosus patients with renal involvement) or who receive large citrate loads (eg, TTP patients receiving FFP as replacement fluid), significant metabolic alkalosis

can occur. This can result in respiratory depression and further electrolyte abnormalities, and dialysis may be necessary.
- Because of the metabolic alkalosis, hypokalemia occurs. As intracellular protons buffer the bicarbonate, potassium enters the cells to maintain electrical neutrality. Significant reductions in potassium blood levels with the development of symptoms can occur, especially in patients who were hypokalemic before administration of citrate.
- As a divalent cation, magnesium is chelated by citrate. Hypomagnesemia is caused by citrate anticoagulant.
- Apheresis procedures have limited to no effects on sodium levels. Hyponatremia is not caused by citrate anticoagulant.

REFERENCES

1. Winters JL, Pineda AA. Hemapheresis. In: McPherson RA, Pincus MR, eds. Henry's clinical diagnosis and management by laboratory methods. 21st ed. Philadelphia: Saunders Elsevier, 2006:685-715.
2. Szczepiokkowski ZM, Bandarenko N, Kim HC, et al. Guidelines on the use of therapeutic apheresis in clinical practice—Evidence-based approach from the Clinical Applications Committee of the American Society for Apheresis. J Clin Apher 2007;22:106-75.
3. Winters JL, Gottschall J, eds. Therapeutic apheresis: A physician's handbook. 2nd ed. Bethesda, MD: AABB, 2008.
4. Szczepiokkowski ZM, Shaz BH, Bandarenko N, Winters JL. The new approach to assignment of ASFA categories—Introduction to the fourth special issue: Clinical applications of therapeutic apheresis. J Clin Apher 2007;22:96-105.

14

The HLA System

QUESTIONS

Question 1: The most highly polymorphic antigen system in humans is:

A. MNSs.
B. Rh.
C. ABO.
D. HLA.
E. HTLA.

Question 2: HLA antigens are glycoprotein molecules found on cell surface membranes; they are products of genes located on:

A. The short arm of chromosome 1.
B. The short arm of chromosome 6.
C. The long arm of chromosome 1.
D. The long arm of chromosome 6.
E. The long arm of chromosome 19.

Question 3: Class II HLA antigens are *not* expressed in:

A. Spermatozoa.
B. Resting T lymphocytes.

C. Macrophages.
D. B lymphocytes.
E. Langerhan cells of the skin.

Question 4: Which of the following donors would most likely be the best source of HLA-identical hematopoietic progenitor cells (HPCs) for a recipient requiring transplantation?

A. Mother.
B. Father.
C. Siblings.
D. Cousins.
E. Aunts or uncles.

Question 5: A family has been HLA-typed because one of the children needs an HPC transplant. Typing results are as follows:

Father: A1,A3;B8,B35
Mother: A2,A23;B12,B18
Child #1:   A1,A2;B8,B12
Child #2:   A1,A23;B8,B18
Child #3:   A3,A23;B18,BY
Antigen Y in child #3 is:

A. B1.
B. B8.
C. B12.
D. B18.
E. B35.

Question 6: A patient (sibling 1) from a family with eight siblings requires HPC transplantation. Table 14-6 identifies the HLA typings of the patient and the seven siblings. The parents are deceased.

Table 14-6.

Siblings	HLA Type
1, 3, 7	A1,AX;B35,B70
2, 5	A1,A2;B45,B70
6	A1,AX;B35,B58
4, 8	A1,A2;B45,B58

The unidentified antigen X is:

A. 1.
B. 2.
C. 35.
D. 45.
E. 70.

Question 7: As shown below, the identification of the missing antigens (-) is required to determine if there is an HLA-identical sibling who could serve as an HPC donor for the recipient. The parents are deceased. The phenotypes of the recipient and five siblings are as follows:

Recipient: A2,A3;B35,-
Sibling #1:   A2,A11;B7,B35
Sibling #2:   A3,A11;B35,B44
Sibling #3:   A2,A3;B35,-
Sibling #4:   A11,-;B7,B44
Sibling #5:   A2,A11;B7,B35

The missing antigen in the recipient and in sibling #3 at the X locus is:

A. The same.
B. Different.
C. 7.
D. 11.
E. 44.

Question 8: A diabetic patient in a family of six siblings requires a combined renal and islet cell transplant for end-stage renal disease. Table 14-8A shows the ABO and HLA typings of the family.

Table 14-8A.

Family Member	ABO	HLA			
Father	A	A4	A28	B22	B35
Mother	B	A8	A11	B7	B44
Patient	B	A4	A11	B7	B35
Sibling 1	AB	A4	A11	B7	B35
Sibling 2	B	A4	A8	B22	B44
Sibling 3	B	A4	A11	B7	B35
Sibling 4	A	A11	A28	B7	B22
Sibling 5	O	A4	A11	B7	B35

The patient's genotype is:

A. A4,B35;A11,B7.
B. A4,B35;A11,B7.
C. A8,B7;A28,B22.
D. A11,B7;A22,B22.
E. A4,B44;A11,B35.

Question 9: The genotype of sibling #2 in Question 8 is the result of:

A. Crossover and recombination of the mother's chromosomes.
B. Crossover and recombination of the father's chromosomes.
C. Translocation of the mother's chromosomes.
D. Translocation of the father's chromosomes.
E. A random segregation event.

Question 10: Based on the information provided in Question 8, the best possible kidney and islet cell donor for the patient is:

A. Sibling #1.
B. Sibling #2.
C. Sibling #3.
D. Sibling #4.
E. Sibling #5.

Question 11: Based on the information provided in Question 8, the best possible HPC donor for the patient would be:

A. Sibling #1.
B. Sibling #2.
C. Sibling #3.
D. Sibling #4.
E. Sibling #5.

Question 12: The least important test for matching a kidney donor with a recipient is:

A. ABO typing.
B. Rh typing.
C. Serologic typing for Class I antigens.
D. Molecular typing for Class II antigens.
E. HLA crossmatching.

Question 13: Solid organ rejection in transplantation can be caused by which of the following?

A. T-cell inactivation.
B. Adequate treatment with cyclosporine.
C. Pretransplantation transfusions.

D. Compatibility of non-HLA, minor histocompatibility genes.
E. HLA crossmatch testing by flow cytometry.

Question 14: An HLA antibody screen was performed via microlymphocytotoxicity testing. The panel reactive antibody (PRA) was 95%. The patient underwent HLA typing. An apheresis product from a donor who is an A match was transfused. The patient had a poor 10-minute post-transfusion platelet count increment. Which of the following is the best explanation for this finding?

A. The platelets were incompatible at the *HLA-DR* locus.
B. The patient had an antibody toward HPA-1a (Pl^{A1}).
C. The platelets were ABO-compatible.
D. The patient was afebrile.
E. The patient was bleeding.

Question 15: A 28-year-old woman received chemotherapy for acute myelocytic leukemia diagnosed 4 weeks ago. She is afebrile and has no lymphadenopathy or hepatosplenomegaly. Her platelet count is 8000/µL. She is group AB, D negative. She has received multiple platelet and red cell transfusions since her diagnosis. Anti-D has been found in her serum by the blood bank. One hour after transfusion of 8 units of pooled platelet concentrates, her platelet count is 12,000/µL. The next day, her platelet count is 8500/µL. Transfusion of 8 units of pooled platelet concentrates produces a 1-hour posttransfusion count of 8600/µL. These findings indicate that the patient most likely needs to receive:

A. D-negative platelets of any ABO type.
B. Group AB, D-negative platelets.
C. An adequate dose of platelets.
D. HLA-matched platelets.
E. Group AB, D-positive platelets.

Question 16: A 58-year-old man with hairy cell leukemia has received a transfusion of pooled platelet concentrates (6 units) for the first time.

This produced an increase in his platelet count from 20,000/μL to 25,000/μL on a blood sample drawn 5 hours after completion of the transfusion. You should:

A. Suspect HLA alloimmunization and recommend switching to HLA-matched platelets.
B. Suspect hypersplenism and advise emergency splenectomy.
C. Suspect HLA alloimmunization and recommend treatment with intravenous gamma globulin.
D. Suspect HLA alloimmunization and recommend leukocyte-reduced platelets.
E. Suspect hypersplenism and recommend giving a second transfusion of 6 units followed by a 1-hour posttransfusion platelet count.

Question 17: Which of the following statements regarding antibodies directed against HLA antigens is correct?

A. They are naturally occurring.
B. Their titers are reduced by transfusion.
C. They are an important cause of hemolytic transfusion reactions.
D. They are important in the pathogenesis of hemolytic disease of the fetus and newborn (HDFN).
E. Multiparous women may have high-titer HLA antibodies.

Question 18: HLA antibodies are associated with which of the following clinical conditions?

A. Acute hemolytic transfusion reactions.
B. Delayed hemolytic transfusion reactions.
C. Anaphylactic transfusion reactions.
D. HDFN.
E. Transfusion-related acute lung injury (TRALI).

Question 19: Which of the following statements is *true* regarding Bg (Bennett-Goodspeed) antigens?

A. Standard lymphocytotoxicity tests detect anti-Bg.
B. Anti-Bg^c is directed against HLA-A7.
C. Anti-Bg causes hemolytic transfusion reactions.
D. Reagent red cells expressing Bg antigens are required in pretransfusion antibody detection tests.
E. Anti-Bg can be present in multiparous women and multitransfused patients.

Question 20: The observed frequency of two genes occurring together more than expected by chance alone is the definition of:

A. Linkage disequilibrium.
B. Genetic anticipation.
C. Genetic imprinting.
D. The Hardy-Weinberg principle.
E. Lyonization.

Question 21: The HLA type of a patient suffering from immune-mediated platelet refractoriness caused by HLA antibodies is A1,A23;B7,B27. Which of the following donors is a B2U HLA match?

A. A11,A19;B7,B8.
B. A1,A23;B7,B27.
C. A1,-;B7,-.
D. A3,-;B7,B27.
E. A1,A10;B7,-.

Question 22: Which of the following statements concerning cross-reactive groups (CREGs) is *true*?

A. Class I molecules in a CREG share one or more determinants that are also shared by molecules in another CREG.
B. CREGs were identified initially by finding alloantisera that bind to one HLA allele alone.
C. A CREG specificity can result from shared amino acid sequences between HLA antigens.
D. CREG groups are highly standardized.
E. An epitope shared among members of a CREG is called a private antigen.

Question 23: Which of the following HLA disease association pairs is correct?

A. Ankylosing spondylitis—B7.
B. Celiac disease—DQ2.
C. Narcolepsy—DR5.
D. Subacute thyroiditis—B27.
E. Rheumatoid arthritis—DR3.

Question 24: Which of the following statements is *true* regarding the HLA allele designated by *A*0201*?

A. It is an allele of the *HLA-B* locus.
B. The first two digits represent the serologic specificity.
C. The third and fourth digits represent the designation of an allele with a similar amino acid sequence.
D. It bears the serologic specificity of A3.
E. The first two digits refer to the order in which the allele was described.

Question 25: Which of the following statements is *true* regarding soluble HLA Class I and Class II antigens?

A. Levels fall with infection and inflammatory disease.
B. Levels rise as malignancies progress.

C. Levels in blood components are proportionate to the number of residual donor leukocytes.
D. Levels in blood components fall throughout the length of storage.
E. Soluble HLA in blood components enhances the immune responsiveness of recipients.

ANSWERS

Question 1: D

Explanation:

- The HLA genes are the most polymorphic loci in humans.
- The extreme polymorphism of the HLA system results from the existence of multiple alleles at several loci.
- It is estimated that more than 100 million different phenotypes can result from all of the combinations of alleles found in the HLA system.
- The HLA genes and their antigen products are the primary contributors to the recognition of self and non-self, the immune responses to antigenic stimuli, and the coordination of cellular and humoral immunity.

Question 2: B

Explanation:

- Band 21.3 on chromosome 6p (petit = short) is the location of the α chain gene of HLA Class I molecules.
- Nonpolymorphic genes encoding the β chain of HLA Class I molecules are located on chromosome 15. The gene product is β_2-microglobulin and is required for the stability of Class I molecules. The two noncovalently linked polypeptides that form the Class I HLA antigens are produced independently and are associated, posttranslationally, to produce the final Class I HLA molecule.
- Band 21.1 on chromosome 6p is the location of the α and β chain genes of HLA Class II molecules.
- The *Rh* genes are located on chromosome 1p. The *RHD* gene determines D antigen expression, and the *RHCE* gene determines C, c, E, and e antigen expression.
- The closely linked *H*, *Le*, and *Se* genes are located on chromosome 19.

Question 3: B

Explanation:

- Class II antigens are present on B lymphocytes, monocytes, macrophages, dendritic cells, intestinal epithelium, early hematopoietic cells, epithelial cells, spermatozoa, and *activated* T lymphocytes. The antigens are not present on resting T lymphocytes.
- Class II antigens are expressed nonconstitutively on resting T lymphocytes but can be induced in conjunction with an immune response by lymphokines such as IL-2, interferon-γ, IL-4, TNF-β, and prostaglandins.
- Class II HLA antigens may also be induced by cytokines on other cell types, including renal epithelial cells and pancreatic β cells. This represents a possible mechanism for autoimmunization and graft rejection.
- Class I HLA antigens are expressed on the surface of platelets and most nucleated cells in the body including lymphocytes, monocytes, granulocytes, and constituents of solid tissues. Nucleated immature red cells express Class I molecules, but mature red cells usually lack Class I HLA antigens when conventional typing methods are used.

Question 4: C

Explanation:

- In the HLA system, individuals inherit one HLA haplotype from each parent.
- 25% of siblings have two identical haplotypes.
- 50% of siblings have one identical haplotype.
- 25% of siblings have no identical haplotypes.
- Parents and their children share one identical haplotype.
- Cousins, aunts, and uncles may or may not share one identical haplotype.
- A patient (transplant recipient) with "n" siblings has a $1-(3/4)^n$ chance of having one HLA- identical sibling. However, the chance of having one HLA-identical sibling is never 100%, no matter how many siblings are available for typing. The exception to this rule is identical twins which, by their genetic nature, are HLA-identical.

Question 5: E

Explanation:

- The HLA gene region on chromosome 6 is composed of a set of closely linked loci of three classes. The antigens are expressed codominantly and are inherited en bloc from each parent as a unit called a haplotype. In parentage testing, the Class I HLA antigens (HLA-A, -B, and -C) are defined serologically for each family member.
- A person's genotype can be deduced by phenotyping the family unit. A missing or unidentified antigen can also be determined by genotypic determination of the family unit.
- The phenotypes and possible genotypes of the family in this question are listed in Table 14-5A.

Table 14-5A.

	Phenotype	Possible Genotypes
Father	A1,A3;B8,B35	*A1,B8;A1,B35* and *A3,B8;A3,B35*
Mother	A2,A23;B12,B18	*A2,B12;A2,B18* and *A23,B12;A23,B18*
Child #1	A1,A2;B8,B12	*A1,B8;A1,B12* and *A2,B8;A2,B12*
Child #2	A1,A23;B8,B18	*A1,B8;A1,B18* and *A23,B8;A23,B18*
Child #3	A3,A23;B18,BY	*A3,B18;A3,BY* and *A23,B18;A23,BY*

- Genotypes are deduced by the identification of common haplotypes, as shown in Table 14-5B.
- Child #3 inherited A3,BY from the father. The father could pass A3,B35.
- Antigen B8, and hence haplotype A3,B8, is not present in the father.
- Antigen B8 travels with the haplotype A1,B8, which the father has transmitted to child #1 and child #2.
- Child #3 must inherit A3,BY = A3,B35 from the father.
- The missing antigen Y in child #3 is B35.

Table 14-5B.

	Haplotype Inherited from the Mother	Haplotype Inherited from the Father	Confirmed Genotype
Child #1	A2,B12	A1,B8	*A1,B8;A2,B12*
Child #2	A23,B18	A1,B8	*A1,B8;A23,B18*
Child #3	A23,B18	?	*A23,B18; ?*

Question 6: A

Explanation:

- A1,B58 is a common haplotype among siblings 4, 6, and 8. The siblings inherited A1,B58 from the first parent.
- AX,B35 is the second haplotype in sibling 4 and A2,B45 is the second haplotype in siblings 6 and 8.
- The genotype of the second parent is *AX,B35;A2,B45*.
- Analysis of the HLA types of siblings 1, 2, 3, 5, and 7 reveals that A1,B70 is a common haplotype. The siblings inherited A1,B70 from the first parent.
- The genotype of the first parent is: *A1,B70;A1,B58*.
- The first parent is homozygous for A1 at the *A* locus.
- The unidentified antigen X is 1.
- The patient and siblings 3 and 7 have identical HLA phenotypes: A1,A-; B35,70.

Question 7: A

Explanation:

- Phenotype of the recipient: A2,A3; B35,-
- Possible genotypes of the recipient: A2,B35;A3,Y and
                                                               A3,B35;A2,Y
- Phenotype of sibling #1:   A2,A11;B7,B35
- Possible genotypes of sibling #1:   A2,B7;A11,B35 and
                                                                A11,B7;A2,B35
- A2,B35 is the common haplotype.
- Confirmed genotype of the recipient: A2,B35;A3,Y
- Confirmed genotype of sibling #1:   A2,B35;A11,B7
- One haplotype of parent #1:   A2,B35; ?
- Genotype of parent #2:   A3,Y;A11,B7
- Phenotype of sibling #2:   A3,A11;B35,B44
- Possible genotypes of sibling #2:   A3,B35;A11,B44 and
                                                                A11,B35;A3,B44
- Sibling #2 has inherited either *A11,B35* or *A11,B44* from parent #1.
- Confirmed genotype of parent #2:   A3,B35;A11,B7
- The missing antigen in sibling #4 at the *A* locus is X.
- Phenotype of sibling #4:   A11,X;B7,B44
- Genotype of sibling #4:   A11,B44;X,B7
- Antigen B7 travels with A11.
- Genotype of sibling #4:   A11,B44;A11,B7
- X = A11
- Sibling #4 is homozygous for A11.
- Genotype of parent #1:   A2,B35;A11,B44
- Genotype of parent #2:   A3,B35;A11,B7
- The parents share B35 and A11
- Sibling #2 has inherited *A11,B44* from parent #1.
- Genotype of sibling #2:   A11,B44;A3,B35
- Sibling #2 has inherited the haplotype *A3,Y* (i.e. *A3,B35*) from the second parent.
- Antigen A3 travels with B35. Y = B35.
- Confirmed genotype of the recipient and sibling #3: A2,B35;A3,B35
- The recipient and sibling #3 are homozygous for B35 and are HLA identical.
- Phenotype of sibling #5:   A2,A11;B7,B35
- Confirmed genotype of sibling #5:   A2,B35;A11,B7

Questions 8: B

Explanation:

- Possible genotypes and confirmed genotypes of family members are listed in Table 14-8B.

Table 14-8B.

Family Members	Possible Genotypes	Confirmed Genotypes
Father	*A4,B22;A4,B35* and *A28,B22;A28,B35*	*A4,B35;A28,B22*
Mother	*A8,B7;A8,B44* and *A11,B7;A11,B44*	*A8,B44;A11,B7*
Patient	*A4,B7;A4,B35* and *A11,B7;A11,B35*	*A4,B35;A11,B7*
Sibling 1	*A4,B7;A4,B35* and *A11,B7;A11,B35*	*A4,B35;A11,B7*
Sibling 2	*A4,B22;A4,B44* and *A8,B22;A8,B44*	*A4,B22;A8,B44*
Sibling 3	*A4,B7;A4,B35* and *A11,B7;A11,B35*	*A4,B35;A11,B7*
Sibling 4	*A11,B7;A11,B22* and *A28,B7;A28,B22*	*A11,B7;A28,B22*
Sibling 5	*A4,B7;A4,B35* and *A11,B7;A11,B35*	*A4,B35;A11,B7*

- The patient and the HLA-identical siblings 1, 3, and 5 have received haplotype A4,B35 from the father and haplotype A11,B7 from the mother.

Question 9: B

Explanation:

- Sibling #2 received the haplotype A4,B22 from the father, a result of crossover and recombination of antigens A4 and B22 on the HLA loci of the father's homologous chromosomes.

- The father has the haplotype A4,B35; *not* the haplotype A4,B22. However, he does have the antigens A4 and B22.
- The individual loci of the HLA complex are tightly linked. Thus, genetic recombination or crossing over is a rare event.
- The frequency of genetic recombination between different loci is given in Table 14-9.
- Genetic recombination has important implications in transplantation and parentage testing.

Table 14-9.

Genetic Recombination between Different Loci	Frequency (%)
A and *B*	0.8
B and *DR*	0.5
A and *C*	0.06
B and *C*	0.02

Question 10: C

Explanation:

- ABO antigens are the most important antigens in solid organ transplantation. These antigens are present on all tissues of the body with the exception of the central nervous system. Antibodies recognizing these antigens are naturally occurring, meaning that they arise secondary to the exposure of antigens found in nature (rather than via red cell exposure).
- In ABO-incompatible grafts, the recipient's ABO antibodies react with ABO antigens found on the vascular endothelium of the transplanted graft. The risk is hyperacute rejection.
- Class I and Class II HLA antigens continue to have a significant influence on graft survival.

- Pancreatic tissue can be transplanted as a solid organ or as dissociated islet cells. Both of these are exceptionally susceptible to injury via HLA antibodies.
- ABO- and HLA-identical sibling #3 is the best possible combined renal and islet cell donor for the patient.
- ABO-compatible group O and HLA-identical sibling #5 is the second choice, as there are no A or B antigens on the vascular endothelium of this sibling.
- The group B, HLA haploidentical mother is the third choice for transplantation.
- Group B sibling #2, who shares only one HLA antigen with the patient (A4), is *not* a good choice.
- Sibling #1 is also not a good choice. Although this sibling is HLA-identical, there is ABO incompatibility (sibling #1 is group AB).

Question 11: C

Explanation:

- The prevention of graft-vs-host-disease (GVHD) is the most important consideration in HPC transplantation. Complete (6/6) matching of the HLA Class I (A and B loci) and HLA Class II (DR loci) antigens is the most important factor in minimizing GVHD. DNA-based typing is the preferred method for typing HLA Class II antigens. DNA-based typing for HLA Class I antigens is being incorporated by many centers, though serologic testing methods are still being employed.
- Most patients requiring HPC transplantation have a nonfunctioning or dysfunctional immune system. Reasons for this include the following:
  - Underlying disease.
  - Cytoreductive chemotherapy.
  - Pretransplantation irradiation.
- Although minimal, the reactivity of the recipient's immune system against the donor progenitor cells can manifest as graft rejection or failure of engraftment. Preformed HLA antibodies, produced as a result of pretransplantation transfusion or pregnancy, can also result in rejection or failure to engraft.
- ABO- and HLA-identical sibling #3 is the best possible HPC donor for the patient.

- Group O and HLA-identical sibling #5 is the second choice as the HPC donor for the patient.
- Group AB and HLA-identical sibling #1 would be the third choice for consideration.
- Minor histocompatibility genes are non-HLA genes that are not well defined. These genes are believed to affect transplantation success. The use of sibling donors increases the probability of matching these genes.

Question 12: B

Explanation:

- ABO compatibility is the most important factor determining the immediate survival of solid organ transplants.
- The HLA system is second in importance in determining the long-term survival of transplanted solid organs.
- For renal transplant evaluation, the donor and recipient are typed for ABO, HLA-A, HLA-B, and HLA-DR antigens.
- HLA-C and HLA-DQ testing is usually not performed.
- Serologic assays (eg, lymphocytotoxicity testing) are commonly used to detect Class I HLA antigens.
- Mixed lymphocyte culture testing, for the detection of HLA Class II antigens, was used in the past. Now it is seldom performed, as molecular testing is the preferred method for typing HLA Class II antigens.
- The sera of patients awaiting renal transplantation is tested for the presence of HLA antibodies, as these antibodies could cause hyper-acute rejection.
- A method more sensitive than routine lymphocytotoxicity testing is required to detect crossmatch incompatibility between the recipient's serum and donor's lymphocytes before surgery. Flow cytometry is the most sensitive method for this detection.
- Rh compatibility is not an important consideration in the setting of renal transplantation because Rh antigens are expressed only on red cells, not on endothelium.

Question 13: C

Explanation:

- Pretransplantation transfusions have a weak immunosuppressive effect that may enhance graft survival. The negative aspect of this is that multiple transfusions result in the exposure to HLA antigens. Alloimmunization can then occur with associated difficulty in finding a compatible organ.
- The compatibility of non-HLA, minor histocompatibility genes has a positive influence on graft survival.
- The treatment of transplanted patients with the immunosuppressive drug cyclosporin A is associated with improved graft survival on the order of 10% to 15%. A disadvantage of this therapy is that renal transplant patients treated with cyclosporine A are more likely to develop squamous cell and basal cell cancers of the skin, compared with the general population.
- Flow cytometry is an extremely sensitive, complement-independent technique used for crossmatching donors and recipients; however, expertise in flow cytometry is required for the proper interpretation of results.
- Cytokine-induced T-cell *activation* can cause graft rejection.

Question 14: B

Explanation:

- Lymphocyte microcytotoxicity assays test a patient's serum with panels of lymphocytes of known HLA type in the presence of complement and a dye, which is taken up by lysed cells. Based upon the pattern of lysis, specificity of the HLA antibodies can be determined.
- The percent of the panel cells to which the recipient has formed cytotoxic antibodies is referred to as the PRA level. The specificity of the antibodies is also identified.
- This assay will only identify antibodies to HLA antigens, not antibodies directed toward other antigens present on platelets, including antibodies to platelet-specific antigens (eg, HPA-1a), drug-depen-

dent antibodies (eg, quinidine), and autoantibodies. All of these antibodies can cause immune-mediated platelet refractoriness and should be considered when the HLA antibody results and the clinical picture do not agree.
- ABO incompatibility, while usually clinically insignificant in platelet transfusion, has been reported to contribute to immune refractoriness among alloimmunized patients. Platelets weakly express ABH antigens.
- It is important to remember that platelets do not express HLA Class II molecules (HLA-DR, -DQ, and -DP). Therefore, antibodies directed against these antigens are not important with respect to platelet refractoriness. In addition, HLA-C antigens are very weakly expressed on platelets. Because of this, matching for the *HLA-C* locus is not necessary when providing HLA-matched platelets.
- In addition to immune-mediated platelet refractoriness, the refractory state may be caused by clinical factors such as sepsis, fever, disseminated intravascular coagulation (DIC), and hypersplenism.
- Bleeding can be associated with a falling platelet count, but a poor platelet increment, as assessed by an immediate posttransfusion platelet count, would not be expected.
- The degree of matching for HLA antigens (HLA Class I, *A* and *B* loci) is shown in Table 14-14.

Table 14-14.

A	4 antigens match
B1U	3 antigens detected in the donor, all match
B1X	3 donor antigens match, 1 cross-reactive
B2U	2 antigens detected in the donor, both match
B2UX	3 antigens detected in the donor, 2 match and 1 cross-reactive
B2X	2 donor antigens match, 2 cross-reactive
C	1 antigen in donor not present in recipient and not cross-reactive
D	2 antigens in donor not present in recipient and not cross-reactive

Question 15: D

Explanation:

- A significant number of patients who receive multiple transfusions develop immune-mediated platelet refractoriness. Other routes of exposure to foreign HLA antigens include pregnancy and transplantation.
- Failure to obtain an appropriate increment on a 1-hour posttransfusion platelet count (count drawn between 10 minutes and 1 hour after the completion of the platelet transfusion) suggests an immune-mediated cause of platelet refractoriness. This could result from the presence of HLA antibodies (most common cause), antibodies toward platelet-specific antigens (eg, HPA-1a), or autoantibodies.
- If immune refractoriness is suspected, testing for the presence of HLA antibodies is indicated. If present, possible options for treatment include:
  - Transfusion of HLA-matched platelets.
  - Transfusion of HLA antigen-negative platelets (platelets lacking the HLA antigens to which the patient's antibodies are directed).
  - Crossmatch-compatible platelets.
- A low platelet count determined hours after transfusion, in the presence of an adequate 1-hour posttransfusion count, suggests nonimmune platelet refractoriness.
- There is no need to give D-negative platelets because the D antigen is not expressed on platelets.
- Sensitization to the D antigen should be avoided in women of childbearing potential. This can be done by transfusing only D-negative cellular blood components or through the administration of Rh Immune Globulin when Rh-positive components cannot be avoided. However, it is important to recognize that it is uncommon for Rh-negative oncology patients to form anti-D, especially when apheresis platelets are transfused.
- When anti-D is present, hemolysis of the small volume of red cells in D-positive platelet products will have no ill effect on the patient.

Question 16: E

Explanation:

- Failure to obtain an adequate posttransfusion platelet increment could result from a platelet product of poor quality, alloimmunization, or splenic sequestration, among other causes (eg, fever, sepsis, DIC). In this case, splenic sequestration is most likely. To help eliminate other options, transfusing an additional 6 units of platelets followed by a 1-hour posttransfusion platelet count would be useful. An appropriate increment on a 1-hour count coupled with a failure to maintain the increment suggests a nonimmune cause such as splenic sequestration. In the presence of splenic sequestration, higher doses of platelet concentrates may be necessary to achieve the desired posttransfusion increment.
- The clinical manifestations of hairy cell leukemia (HCL) are mostly caused by leukemic cell infiltration of the marrow, spleen, and liver. Splenomegaly, often massive, is a common feature of HCL. Pancytopenia, resulting from splenic sequestration and marrow failure, is seen in more than 50% of cases. Treatment options in HCL include splenectomy, α-interferon, chemotherapy, and local radiation to osteolytic bone lesions (a rare finding). Splenectomy is beneficial in most patients. Platelet count, hemoglobin levels, and granulocytes are increased within days to months.
- Immune platelet refractoriness (HLA alloimmunization) is a common problem in patients who are chronically transfused. This is caused by leukocytes in the transfused product that induce HLA antibodies in the recipient. After evaluating the transfusion history of the patient, if HLA alloimmunization is suspected, further workup to identify the presence of HLA antibodies is warranted. If present, treatment with HLA-matched, antigen-negative, or crossmatch-compatible platelets is indicated. In this patient, HLA alloimmunization is unlikely because the patient is a man who has no history of transfusion.
- Intravenous gamma globulin is not first-line therapy for HLA alloimmunization. This option has been reported to be successful in some case series and can be considered in the severely alloimmunized patient for whom appropriate platelets cannot be identified.
- Alloimmunization can be delayed or reduced through the transfusion of leukocyte-reduced cellular blood components.

Question 17: E

Explanation:

- HLA antibodies are IgG and IgM immunoglobulins that are induced by pregnancy, transfusion, or previous organ transplantation.
- Pregnancy is the strongest stimulus, and the antibody response is sharp and well defined. Multiparous women may have high-titer HLA antibodies. Their serum is often used for lymphocytotoxicity testing.
- Transplantation is the weakest stimulus for the induction of antibodies. The underlying disease process and iatrogenic immunosuppressive therapy compromise the immune system of these patients.
- The quality of the antibody response accompanying transfusion falls between that of pregnancy and transplantation.
- HLA antibodies in transfusion recipients may bind to white cells in a blood component, resulting in cytokine-mediated febrile, non-hemolytic transfusion reactions. However, HLA incompatibility has rarely been implicated as a cause of hemolytic transfusion reactions.
- HLA antibodies are implicated in rare cases of neonatal alloimmune thrombocytopenia, although this is controversial and not accepted by all. However, HLA antibodies are not important in the pathogenesis of HDFN.

Question 18: E

Explanation:

- HLA antibodies are not implicated in either acute or delayed hemolytic transfusion reactions, although they are rare causes of shortened red cell survival in patients with antibodies to HLA antigens such as B7 (Bg^a), B17 (Bg^b), and A28 (Bg^c) that are expressed weakly on red cells.
- HLA antibodies are not implicated in cases of HDFN and are not important in the pathogenesis of anaphylactic transfusion reactions.
- HLA antigens and antibodies are associated with each of the following clinical conditions:
  - Febrile, nonhemolytic transfusion reactions.

THE HLA SYSTEM 529

- TRALI.
- Immune platelet refractoriness.
- Solid organ and HPC transplant rejection.

Question 19: E

Explanation:

- Bg antibodies react with HLA remnants on the *mature* red cell membrane, whereas most HLA antigens are present on immature red cells only. The Bg antigens are as follows:
  - Bg^a = HLA-B7.
  - Bg^b = HLA-B17.
  - Bg^c = HLA-A28.
- Bg antibodies are detected using an antihuman globulin reagent.
- Bg antibodies are clinically insignificant and are not implicated in hemolytic transfusion reactions or cases of HDFN.
- Immune IgG anti-Bg can be present in multiparous women and multitransfused patients.
- Reagent red cells with a *weaker* expression of Bg antigens are desired in pretransfusion antibody detection tests. This avoids expensive and fruitless testing for antibodies that are not clinically significant.
- Bg antigens are not present in body fluids and plasma.

Question 20: A

Explanation:

- Genetic disequilibrium, gametic association, and linkage disequilibrium are all terms that describe an association of certain genes more frequently than would be expected on the basis of individual gene frequencies.
- Genetic anticipation is the progressive increase in severity and/or the earlier age of onset of a genetic disorder in subsequent generations of a kindred (eg, myotonic dystrophy and fragile X syndrome).

- Genetic imprinting is the differential expression of a gene, depending on which parent the gene was inherited from (eg, Prader-Willi and Angelman syndromes).
- The Hardy-Weinberg principle suggests that different alleles of the HLA antigens are associated with each other roughly in proportion to their frequencies in the population as a whole, assuming random mating, a low mutation rate, and no emigration or immigration from the population.
- Lyonization is the inactivation of one of the X chromosomes in a female subject.

Question 21: C

Explanation:

- The nomenclature for expressing the degree of HLA-matching between platelet donors and transfusion recipients is given in Table 14-21.

Table 14-21.

A	4 antigens match
B1U	3 antigens detected in the donor, all match
B1X	3 donor antigens match, 1 cross-reactive
B2U	2 antigens detected in the donor, both match
B2UX	3 antigens detected in the donor, 2 match and 1 cross-reactive
B2X	2 donor antigens match, 2 cross-reactive
C	1 antigen in donor not present in recipient and not cross-reactive
D	2 antigens in donor not present in recipient and not cross-reactive

- Answer C (A1,-;B7,-) is a B2U match. Only two antigens are identified in the donor, both of which are present in the recipient. The unidentified (U) antigens suggest that the donor is homozygous for A1 and B7.

- Answer A is a D match, as A11 and A19 are not present in the recipient and do not belong to cross-reactive antigen groups for the patient's HLA-A antigens.
- Answer B is a C match, as A23 is not present in the recipient and does not belong to a cross-reactive antigen group.
- Answer D is a B2UX match, as B7 and B27 are present in the recipient, A3 is cross-reactive with A1, and an antigen is missing.
- Answer E is a C match, as A10 is not present in the recipient and does not belong to a cross-reactive antigen group.
- The following are reasons why an individual may test positive for only one antigen at a given locus (ie, have a "blank" or "-"):
  - The individual is homozygous for the detected allele.
  - The individual expresses an antigen for which appropriate antisera are unavailable.
  - There is a technical failure in testing (ie, a false negative).
  - There is a null (unexpressed) gene; this is very rare.

Question 22: C

Explanation:

- CREGs are groups of HLA antigens that share antigenic determinants and, as a result, will react with alloantisera that recognize these determinants.
- The shared epitopes in CREGs result from shared amino acid sequences.
- Public antigens are epitopes with common amino acid sequences found among many different HLA specificities. These appear to represent the less variable portion of the HLA molecule.
- CREGs are not standardized because different antisera produce unique reaction patterns. There is, however, considerable overlap between reported CREGs.

Question 23: B

Explanation:

- Celiac disease is associated with HLA-DQ2. The relative risk of disease in an individual with DQ2 is >250.
- Some diseases demonstrate associations with HLA antigens. These associations frequently occur with autoimmune diseases and may represent a relationship between the antigens and a faulty immune response, linkage disequilibrium between the HLA antigen and susceptibility genes for the disease, or antigenic mimicry.
- HLA disease associations:
  - Ankylosing spondylitis—B27.
  - Postgonococcal arthritis—B27.
  - Acute anterior uveitis—B27.
  - Rheumatoid arthritis—DR4.
  - Chronic active hepatitis—DR3.
  - Sjögren syndrome—DR3.
  - Type I diabetes mellitus—DR3, DR4.
  - 21-hydroxylase deficiency—BW47.
  - Idiopathic hemochromatosis—A3.
  - Subacute thyroiditis (de Quervain)—B35.
  - Psoriasis vulgaris—Cw6.
  - Narcolepsy—DQ6.
  - Pernicious anemia—DR5.
  - Juvenile rheumatoid arthritis—DR8.
  - Pemphigus vulgaris—DR4.
  - Goodpasture disease—DR3.
  - Systemic lupus erythematosus—DR3.
- Despite strong disease associations, HLA typing is of only limited value in the diagnosis of most diseases because the association is incomplete, being prone to false-positive and false-negative results. For example, more than 90% of people of European ethnicity with ankylosing spondylitis are HLA-B27-positive; however, only 20% of individuals with the B27 antigen develop ankylosing spondylitis.

THE HLA SYSTEM

Question 24: B

Explanation:

- A serologic specificity may be described by more than one nucleotide sequence.
- The nomenclature for the gene locus consists of the name of the gene locus followed by 4 to 7 digits representing the following:
  - Digits 1 and 2 represent the serologic specificity (eg, *A*0101* and *A*0102* both appear serologically to be A1 though they have different nucleotide sequences).
  - Digits 3 and 4 represent the order in which the unique variants of the allele was described.
  - Digit 5 is used to distinguish unique nucleic acid sequences in alleles when the predicted amino acid sequence is the same.
- In this case:
  - A identifies the allele as being located at the *HLA-A* locus.
  - The first two digits represent the serologic specificity; in this case it is A2.
  - The last two digits represent the order in which the variant allele was identified; in this case it is the first.

Question 25: C

Explanation:

- Soluble Class I and Class II HLA antigens are shed from cells and are found in blood and other body fluids.
- Soluble HLA may play a role in modulating immune reactivity.
- Levels of soluble HLA rise with infection (eg, HIV), inflammatory disease, and transplant rejection, and levels decline as malignancies progress.
- HLA antigens are shed from the residual donor leukocytes in blood components. Soluble antigen levels are proportionate to both the number of residual donor leukocytes and the length of storage.
- Soluble HLA antigens in blood components may play an important role in the immunomodulatory effect of blood transfusion.

REFERENCES

1. Gebel H, Pollack M, Bray R. The HLA system. In: Roback JD, Combs MR, Grossman BJ, Hillyer CD, eds. Technical manual. 16th ed. Bethesda, MD: AABB, 2008:547-68.
2. Roitt IM, Delves PJ. Roitt's essential immunology. 10th ed. Malden, MA: Blackwell Scientific, 2005.

15

Tissue Banking and Organ Transplantation

QUESTIONS

Question 1: Code of Federal Regulations, Title 21, Part 1271 (21 CFR 1271), referred to as good tissue practice, is concerned with:

A. Reducing the infectious complications of tissue transplantation.
B. Increasing donation of tissues for transplantation.
C. Improving indications for tissue use in transplantation.
D. Reducing wastage of tissue during transplantation.
E. All of the above.

Question 2: Which of the following tissues is regulated under 21 CFR 1271?

A. Heart.
B. Lung.
C. Pancreas.
D. Semen.
E. Kidney.

Question 3: Which of the following donors would be considered *eligible* to donate hematopoietic progenitor cells (HPCs) according to Food and Drug Administration (FDA) guidance?

A. A male who had sex with another male 10 years ago.
B. A female whose husband has received injections of live monkey brain cells to treat his Parkinson's disease.
C. A female who received a blood transfusion while in France in 1998.
D. A donor with a history of hepatitis 1 year ago at age 25. The cause of the hepatitis is unknown.
E. None would be eligible to donate.

Question 4: Which of the following donors would be *ineligible* to donate bone according to FDA guidance?

A. Donor has a porcine artificial heart valve.
B. Donor is a former prostitute and has not exchanged sex for money in the last 15 years.
C. Donor lives with a brother who has asymptomatic hepatitis C virus (HCV).
D. Donor received a dura mater graft during surgical repair of an aneurysm.
E. Donor was vaccinated for smallpox 30 days ago; the scab fell off spontaneously.

Question 5: According to FDA guidance, which of the following must be performed to determine whether a donor is eligible to donate nonvascular tissue and cells?

A. Review available medical records for infectious disease risks.
B. Test the donor for relevant communicable diseases.
C. If the donor is deceased, review the autopsy findings, if available.
D. If the donor is deceased, review police reports, if available.
E. All of the above.

Question 6: For which of the following tissues is testing of the donor for human T-cell lymphotropic virus, types I and II (HTLV-I/II) required according to FDA guidance?

A. Tendon.
B. Bone.
C. Semen.
D. Heart valve.
E. All of the above.

Question 7: Which of the following statements is *true* concerning serologic testing of tissue donors for relevant communicable diseases according to FDA guidance?

A. A cadaveric donor who has been transfused or undergone volume resuscitation requires no special handling with regard to testing.
B. Serologic tests licensed by the FDA for use in donors can always be used to test cadaveric donors.
C. Serologic tests used for the diagnosis of diseases can be used to determine donor eligibility, even if they are not licensed for donor testing as long as they are FDA licensed.
D. Testing of HPC donors can occur up to 30 days before the collection of the progenitor cell product.
E. Testing of donors of therapeutic T cells (also called donor lymphocytes) can be performed up to 30 days before the collection of the product.

Question 8: Which of the following statements concerning the shelf life of tissues is *true*?

A. Frozen bone stored at −40 C has a shelf life of 10 years.
B. Bone stored at 1 to 10 C has a shelf life of 7 days.
C. Frozen bone stored at −20 C has a shelf life of 6 months.
D. Lyophilized fascia stored at room temperature has a shelf life of 10 years.
E. Skin stored at 1 to 10 C has a shelf life of 3 weeks.

Question 9: Which of the following information is included on the label of the tissue package?

A. Descriptive name of the tissue.
B. Name and address of the tissue bank(s) responsible for determining donor eligibility, processing, and distribution.
C. Expiration date.
D. Quantity of tissue.
E. All of the above.

Question 10: Of the following organizations that accredit for or regulate tissue handling, which focuses *only* on hospitals that use tissues for transplantation?

A. Eye Bank Association of America (EBAA).
B. American Association of Tissue Banks (AATB).
C. The Joint Commission.
D. AABB.
E. FDA.

Question 11: Which of the following statements is *true* concerning bone grafting?

A. Graft revascularization and remodeling takes longer with autologous bone than frozen or lyophilized bone.
B. Cortical bone induces a greater inflammatory response and more rapid revascularization than cancellous bone.
C. Cancellous bone grafts tend to require less protection from mechanical stress than cortical bone grafts.
D. ABO and HLA type of the donor must be considered when selecting frozen bone grafts, and the grafts must be matched accordingly.
E. Immunization to the D blood group antigen has not been reported when using fresh bone grafts.

Question 12: Which of the following statements is *true* concerning frozen or lyophilized bone grafts?

A. Donor-derived osteoblasts and osteoclasts are important in the incorporation of the graft into the defect.
B. The calcium present in the graft is essential for incorporation of the graft and bone formation.
C. Freezing and thawing of bone is not associated with adverse effects on mechanical properties.
D. Lyophilized bone is preferred over frozen bone because it does not need to be thawed and can be implanted directly from the package.
E. All of the above.

Question 13: Which of the following statements about the processing, storage, and distribution of bone and soft tissue grafts is *true*?

A. Tissues from multiple donors can be pooled during processing.
B. Tissues, such as tendons and fascia, can be sterilized using ethylene oxide or gamma irradiation.
C. A "lot" is defined as grafts from multiple donors that were produced at one time using one set of instruments and supplies.
D. Tissues received by a hospital need to be logged in only if they are transplanted to a patient.
E. Upon receipt of the tissue by the hospital, the package should be inspected. This is the only time this is necessary.

Question 14: Which of the following statements concerning cardiac valvular grafts is *true*?

A. Tissue can be harvested from donors ranging from newborns to 60-year-olds.
B. A history of endocarditis is not grounds for donor deferral.
C. Valvular tissue can be harvested up to 72 hours after death.

D. Cardiac valvular grafts are lyophilized and have a shelf life of 5 years at room temperature.
E. Patients do not require systemic anticoagulation, and the grafts survive longer than mechanical heart valves.

Question 15: Which of the following is an essential function of a hospital-based tissue service?

A. Investigating and reporting adverse outcomes.
B. Screening the donors before tissue harvest.
C. Validating the storage conditions for a tissue graft.
D. Testing the donor for relevant communicable diseases.
E. Packaging the tissue product.

Question 16: Blood vessels are frequently harvested with vascular organs such as the liver. These vessels are provided to the transplant center receiving the vascular organ and may be used to create a vascular anastomosis between the recipient and the donor organ. Which of the following statements concerning these vessels is *true*?

A. As a tissue, they are regulated by the FDA under 21 CFR 1271.
B. They are typically either cryopreserved or lyophilized.
C. They can be used by the transplant center to create a vascular anatomosis in a patient other than the one who received the organ.
D. Transmission of viral infection has not been reported with these vessels.
E. All of the above.

Question 17: Which of the following statements concerning the clinical use of allogeneic skin grafts is *true*?

A. Used to cover extensive wounds when sufficient autologous tissue is not available.
B. Test the ability of a wound to accept an autograft.

C. Use as a biologic dressing to cover a meshed autograft.
D. Used in extensive epidermal sloughing such as in Stevens-Johnson syndrome.
E. All of the above.

Question 18: Which of the following is *true* about the use of human skin allografts to cover a wound?

A. It does not suppress bacterial growth to the same extent as standard dressings.
B. It is associated with increased pain compared to standard dressings.
C. It is associated with decreased water, electrolyte, and protein loss compared to standard dressings.
D. It requires greater metabolic energy requirements by the patient than standard dressings.
E. All of the above.

Question 19: Which of the following diseases have been transmitted by allogeneic skin grafts?

A. Human immunodeficiency virus (HIV).
B. Cytomegalovirus (CMV).
C. Pathogenic bacteria.
D. Pathogenic fungi.
E. All of the above.

Question 20: Which of the following statements is *true* concerning fresh allogeneic skin grafts?

A. They are equivalent to frozen allograft skin with regard to viability.
B. Fresh allogeneic skin does not express HLA antigens and does not undergo rejection.
C. Fresh allogeneic skin is stored in tissue media at 1 to 10 C.

D. Donor age is associated with viability; the younger the donor, the more viable the tissue.
E. The time between death of the donor and harvest does not affect viability.

Question 21: Corneal tissue is the second most commonly transplanted tissue after bone. Which of the following diseases has been transmitted by corneal tissue?

A. Creutzfeldt-Jakob disease (CJD).
B. Rabies.
C. CMV.
D. Hepatitis B virus (HBV).
E. All of the above.

Question 22: Which of the following tests is not required for anonymous and directed oocyte donors according to AATB standards?

A. *Neisseria gonorrhea.*
B. *Chlamydia trachomatis.*
C. Syphilis.
D. HTLV-I/II.
E. HIV-1/2.

Question 23: A 30-year-old female with a 25-year history of type I diabetes and associated renal failure undergoes a combined kidney and pancreas transplant. The recipient is A, Rh positive with a negative antibody screen, and the donor was O, Rh negative with a negative antibody screen. Both are CMV seropositive. On post-op day 8, she is found to have a hemoglobin of 6 g/dL with a positive polyspecific direct antiglobulin test (DAT). Antibody screen and eluate are negative. The hemoglobin on the preceding day was 13 g/dL. The most likely explanation for the fall in hemoglobin is:

A. Cytopathic effect of CMV on her marrow.

B. Hemolysis as a result of the effects of anti-rejection drugs.
C. Hemorrhage as a result of thrombocytopenia from antibodies to human platelet antigen (HPA)-1a produced by passenger lymphocytes from the transplanted organs.
D. Hemolysis as a result of anti-A produced by passenger lymphocytes from the transplanted organs.
E. Hemolysis as a result of anti-D produced by passenger lymphocytes from the transplanted organs.

Question 24: Which of the following statements concerning ABO blood group and solid organ transplantation is *true*?

A. ABO compatibility is not important with regard to heart transplantation.
B. ABO-incompatible renal transplants have never been successful because of hyperacute rejection.
C. The United Network for Organ Sharing (UNOS) requires that the ABO typing be performed a minimum of two times on a recipient before entry of the recipient or organ into the UNOS registry.
D. UNOS requires that the ABO typing be performed a minimum of three times on a donor before entry into the UNOS registry.
E. All of the above.

Question 25: Which of the following statements concerning transfusion support of organ recipients and potential organ recipients is *true*?

A. CMV-seropositive donors receiving CMV-seropositive organs require transfusion with CMV-safe blood components (CMV seronegative or leukocyte reduced).
B. Transfusion-associated graft-versus-host disease (TA-GVHD) is common, and irradiated blood components are required.
C. When ABO-incompatible renal transplants are performed and plasma is infused, it should be of recipient ABO type.
D. Before and after transplantation, patients should receive leukocyte-reduced blood components in order to avoid HLA alloimmunization.
E. All of the above.

ANSWERS

Question 1: A

Explanation:

- 21 CFR 1271 focuses on reducing the risks of infectious disease transmission only.
- In response to numerous cases of disease transmissions by tissue, both bacterial and viral transmissions, the Food and Drug Administration (FDA) created the good tissue practice (GTP) outlined in Part 1271. These federal rules govern the registration of facilities involved in the procurement and processing of tissues as well as the determination of donor eligibility.
- The Centers for Medicare and Medicaid Services (CMS) rules for participation address some of the other areas, including increasing tissue donation by requiring participating health-care facilities to have policies and systems that require notification of organ procurement agencies when deaths are imminent, provision of information concerning organ and tissue donation, and a memorandum of understanding between health-care facilities and organ, tissue, and eye procurement agencies.

Question 2: D

Explanation:

- 21 CFR 1271 concerns only nonvascularized tissues.
- Vascular organs such as the heart, lung, kidney, pancreas, liver, etc, are regulated by the Health Resources and Services Administration (HRSA), a unit of the Department of Health and Human Services.
- HRSA issues contracts to organizations to provide nationwide services with regard to tissue and organ transplantation. For example, HRSA has issued contracts to the National Marrow Donor Program (NMDP) to manage the US marrow and cord blood transplantation program and to the United Network for Organ Sharing (UNOS) to run the Organ Procurement and Transplantation Network (OPTN).

- Tissues covered by 21 CFR 1271 are bone, ligaments, tendon, fascia, cartilage, cornea, sclera, skin, arteries, veins (except umbilical cord veins), pericardium, amniotic membrane, dura mater, heart valves, peripheral blood stem cells, cord blood stem cells, bone marrow, donor oocytes, donor embryos, and donor semen.

Question 3: A

Explanation:

- The rules for determining donor eligibility are outlined in FDA guidance.
- The rules are similar to those used in determining blood donor eligibility in many ways, but there are significant differences.
- HPC donor criteria that differ from blood donor criteria:
  - Males who have had sex with a male in the preceding 5 years are deferred.
  - Persons with a history of injection drug use in the preceding 5 years are deferred.
  - Persons with hemophilia or other related clotting abnormalities who have received factor concentrates in the preceding 5 years are deferred. A person who received a factor concentrate for an acute bleeding event within 12 months is deferred.
  - Persons who have engaged in the exchange of sex for money or drugs in the preceding 5 years are deferred.
  - Children born to mothers with HIV infection or at risk of HIV infection are deferred if they are 18 months of age or younger or have been breast fed in the preceding 12 months.
  - Persons with a past diagnosis of clinical, symptomatic, viral hepatitis after their 11th birthday are deferred unless evidence from the time of illness documents it was caused by hepatitis A virus (HAV), cytomegalovirus (CMV), or Epstein-Barr virus.
  - Persons who are deceased and have a documented medical diagnosis of sepsis or have documented clinical evidence consistent with a diagnosis of sepsis are deferred.
  - Donors of reproductive human cells, tissues, and cellular and tissue-based products (HCT/Ps) who have been treated for or had *Chlamydia trachomatis* or *Neisseria gonorrhea* infection in the preceding 12 months are deferred.

- Persons who have been diagnosed with dementia or any degenerative or demyelinating disease of the central nervous system or other neurologic disease of unknown etiology are deferred.
- Persons who are xenotransplantation product recipients or intimate contacts of a xenotransplantation product recipient are deferred. These people may be at risk of transmitting animal viruses to the recipients. Of note, a xenotransplantation involves the transplantation of *living* cells, tissues, or organs.
- HPC donor criteria that are identical to blood donor criteria:
  - Persons who have engaged in sex with any of the types of people in the first four criteria above or with a person with human immunodeficiency virus (HIV) or a positive test for HIV, hepatitis B virus (HBV), or symptomatic hepatitis C virus (HCV) in the preceding 12 months are deferred.
  - Persons exposed to blood known or suspected to be infected with HIV, HBV, or HCV through percutaneous inoculation, open wound contact, nonintact skin contact, or mucous membrane contact in the preceding 12 months are deferred.
  - Persons who have been in juvenile detention, lockup, jail, or prison for more than 72 consecutive hours in the preceding 12 months are deferred.
  - Persons who have lived with someone with HBV or symptomatic HCV in the preceding 12 months are deferred.
  - Persons for whom sterile procedures were not used while undergoing tattooing, ear piercing, or body piercing in the preceding 12 months are deferred.
  - Persons with smallpox vaccination in the preceding 8 weeks are handled as follows:
    - Deferred 21 days from the date of vaccination or until the vaccination site scab falls off, whichever is later (if no complications have occurred); 2 months from the date of vaccination if the scab was removed (did not fall off); or 14 days after resolution of complications in those with vaccine-related complications.
    - Persons with clinically recognizable vaccinia infection from exposure to a person receiving the smallpox vaccine are deferred as follows:
      - No deferral if 1) there is no scab in a cadaveric donor, 2) a living donor's scab has spontaneously separated, or 3) it has been 3 months from the time of vaccination of the person

that the potential donor came in contact with and the scab was removed (did not fall off).
- Deferral if a scab is present in a cadaveric donor, or until the scab falls off in a living donor.
○ Persons who have had a medical diagnosis or come under suspicion of having West Nile virus (WNV) infection (based on symptoms and/or laboratory results, or confirmed WNV viremia) should be deferred for 120 days following diagnosis or onset of illness, whichever is later.
○ Persons who have tested positive or reactive for WNV infection using an FDA-licensed or investigational WNV nucleic acid testing (NAT) donor screening test in the preceding 120 days are deferred.
○ Persons who have been treated for or had syphilis within the preceding 12 months are deferred.
○ Persons who have been diagnosed with variant Creutzfeldt-Jakob disease (vCJD) or any other form of CJD are deferred.
○ Persons who are recipients of human-derived growth hormone or dura mater grafts are deferred.
○ Persons who have one or more blood relatives with CJD are deferred.
○ Persons who have resided in Great Britain (England, Wales, Scotland, Northern Ireland, the Isle of Man, Channel Islands, Gibraltar, Falkland Islands) for a total of 3 months between 1980 and 1996 are deferred.
○ Persons who have received transfusion of blood or blood components in the United Kingdom or France since 1980 are deferred.
○ Persons who have lived 5 or more cumulative years in Europe since 1980 are deferred.
○ Former or current US military personnel, civilian employees, or dependents associated with a US military base in Northern Europe (Germany, United Kingdom, Belgium, the Netherlands) for 6 months or more between 1980 and 1990 are deferred.
○ Former or current US military personnel, civilian employees, or dependents associated with a US military base in Southern Europe (Greece, Turkey, Spain, Portugal, Italy) for 6 months or more between 1980 and 1996 are deferred.
○ Persons are deferred who were born in, lived in, visited and received blood products in, or had sex with someone who was born in, lived in, or received blood components in Cameroon, Central African Republic, Chad, Congo, Equatorial Guinea, Gabon, Niger, or Nigeria. (Deferral is because of the presence of HIV-1 group O in

these countries. HIV-1 group O is not detected by all HIV assays. If an assay that detects HIV-1 group O is used to test the donor, these questions need not be asked and there is no reason for deferral.)

Question 4: E

Explanation:

- See the explanation for Question 3 for deferral criteria.
- Porcine cardiac valves are *not* considered a xenotransplant; only *living* cells, tissue, and organs from animals are considered to be xenotransplants. Bovine bone for dental or orthopedic repair would also not be categorized as a xenotransplant.

Question 5: E

Explanation:

- In order to determine the eligibility of a donor, the following must be performed to look for risk factors for relevant communicable diseases:
  - A donor medical history interview with the donor (if a living donor) or with one or more of the following if a deceased donor:
    - Next of kin.
    - Nearest available relative.
    - Member of donor's household.
    - An individual with a relationship with the donor.
    - Donor's primary treating physician.
  - Physical assessment of a cadaveric donor or the physical examination of a living donor to look for signs of relevant communicable disease and for signs suggestive of any risk factors for such disease.
  - Review of the following:
    - Laboratory test results (other than the results of testing required for the donor eligibility determination).
    - Medical records.

- Coroner and autopsy reports.
- Records or other information pertaining to risk factors for relevant communicable disease, such as medical examiner reports and police records, if available.
  - Performance of testing for relevant communicable disease.

Question 6: C

Explanation:

- FDA guidance requires testing for HTLV-I/II and CMV when the tissue is leukocyte rich because these viruses are transmitted by leukocytes.
- Leukocyte-rich tissues are hematopoietic stem/progenitor cells and semen.
- The American Association of Tissue Banks (AATB) standards require testing for all donors for both HTLV-I/II and CMV, except for oocyte donors.

Question 7: D

Explanation:

- Volume resuscitation with blood components, colloid solutions, or crystalloid solutions may dilute donor plasma and result in unreliable test results. Transfusion/infusion of more than 2 L of blood components or crystalloid/colloid solutions in the 48 hours or the hour before sample collection makes the sample invalid. If a pretransfusion or preinfusion sample is not available, the donor cannot be used for tissue harvest. Samples taken before the transfusion/infusion, for up to 7 days before the tissue collection, can be used for testing.
- Serologic tests may be licensed for general donor testing or for cadaveric donor testing. Only tests licensed specifically for cadaveric donor testing can be used to determine eligibility in cadaveric donors.
- Diagnostic testing is not the same as donor testing. Only tests licensed for donor testing can be used to determine donor eligibility.

- FDA guidance allows testing to be performed up to 30 days before collection or up to 7 days after collection for HPCs (either marrow or peripheral blood HPCs) and oocytes. For all other tissues, including therapeutic T-cells (donor lymphocytes), testing must be performed within 7 days before collection or within 7 days after collection of the product.

Question 8: C

Explanation:

- See Table 15-8A for tissues and storage conditions for which shelf life has been defined.

Table 15-8A.

Tissue	Storage Condition	Shelf Life
Bone	–40 C	5 years
	–20 C	6 months
	1 to 10 C	5 days
	Lyophilized, room temperature	5 years
Tendon	–40 C	5 years
Fascia	–40 C	5 years
	Lyophilized, room temperature	5 years
Cartilage	–40 C	5 years
	1 to 10 C	5 days
Skin	1 to 10 C	14 days
Cornea	2 to 6 C	14 days

- See Table 15-8B for tissues and storage conditions for which a maximum shelf life has not been defined.

Table 15-8B.

Tissue	Storage Condition
Bone	Liquid nitrogen
Cartilage	Liquid nitrogen
Skin	–40 C
	Lyophilized, room temperature
Hematopoietic progenitor cells	Liquid nitrogen (immersed or vapor phase)
Semen	Liquid nitrogen (immersed or vapor phase)
Heart valve	Liquid nitrogen (immersed or vapor phase)
Dura mater	Lyophilized, room temperature

Question 9: E

Explanation:

- All of the items listed are essential elements of the package label.
- Items on the label include the following:
    - Descriptive name of the tissue.
    - Name and address of the tissue bank(s) responsible for determining donor eligibility, processing, and distribution.
    - Expiration date.
    - Quantity of tissue.
    - Storage conditions.
    - Disinfection or sterilization procedure.
    - Preservative.
    - Potential residues of processing agents/solutions.
    - Reference to the package insert.

Question 10: C

Explanation:

- EBAA standards cover all aspects of tissue banking except those associated with the institutions that dispense the tissue (hospitals).
- AATB's *Standards for Tissue Banking* provide a comprehensive foundation for guiding tissue banking activities, including the organizational requirements of a tissue bank, records management, procedure manuals, quality assurance, consent, donor screening, tissue recovery and collection, donor and tissue testing, processing and preservation, labeling, storage, release, distribution, and dispensing (hospitals).
- Both New York State and the State of Florida license and inspect tissue banks that provide tissue to facilities within their state. They inspect such facilities even if they are not located within their respective states. California, Georgia, and Maryland license facilities that procure and process tissue that may be used within their respective states, but they do not have inspection programs for these facilities.
- AABB's *Standards for Blood Banks and Transfusion Services* applies standards for blood components to tissues, including standards on sterility, receipt and inspection, and traceability. AABB's *Standards for Cellular Therapy Product Services* covers not only the dispensing (hospital) but also the procurement and processing aspects of HPCs and other cellular-based therapies.
- The Joint Commission's standards focus on the dispensing institution and lack requirements concerning procurement. Standards require designated oversight and responsibility for tissues at an institution and identification of the positions responsible for compliance, accreditation, and regulatory requirements.
- The College of American Pathologists also focuses solely on dispensing institutions.
- The FDA regulates donor eligibility with regard to infectious disease as well as all other aspects of tissue manufacturing. They do not have requirements for hospitals who obtain tissue from outside suppliers. Also, a hospital that acquires tissue for use within the same facility does not need to register with the FDA. If, however, the hospital distributes tissue to other unaffiliated facility, it must register with the FDA.

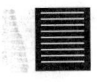

Question 11: C

Explanation:

- Autologous bone, usually harvested from the iliac crest, has more rapid revascularization and remodeling. Unfortunately, the disadvantages of this material include lack of adequate bone volume required to fill large defects and increased morbidity associated with the harvesting, such as greater time for surgical recovery, increased blood loss, more complex surgery, etc. As a result, allogeneic bone has become the preferred alternative in many cases.
- Because of its greater surface area, cancellous bone induces a greater inflammatory response and more rapid vascularization. This means that there is a greater osteoblast response.
- With cortical bone, there is slower vascularization and a predominant osteoclastic response, resulting in an early phase of bone weakening compared with cancellous bone. The result is that while it is being incorporated, greater protection from mechanical stress is needed with cortical bone compared to cancellous bone.
- HLA antigens and ABO antigens are not important with regard incorporation of the bone, and matching is not necessary.
- Immunization to the D, Fy^a, and Jk^b antigens have been reported with the implantation of fresh as well as frozen unprocessed bone. This is caused by red cells present in the bone. Lyophilized bone has not been reported to result in alloimmunization. Fresh or frozen unprocessed bone implanted into an Rh-negative woman of childbearing potential should be Rh negative.

Question 12: C

Explanation:

- Viable cells are not present in frozen or lyophilized bone. Donor cells are not involved in the incorporation process.
- Calcium is not essential for bone graft incorporation. Demineralized bone matrix is cortical bone that has been ground and had the calcium removed with hydrochloric acid. This putty of matrix proteins

can be used to fill defects and is preferred by periodontists and oral surgeons to augment bone growth around teeth or fill defects in facial bones. It is also used by spinal surgeons.
- Freezing bone does not alter its mechanical properties.
- Lyophilized bone is very brittle and most be rehydrated before use. This involves soaking the bone in a sterile solution for 2 to 4 hours before implantation. Frozen bone is thawed by soaking in a sterile solution, but the length of time required is much less.

Question 13: B

Explanation:

- Tissues from multiple donors *cannot* be pooled during processing as it can lead to contamination of tissue derived from one donor with infectious agents from another. This is defined in AATB standards.
- Tissues can be sterilized with ethylene oxide or gamma irradiation. Ethylene oxide-sterilized tissues may contain toxic metabolites and have higher failure rates. Gamma irradiation up to 25 kGy is used without adversely affecting the tissue.
- A "lot" is defined as the tissue from *one* donor produced at one time using one set of instruments and supplies.
- The Joint Commission requires that tissues are logged in and records kept when they are received, regardless of whether the tissue is transplanted or not.
- Packaging should be inspected at receipt, but also at the time of use. If integrity of the packaging is compromised or labeling is not correct, the tissue should not be used, it should be quarantined, and the problem should be reported to the manufacturer. This is required by AABB, AATB, and Joint Commission standards.
- According to AATB standards, the following diseases are grounds for deferral from musculoskeletal tissue donation: rheumatoid arthritis, systemic lupus erythematosus, polyarteritis nodosa, and clinically significant metabolic bone disease.

Question 14: A

Explanation:

- Donors from newborns to 60 years of age can be cardiac valvular tissue donors according to AATB standards. Tissue from donors older than 55 are associated with increased allograft incompetence.
- AATB standards state that a history of the following is grounds for deferral of the donor from heart donation: endocarditis, rheumatic fever, viral or idiopathic cardiomyopathy, and prior coronary artery bypass grafting.
- AATB standards require the following:
  - Warm ischemic time should not exceed 24 hours if the body was cooled or refrigerated within 12 hours of asystole or 15 hours if the body was not cooled.
  - Total warm and cold ischemic time should not exceed 48 hours.
- The harvested heart is transported at 1 to 10 C to a processing center for removal of the valves.
- Valvular grafts are harvested under clean room conditions in laminar flow hoods at 1 to 10 C. The tissue is disinfected using antibiotic solutions. The use of ethylene oxide or gamma irradiation used with other tissues results in a high frequency of graft failure.
- Cardiac valvular grafts are cryopreserved in 10% dimethyl sulfoxide. They are frozen at a controlled rate to -100 C and stored in liquid- or vapor-phase nitrogen. They are slowly thawed at 15 C per minute. Rapid thawing is associated with fracturing of the graft.
- Bioprosthetic heart valves do not require systemic anticoagulation, but they have a higher risk of structural failure and reoperation. As a result, bioprosthetic valves are reserved for individuals who cannot tolerate anticoagulation and/or have a life expectancy less than 10 years.

Question 15: A

Explanation:

- Answers B through D are functions of the tissue procurer and processor. Most hospital tissue services do not procure or process tissues but purchase it from a tissue supplier.
- Essential functions of a hospital tissue service include the following:
  - Qualifying the tissue supplier. This includes determining FDA registration and AATB or EBAA accreditation and monitoring for evidence of noncompliance such as FDA warning letters, recalls, and market withdrawals.
  - Acquiring and storing the tissue according to the manufacturer's instructions and standards.
  - Maintaining records that allow for traceability and documentation of final disposition. This must be bidirectional to allow for the reporting of adverse events to the tissue supplier as well as for determining who received tissue, in the event of a recall.
  - Investigating and reporting adverse events.
  - Providing quality assurance functions.
  - Auditing the use of the allografts.
  - Conducting recalls and look-back investigations.

Question 16: C

Explanation:

- The FDA does not regulate these fresh tissues, which have been specifically excluded from regulation by 21 CFR 1271.
- These vessels are shipped fresh with the organ in a sterile solution. They are not processed or preserved in any way.
- These vessels have been used to perform surgical repairs and anastomoses in patients who have not received the organ that they accompanied. This practice is common and is not prohibited. This practice points to the need for appropriate labeling, storage, and, most of all, traceability of tissues.

TISSUE BANKING AND ORGAN TRANSPLANTATION   557

- These vessels *have* transmitted viral infections, including one case where rabies was transmitted by iliac veins that accompanied a liver.
- There is no defined shelf life for these vessels and expiration dates need to be determined by the institution that uses them, as guided by 1) regulations and accreditation standards for similar materials, 2) validation of shelf life and storage performed by the institution, and 3) medical judgment.

Question 17: E

Explanation:

- Indications for the use of allogeneic skin grafts include the following:
  - Cover extensive wounds where inadequate amounts of autologous skin are available.
  - Can be used (autologous and allogeneic skin grafts) to cover wider areas by cutting them into a mesh. This is associated with failure of the wound to re-epithelialize in the spaces in the mesh. Allogeneic skin grafts can be placed over these meshed grafts to act as a dressing and enhance epithelialization.
  - Cover extensive partial thickness burns.
  - Cover extensive sloughing of the epidermis.
  - Cover a wound as a test to see if the wound will support a future autologous skin graft. If the allograft adequately adheres and exhibits vascular growth, the wound bed has sufficient blood supply for an autologous graft or flap.
  - Serve as a base for the future application of keratinocytes.

Question 18: C

Explanation:

- Skin allografts function as a biological dressing that is superior to standard surgical dressings. Benefits include the following:
  - Decreased water, electrolyte, and protein loss.
  - Prevents the tissue in the wound from drying out.

- Suppresses bacterial growth.
- Decreases wound pain as it eliminates the need for painful dressing changes.
- Decreases energy requirements by reducing the heat loss seen with severe burns.
- Promotes epithelialization.
- Provides dermis for epidermal grafts.

Question 19: E

Explanation:

- All of the infectious diseases have been transmitted by allogeneic skin grafts.
- Skin banks perform microbial cultures before grafts are released for transplantation in order to minimize disease transmission.
- AATB standards require that skin be discarded if pathogenic fungi or bacteria are present. This includes coagulase-positive *Staphylococci*, group A beta-hemolytic *Streptococci*, *Enterococci*, Gram-negative organisms, *Clostridia* species, yeast, and fungi.

Question 20: C

Explanation:

- Fresh allogeneic skin is harvested from a donor under aseptic conditions. It is processed in a Class 10,000 laminar flow hood. After processing, it is cultured for microbial contamination and stored at 1 to 10 C. The culture medium is changed every 3 days and the skin is stored for up to 14 days.
- Up to 10 days after procurement, skin can be cryopreserved. It is incubated with a cryoprotectant for 30 minutes and frozen at a controlled rate of −1 C per minute to −70 C or −100 C. It is then stored in either a mechanical or liquid nitrogen freezer.
- Fresh skin demonstrates more-rapid adherence and vascularization than cryopreserved or lyophilized skin.
- Donor age and gender are not associated with graft viability.

- The length of time between donor death and harvest predicts graft viability.
- Skin contains Langerhans cells, which express HLA Class II. Immunologic rejection occurs, resulting in marked inflammation and possible wound infection. This occurs 2 to 3 weeks after grafting in burn patients.

Question 21: E

Explanation:

The following have been transmitted by corneal transplants: bacterial infection, fungus, HBV, rabies, herpes simplex virus, CJD, and CMV.

Question 22: D

Explanation:

- AATB standards require that the following testing be performed on tissue donors: HIV-1/2 enyzme immunoassay (EIA), HIV-1 NAT, hepatitis B surface antigen, anti-hepatitis B core antigen, HCV EIA, HCV NAT, syphilis, HTLV-I/II.
- For anonymous or directed semen, CMV is also required.
- For anonymous or directed oocytes, CMV and HTLV-I/II are *not* required.
- For anonymous or directed oocyte donors, testing is required within 30 days of oocyte retrieval. Anonymous or directed semen donors must be tested within 7 days of initial collection.
- Anonymous semen and oocytes are frozen for at least 6 months. After this time, the donors are retested. If the donor cannot be retested, the semen and oocytes cannot be used.
- Anonymous or directed semen donors must be younger than age 40 to minimize genetic diseases. Anonymous or directed oocyte donors must be younger than age 35.

Question 23: D

Explanation:

- Passenger lymphocyte syndrome occurs when organs containing large amounts of lymphoid tissue (liver, lung, heart, pancreas, kidney) are transplanted. Because of the immunosuppressants, the recipient cannot reject these lymphocytes and they begin circulating and producing antibody.
- Passenger lymphocyte syndrome results in the appearance of antibodies directed toward donor red cells, and, in some cases, hemolysis. The most common antibodies are those directed toward ABO antigens when the donor has minor ABO incompatibility with the recipient. Antibodies to other antigens have been reported, including anti-D.
- Anti-D is *not* the cause in this instance as the antibody screen and eluate are negative. The screen and eluate are negative in this case as the screening cells and panel cells used are blood group O and would not detect anti-A.
- Severe thrombocytopenia has been reported because of passenger lymphocyte syndrome when tissues have been transplanted from individuals with immune thrombocytopenic purpura or who had been sensitized to antibodies to the platelet specific antigen HPA-1a.
- Passenger lymphocyte syndrome usually occurs within 14 days of transplantation. Antibodies are usually detectable for 1 to 3 weeks but may persist for up to 1 year. Red cell aplasia has been reported.
- The disorder is usually mild and self-limited. Treatment includes transfusion of compatible red cells. In the presence of severe hemolysis, treatment can consist of plasma exchange, corticosteroids, rituximab, mycophenylate, splenectomy, and red cell exchange. Plasma exchange and red cell exchange for hemolysis from passenger lymphocyte syndrome have not been categorized by the American Society for Apheresis (ASFA). (See Chapter 13.)

Question 24: C

Explanation:

- ABO antigens are expressed on the vascular endothelium of organs. Antibodies to ABO antigens are naturally occurring, present in people without previous blood exposure. The result is that ABO compatibility is required between donor and recipient or else the preformed antibodies will result in endothelial damage and organ ischemia as soon as blood flow is restored. This is called hyperacute rejection.
- ABO-incompatible renal transplants have been performed by two methods. In the first, a kidney from a living donor with a weak subgroup (usually A2) is transplanted into an O individual. Enhanced immunosuppression and, possibly, splenectomy are performed. The second method involves determining the titer of donor-specific antibody. In individuals with low titers, enhanced immunosuppression and intravenous immunoglobulin are used to suppress antibody levels further. In patients with higher titers, plasma exchange is added to the enhanced immunosuppression to reduce antibody levels to the point that hyperacute rejection will not occur. Plasma exchange conditioning for ABO-incompatible renal transplantation is a Category II indication according to ASFA. (See Chapter 13.)
- In heart transplantation, ABO compatibility is almost universal except in the context of pediatric transplantation. Because of difficulties in matching recipient and donor because of chest size, ABO-incompatible transplants have been performed in infants. Plasma exchange before, during, and after transplantation have been used to decrease ABO antibody titers to prevent hyperacute rejection. Plasma exchange conditioning for ABO-incompatible heart transplantation in infants is a Category II indication according to ASFA. (See Chapter 13.)
- UNOS requires that *both* the recipient and the donor have *two* ABO typings before the recipient or the organ are listed. In addition, UNOS requires that separate individuals enter the typings. The same person *cannot* enter both the recipient typing and the donor typing.

Question 25: D

Explanation:

- CMV infection in immunocompromised patients can cause severe infection, and attempts should be made to avoid infection in at-risk recipients such as CMV-seronegative recipients of CMV-seronegative organs. In a CMV-seronegative recipient receiving a CMV-seropositive organ, CMV infection will result from the organ, and some may not provide CMV-safe blood components in this setting.
- Transfusion-associated graft-vs-host disease (TA-GVHD) is an invariably fatal disease similar to GVHD seen in stem cell transplantation. It results from the infusion of viable lymphocytes into a recipient who has compromised cell-mediated immunity such that he or she cannot reject and destroy the cells. It is characterized by diarrhea, hepatitis, and jaundice. In addition, it is characterized by marrow hypoplasia as the infused lymphocytes also attack the marrow, something that does not occur in GVHD in stem cell transplantation, where the marrow is donor derived. Four cases of TA-GVHD have been reported in transplant recipients. Many more cases of transplant-associated GVHD, where the lymphocytes are derived from the organ, have been reported. Irradiated blood components are not routinely provided for transplant recipients because of the extreme rarity of TA-GVHD.
- In ABO-incompatible solid organ transplantation, there is usually major ABO incompatibility between the donor and the recipient (eg, an A kidney into an O recipient). The goal in these transplantations is to *reduce* the antibody titers of antibodies directed toward the donor. Providing recipient-type plasma products and platelets would infuse anti-donor antibodies. These patients should be given plasma products that are compatible with both the recipient and the donor. In the example above, type A Fresh Frozen Plasma (FFP) should be given.
- HLA alloimmunization can result in the development of antibodies that could lead to hyperacute rejection if formed before transplantation (organ never functions, as a result of immediate thrombosis of vasculature caused by complement activation and endothelial injury) or antibody-mediated rejection if formed after (organ functions initially but after some time—days to weeks to months—demonstrates a decline in function as antibody titers rise and damage the graft).

Leukocyte-reduced blood components should be given to patients to help prevent alloimmunization.

REFERENCES

1. Code of federal regulations. Title 21, CFR Part 1271. Washington, DC: US Government Printing Office, 2009 (revised annually).
2. Food and Drug Administration. Guidance for industry: Eligibility determination for donors of human cells, tissues, and cellular and tissue-based products (HCT/Ps). (August, 2007) Rockville, MD: CBER Office of Communication, Training, and Manufacturers Assistance, 2007. [Available at http://www.fda.gov/BiologicsBloodVaccines/GuidanceComplianceRegulatoryInformation/Guidances/Tissue/default.htm (accessed May 30, 2009).]
3. Woll JE. Tissue banking overview. Clin Lab Med 2005;25:473-86.
4. Eisenbrey AB, Frizzo W. Tissue banking regulations and oversight. Clin Lab Med 2005;25:487-98.
5. Woll JE, Smith DM. Bone and connective tissue. Clin Lab Med 2005;25:499-518.
6. Gandhi MJ, Strong DM. Cardiovascular tissues for transplantation. Clin Lab Med 2005;25:571-85.
7. Kagan RJ, Robb EC, Plessinger RT. Human skin banking. Clin Lab Med 2005;25:587-605.
8. Eastlund T. Tissue and organ transplantation and the hospital tissue transplantation service. In: Roback JD, Combs MR, Grossman BJ, Hillyer CD, eds. Technical manual. 16th ed. Bethesda, MD: AABB, 2008:833-64.
9. Pearson KA, Brubaker SA. Standards for tissue banking. 11th ed. McLean, VA: American Association of Tissue Banks, 2006.